Essentials of

Dermatology and Sexually Transmitted Diseases

An Illustrated Synopsis

Second Edition

By the Same Author

- Textbook of Dermatology (with MCQs)
- Leucoderma
- Textbook of Dermatology for Homeopaths (English, Spanish and Hindi Editions)
- Illustrated Textbook of Dermatology
- MCQs in Dermatology and Venereology
- Skin and Hair in Health and Disease (English and Hindi Editions)
- Can We Cure Psoriasis?

Essentials of

Dermatology and Sexually Transmitted Diseases

An Illustrated Synopsis

Second Edition

Ramji Gupta, MD (AIIMS)
Senior Consultant Dermatologist and Professor
Indraprastha Apollo Hospital
New Delhi

Formerly at
Department of Dermatology and Venereology
All India Institute of Medical Sciences
New Delhi

Universities Press

ESSENTIALS OF DERMATOLOGY AND SEXUALLY TRANSMITTED DISEASES: AN ILLUSTRATED SYNOPSIS (SECOND EDITION)

UNIVERSITIES PRESS (INDIA) PRIVATE LIMITED

Registered Office
3-6-747/1/A & 3-6-754/1, Himayatnagar, Hyderabad 500 029, Telangana, India
info@universitiespress.com, www.universitiespress.com

Distributed by
Orient Blackswan Private Limited

Registered Office
3-6-752 Himayatnagar, Hyderabad 500 029, Telangana, India

Other Offices
Bengaluru, Bhopal, Chennai, Guwahati, Hyderabad, Jaipur, Kolkata
Lucknow, Mumbai, New Delhi, Noida, Patna, Vijayawada

First Edition 2010
Second Edition 2018
First published by Universities Press (India) Private Limited 2018

ISBN 978 93 86235 54 1

501422

Typeset in Life 10.5/13.3 *by*
OSDATA, Hyderabad 500 029

Printed in India by
Rasi Graphics Private Limited
Chennai 600 014

Published by
Universities Press (India) Private Limited
3-6-747/1/A & 3-6-754/1, Himayatnagar
Hyderabad 500 029, Telangana, India

To
those undergraduate students
who
motivated me to write this book

Preface to the Second Edition

It is my pleasure to present the revised and updated second edition of the book. It is primarily intended for undergraduate medical students and general practitioners with interest in dermatology.

The bulleted text and numerous tables provide a clear and crisp presentation of content that will be relevant for the undergraduate students to arrive at a diagnosis and understand the treatment protocols to be followed.

A picture is worth a thousand words. This is especially true of a clinical field like dermatology. The USP of this book is that the clinical photographs of a given skin condition are interspersed with the text describing it. This assists in the immediate identification of the skin condition. There are coloured images to clearly demonstrate the results of treatments like cryotherapy, skin excision, grafting, etc.

An additional section on the syndromic management approach for STDs caters to the requirements of the curriculum. It is also useful to the practitioners in a healthcare setting. The appendix provides a consolidated document for management options in dermatology.

This book is a conscious effort to address the syllabus in such a manner as to aid the student in confidently facing the examinations, both in theory and clinical sections.

Comments and criticism are always welcome to improve the book.

Ramji Gupta
email: drramjigupta@yahoo.co.in

Preface to the First Edition

With many advances in the field of dermatology during the recent years, dermatology has emerged as an important field. With good undergraduate teaching and training in almost every medical college, the diagnosis and treatment of common skin diseases have become an integral part of undergraduate teaching. This book has been designed keeping in mind the present undergraduate curriculum.

Comprehensive dermatology and sexually transmitted diseases is concise and limited to common skin and sexually transmitted diseases with their classical presentation and currently used methods of treatment. Most of the diseases have been classified according to their etiological mechanism. The old system of classification based on morphological presentation has been discarded.

I hope this book will fulfill the educational needs of undergraduate students as well as be useful to general practitioners with interest in dermatology and sexually transmitted diseases.

Ramji Gupta

Acknowledgements

Thanks are due to Prof J S Pasricha who is the guiding force behind all my works. I feel indebted to Dr Vikas Khera who spared valuable time from his busy schedule to review this book critically and meticulously.

Dr Sameer Gupta and Dr Charu Gupta of Philadelphia and Dr Sarthak Gupta and Dr Saima of Washington, USA enriched the text with their healthy criticism and suggestions.

I acknowledge the sincere efforts of the medical publishing team of Universities Press—Mr Thomas Mathew Rajesh, Mr Ravi Vishwakarma, Dr Sudha Ganesan, Dr Alpa Agrawal, Mrs Manisha Pant and Mr Nayab—for assisting me in bringing out the second edition of this book. I thank Mr R K Majumdar who has worked on the illustrations and images of this book.

It was impossible to complete such a manuscript without the cooperation and moral support of my wife, Mrs Saroj Gupta.

Ramji Gupta

Contents

Chapter 1

Structure and Functions of Skin

Skin is the outer most part of the body. It covers and protects the internal organs of the body from environmental injuries and harmful organisms. Its surface area is about 1.625 sq metres in an adult male and 1.43 sq metres in an adult female. The outer layer of the skin is made up of dead cells called **stratum corneum**. These cells shed constantly and also interact with the environment.

STRUCTURE

Skin is made up of the following:

1. Three layers of the **tissues:**
   - Epidermis.
   - Dermis.
   - Subcutaneous tissue.
2. Two appendages:
   - Hair.
   - Nail.
3. Two glands:
   - Sweat gland (eccrine and apocrine glands).
   - Sebaceous gland.

Epidermis

Epidermis, the outermost layer of skin, consists of the following:

- Basal cell layer or stratum basale or stratum germinativum.
- Prickle cell layer or stratum spinosum.
- Stratum granulosum.
- Stratum corneum or horny cell layer.

The basal cell layer**,** also known as **stratum germinativum,** is made up of a single layer of columnar epithelial cells which keep on dividing constantly. These cells get gradually displaced outwards by the newly formed cells and transform into polygonal-shaped cells known as **stratum spinosum.** These polygonal cells are attached to each other and to the cells of basal cell layer by a specialised structure called **desmosome**. These cells are also covered with a proteinous substance called intercellular cement. Strata germinativum and spinosum together constitute **stratum malpighii.**

Towards the surface, these cells flatten, lose their prickles and acquire numerous granules in their cytoplasm and are known as granular cells or **stratum granulosum.**

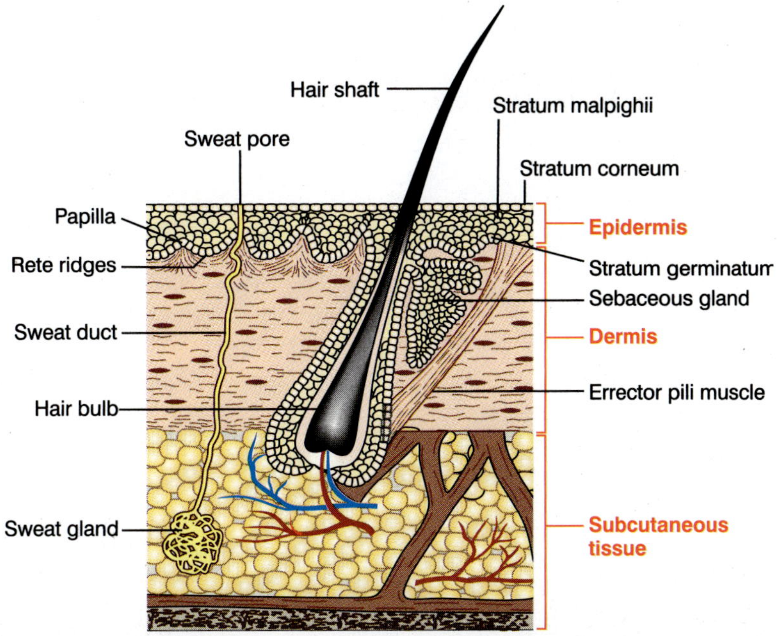

Fig. 1.1 Structure of skin

Table 1.1 Skin structure: At a glance

Epidermis	• Basal cell layer (stratum germinatum) • Stratum malphighii (pickle cell layer) • Stratum granulosum • Stratum lucidum • Stratum corneum
Dermis (3 mm thick)	• Papillary dermis: Upper part • Reticular dermis: Lower part
Fibres: 2	• Collagen fibres • Elastic fibres
Cells: 3	• Fibroblasts • Histiocytes • Mast cells
Subcutaneous Tissue	• Maximum: On palms and soles • Minimum: On eyelids
Appendages: 2	• Hair • Nail
Glands: 2	• Sweat gland • Sebaceous gland
Blood Supply	• Subpapillary • Subdermal
Nerve Supply	• Motor • Sympathetic
Lymphatics	

The **stratum corneum** is the outermost layer of the epidermis and is made up of stratified horn cell layers that forms a tough, elastic and supple surface of the skin

The **horn cells** are dead tissue without any nuclei and are made up of a fibrous protein called keratin. These cells are constantly shed from the surface and are continuously replaced by the newly keratinised cells from the deeper tissues. This process is known as **keratinisation** (Fig. 1.2)

It takes about **28 days** for the basal cell to reach the stage of **mature horn cell.**

Stratum Lucidum

This is an additional layer of nucleated cells with dense homogenous cytoplasm and opaque membranes between the stratum granulosum and corneum in palms and soles.

Stratum corneum
↑
Stratum granulosum
↑
Stratum malpighii
↑
Stratum Germinatum

Fig. 1.2 Keratinisation

Melanocytes

- They are found in the basal cell layer and hair matrix.
- These are responsible for the synthesis of melanin pigment.
- With special stain (DOPA), they show long branching processes called dendrites.
- These cells do not stain with routine haemotoxyline and eosin (H & E) stain.

Langerhans Cells

- These the **dendritic** cells in the epidermis which are responsible for phagocytosis.

Dermis

Dermis is about 3 mm thick and divided into two layers:

- The superficial portion is called papillary dermis.
- Deeper portion is called **reticular dermis.**

Fibres

The fibres are:

Collagen Fibres

They form the bulk of the dermis. Immature collagen fibres are called **reticulum.**

Elastic Fibres

Elastic fibres are present in between the collagen bundles. A gelatinous material called **ground substance** is found in between these fibres.

Cells

Three types of cells are found in the dermis. They are as follow:

Fibroblasts

Fibroblasts are spindle-shaped cells responsible for the production of the following:

- Reticulum
- Collagen
- Possibly elastic fibres.

Histiocytes

Histiocytes are responsible for phagocytosis.

Mast Cells

Mast cells are responsible for the production and release of the following:

- Heparin.
- Histamine.

Subcutaneous Tissue

Subcutaneous tissue consists of fat and the blood vessels and lymphatics. It varies in thickness from place to place, maximum being in palms and soles. It is almost absent in the eyelids.

Blood Supply

Blood supply to the skin is through a large number of arteries which anastomose in the sub-dermal region, from where the arterioles ascend into the dermis and form a second network of sub-papillary capillary plexus in the upper dermis. Terminal arterioles ascend to the papillae forming capillary loops there, which drain into the connecting venules. Blood returns to the large veins in subcutaneous tissue through four venous networks of steadily increasing size lying parallel to the surface. The arterial portion of the vascular system is contractile due to the presence of muscles in its wall, whereas capillaries and small veins are not contractile and are like an inert tube (Fig. 1.3)

Temperature of the skin depends on the rate of blood flow, greater the rate, warmer is the skin.

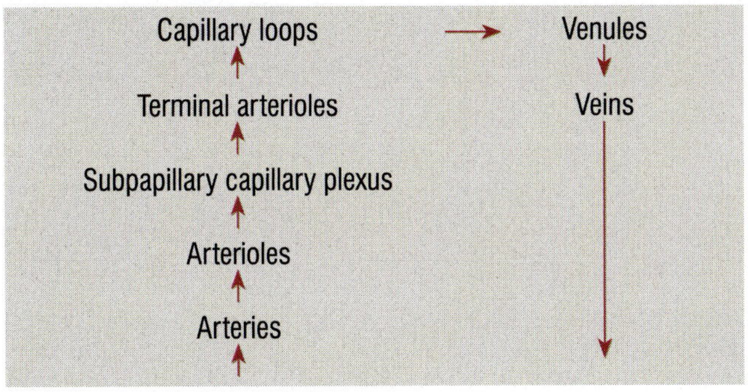

Fig. 1.3 Arterial supply of the skin

Lymphatics

Skin contains a good network of lymphatics which drain into a few large vessels in the subcutaneous tissue.

The main function of the lymphatics is to drain away the protein particles that are too large to be drained by the venous part of the capillary circulation.

Nerve Supply

Motor Component

The nerve supply of the skin consists of a motor component of the autonomic nervous system arising from the sympathetic ganglions.

The motor component has two parts which are as follows:

a) Adrenergic fibers.
b) Cholinergic fibers.

Adrenergic Fibres

Adrenergic fibres innervate the following:

- Blood vessels.
- Erector pilorum muscles.
- Apocrine ducts.

It is responsible for contractions and constriction of the structures supplied

Cholinergic Fibres

The cholinergic fibres supply the sweat glands.

Sensory Component

The Sensory part arises from the dorsal root ganglions and breaks up into numerous fine terminals in between the epidermal cells which present as follows:

- Free nerve endings.
- Specialised nerve endings in the dermis and around cutaneous appendages.

Table 1.2 Functions of skin

Constant shedding of stratum corneum	Acts as a mechanical barrier and does not allow organisms to stay or penetrate into the skin.
Triglycerides free fatty acids	Produced from the breakdown of sebum, act as antibacterial agents.
Sebum	Secreted from sebaceous glands, makes the skin supple.
Melanin	Produced by the melanocytes, protects the body from ultra-violet radiation.
Langerhans cells	Phagocytose agents which invade the skin.
Body temperature	Controlled by sweat glands through secretion and evaporation of sweat.
Vitamin D	Synthesised in the skin in the presence of sunlight.

These nerve endings carry the following sensations:

- Touch.
- Pain.
- Temperature.
- Wetness.
- Itching.

FUNCTIONS OF SKIN

Skin serves a protective function for the body by various means and mechanisms (Table 1.2).

The skin appendages and the glands are described in the respective chapters.

Chapter 2

History and Examination

HISTORY

History taking in dermatology is the same as in any other branch of medicine but still requires some special arts which should be mastered by every dermatologist. Physical examination of the skin is easy because the disease is visible on the surface and one can compare it with adjoining normal skin.

The main aim of history taking is to extract the following useful information:

- Duration of the disease.
- Site of onset.
- Extension.
- Any of the following associated symptoms:
  - i) Itching.
  - ii) Loss of sensation.
  - iii) Burning on exposure to sunlight.
  - iv) Aggravation in sunlight.

In dermatology, it is usually wise to first have a look at the lesion(s), to avoid unnecessary and irrelevant questions. Depending upon the type of lesions and probable diagnosis, further details may be enquired and noted as follows:

Occupation

If the lesions seem to be associated with occupation of the patient, questions may be asked regarding **improvement or worsening** while at work or away at weekend or on holidays.

Drug Reactions

The following details are required in case of drug reactions:

- Intake of any drugs prior to the eruptions.
- Medicines of all systems, be it modern medicine, ayurvedic or homeopathy, are capable of producing drug reactions.

Nutritional Deficiency

Detailed dietary history is taken in cases of diseases occurring due to nutritional deficiency.

Hereditary Diseases

Detailed family history, including maternal uncles and aunts, in case of suspected hereditary diseases.

EXAMINATION

Observe the following precautions during physical examination:

- Patient should be properly exposed in adequate natural light.
- However, undue exposure for prolonged periods should be avoided.
- A female attendant or nurse should always be present during examination of a female patient.

General Examination

Please make a note of the following during a general examination:

- Built.
- State of nutrition.
- Anaemia.
- Jaundice.
- Cyanosis.
- Oedema.
- Lymph nodes.
- Teeth.
- Tonsils.
- Pulse rate.
- Blood pressure.
- Temperature.

Cutaneous Examination

- One should concentrate on the examination of the cutaneous system which includes the examination of the following:
  - Skin.
  - Mucous membranes.
  - Nails and hair.
- For describing the skin lesions, type, distribution and symmetry of the lesions should be noted.

Types of Lesions

Different types (morphology) of skin lesions include:

Macule

Macule is an area of the skin with change in the colour without any change in its consistency (Fig. 2.1).

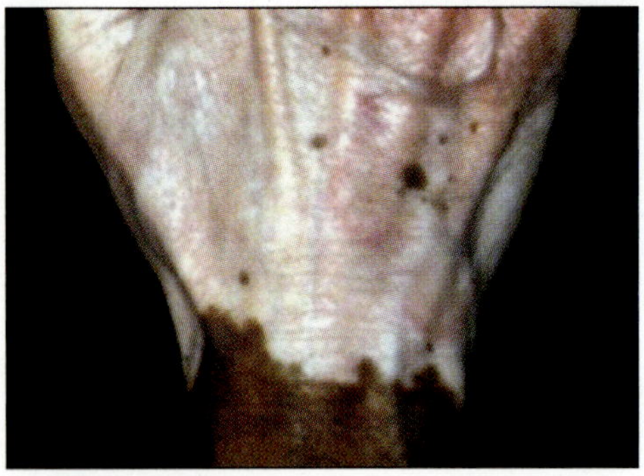

Fig. 2.1 Macule

Papule

It is an indurated lesion that is raised from the surface (Fig. 2.2). A papule is less than 5 mm in diameter.

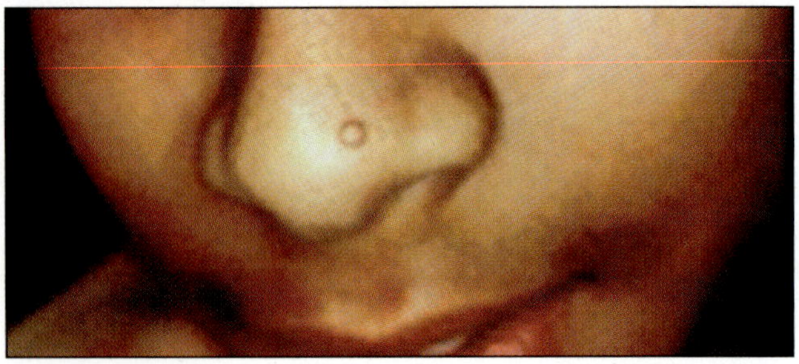

Fig. 2.2 Papule

Micro-papule:

When papules are very small, about 1–2 mm in diameter (Fig. 2.3).

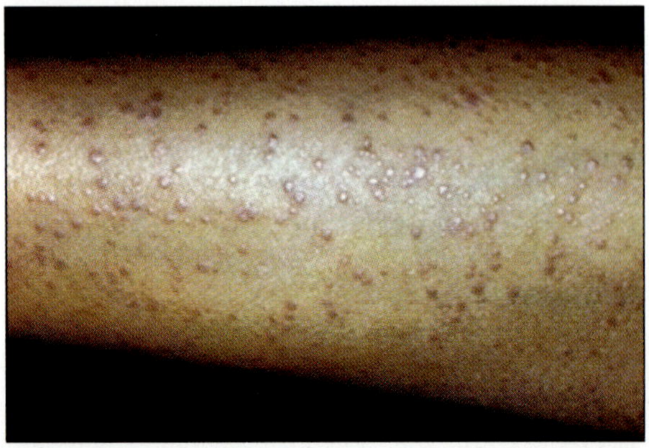

Fig. 2.3 Micro-papule

Nodule

When the lesion is like papule but more than 5 mm (Fig. 2.4).

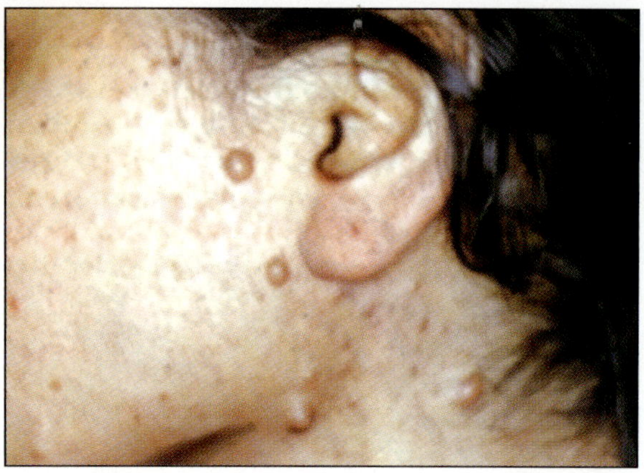

Fig. 2.4 Nodule

Tumour

Lesions that are larger than 10 mm are called tumours (Fig. 2.5).

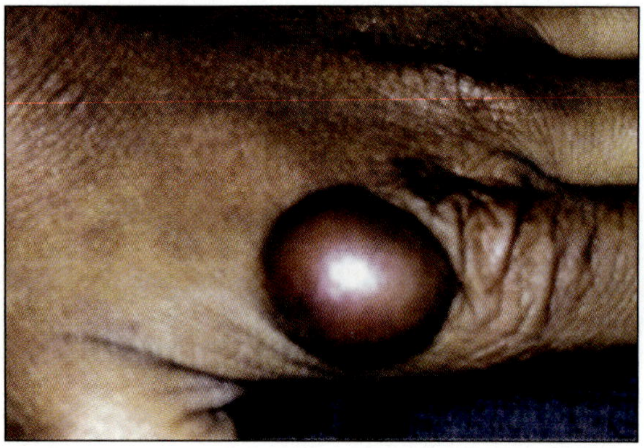

Fig. 2.5 Tumour

Some diseases have characteristic shape of the lesions which is diagnostic (Table 2.1).

Table 2.1 Diagnostic features of different shapes of papules and nodules

Shape	Diagnosis
Dome	Trichoepithelioma
Flat topped	Plane warts
	Lichen planus
Umbilicated	Molluscum contagiosum
Acuminate	Syringoma
Verrucous	Verruca vulgaris
	Tuberculosis verrucosa cuits (TVC)
Pedunculated	Skin tags

Vesicle

It is like a papule but contains fluid (Fig. 2.6).

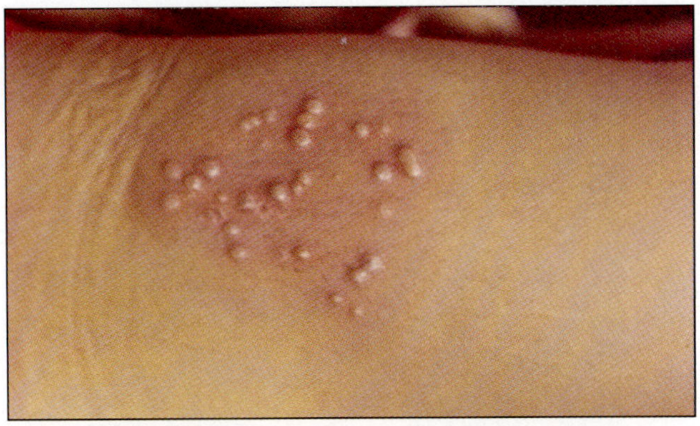

Fig. 2.6 Vesicles

Bullae or blister

When the vesicle is larger than 5 mm (Fig. 2.7)

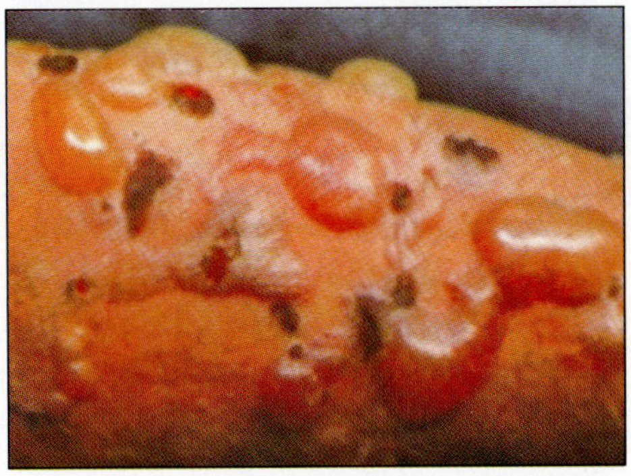

Fig. 2.7 Bullae

Pustule

It is like a vesicle but contains pus in place of serous fluid (Fig. 2.8).

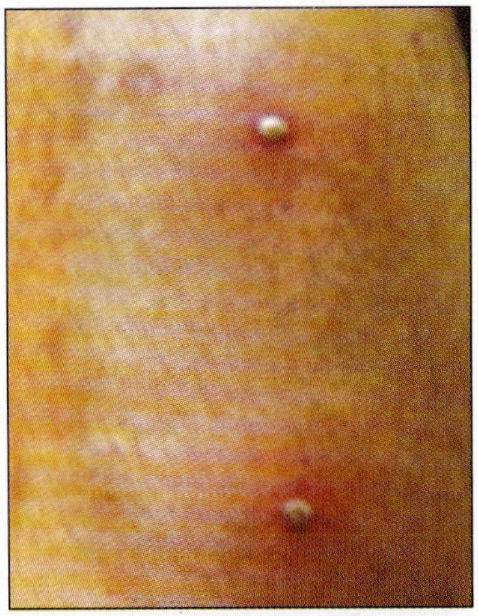

Fig. 2.8 Pustule

Wheal

When there is sudden extravasation of fluid between the fibrous tissues without any definite space, it results in a raised pale area surrounded by a variable degree of erythema (Fig. 2.9).

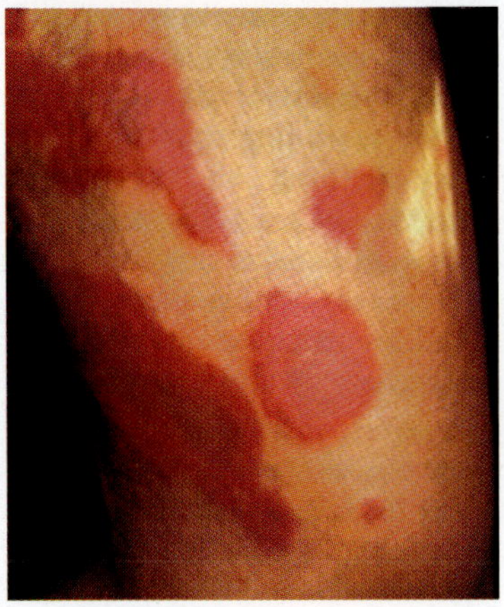

Fig. 2.9 Wheal

This is characteristic of urticaria. The wheal almost always disappears in 24 hours.

Scale

It is a flake-like lesion that occurs due to shedding of the skin (Fig. 2.10). It is generally dry and of skin colour. Diagnostic features of scales in different diseases are given in Table 2.2.

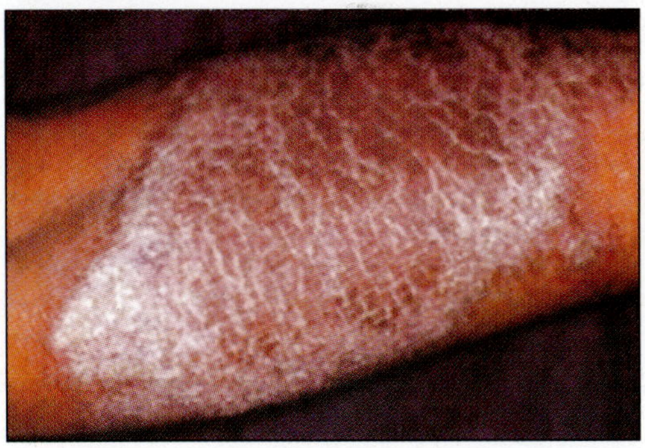

Fig. 2.10 Scale

Table 2.2 Diagnostic features of scales

Type of scale	Disease
Silvery, easily removable	Psoriasis
Fine branny	Pityriasis versicolor
Collarette	Pityriasis rosea
Fish-like	Ichthyosis
Adherent, mica-like	Pityriasis lichenoides chronica
Dirty, stuck-on	Discoid lupus
	Erythematosus

Plaque

It is a flat area which may be raised or depressed from the surface of the skin but it is indurated (Fig. 2.11).

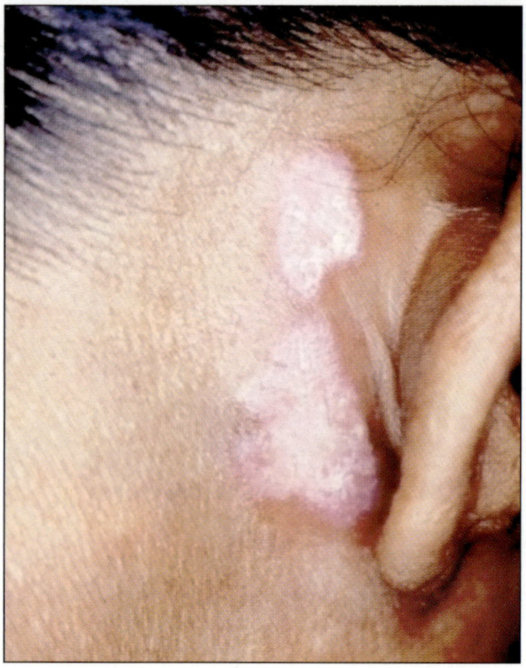

Fig. 2.11 Plaque

Atrophy

It may occur in the epidermis or the dermis. In atrophy of the epidermis (Fig. 2.12), the skin looks shiny and shows fine wrinkles on pressing it between the finger and thumb. Atrophy of dermis presents as an area of depression without any induration (Fig. 2.13).

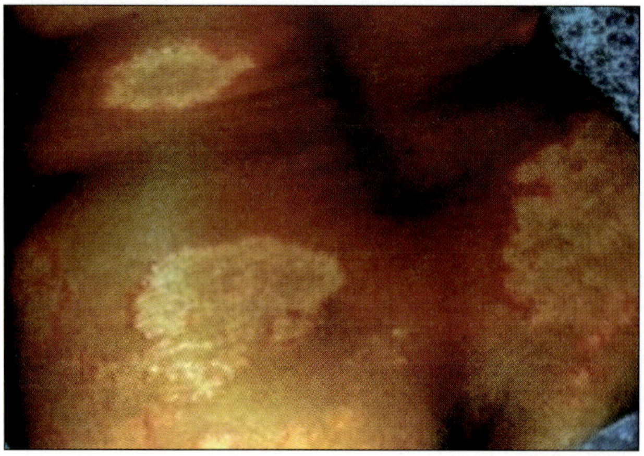

Fig. 2.12 Atrophy epidermis

Fissure

It is due to a crack in the continuity of the skin surface (Fig. 2.14).

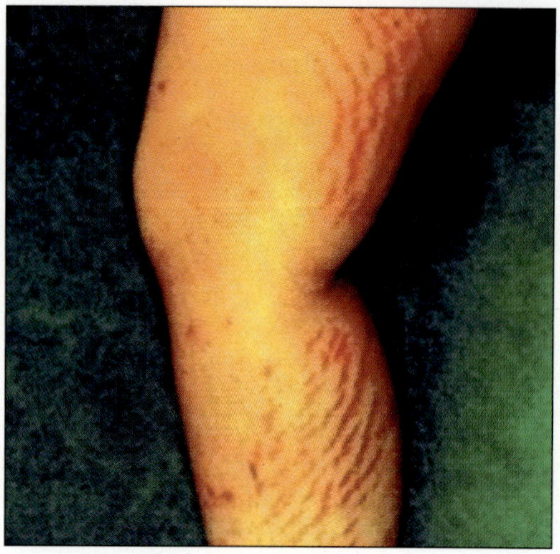

Fig. 2.13 Atrophy dermis

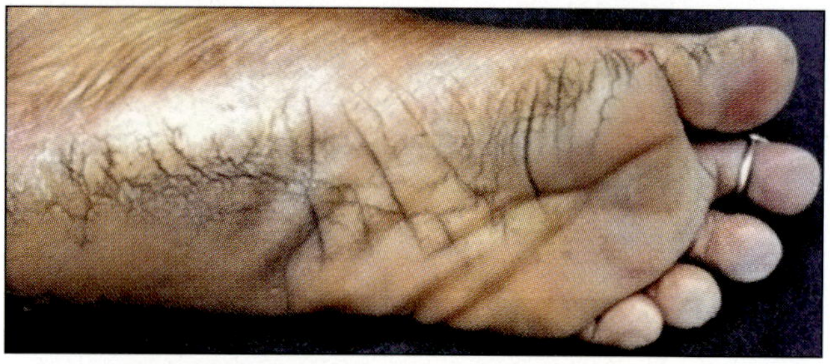

Fig. 2.14 Fissure-Sole

Comedone

It is like a papule with a black plug on the top (Fig. 2.15) which is made-up of keratin.

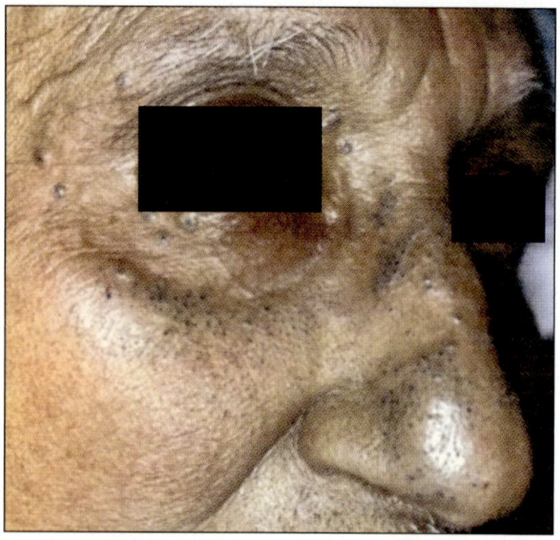

Fig. 2.15 Comedone: black head

This is also called black head or open comedone. Close comedone resembles an ordinary small papule but contains a keratinous plug inside (Fig. 2.16).

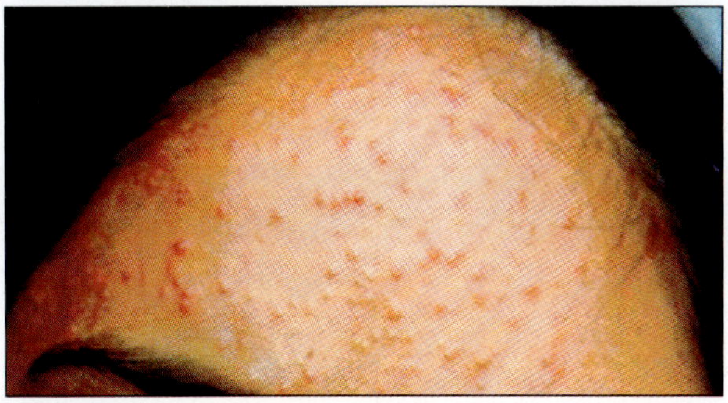

Fig. 2.16 Comedone: close

Burrow

It is formed when a gravid female Acarus penetrates the stratum corneum obliquely for some distance. It is characteristic of scabies.

Hyperkeratosis

Thickened stratum corneum (Fig. 2.17).

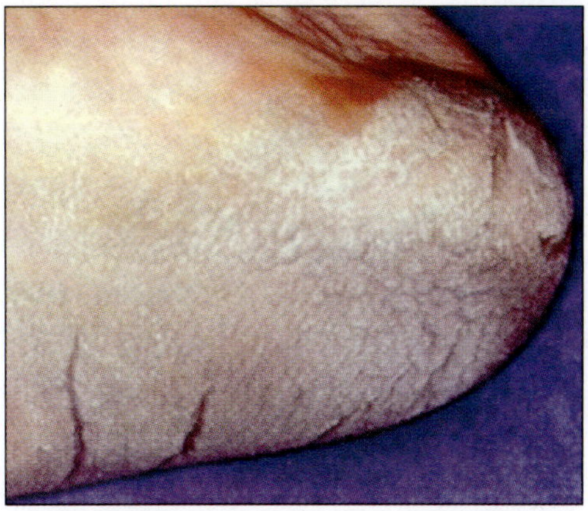

Fig. 2.17 Hyperkeratosis-sole

Excoriation

Lesions associated with severe itching are likely to get excoriated (Fig. 2.18). Thus the excoriation is a sign of itching.

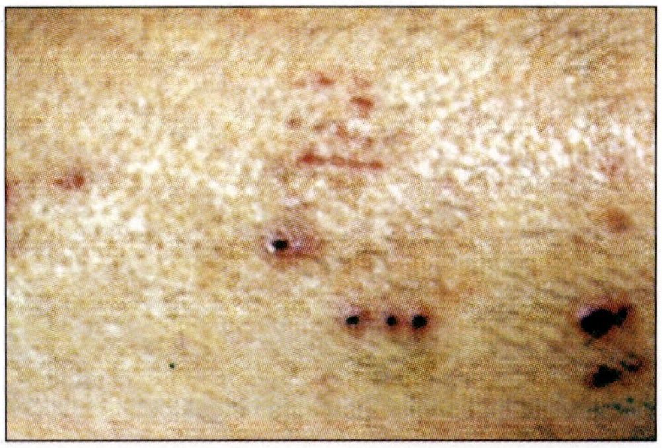

Fig. 2.18 Excoriation

Lichenification

It consists of diffuse thickening of the skin and increased skin marking with hyperpigmentation and itching (Fig. 2.19).

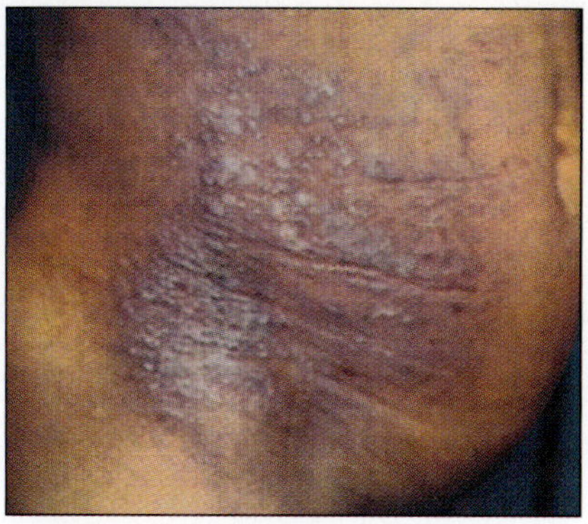

Fig. 2.19 Lichenification: abdomen

Umbilication

Umbilication results in a situation where the centre of the papule gets depressed and forms a crater-like depression (Fig. 2.20).

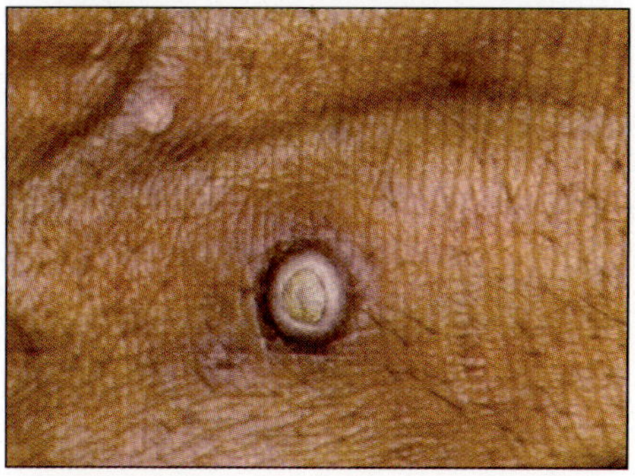

Fig. 2.20 Umbilication

Maceration

Maceration occurs when a lesion associated with hyperkeratosis or scaling, develops a whitish deposit on its surface (Fig. 2.21).

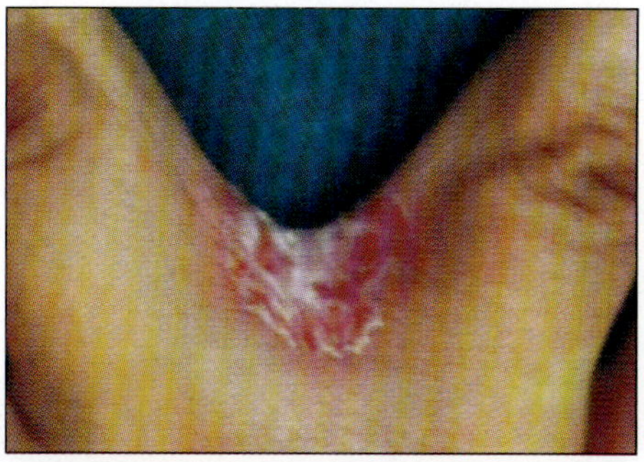

Fig. 2.21 Maceration

Crust

Dried up exudates result in crust formation (Fig. 2.22).

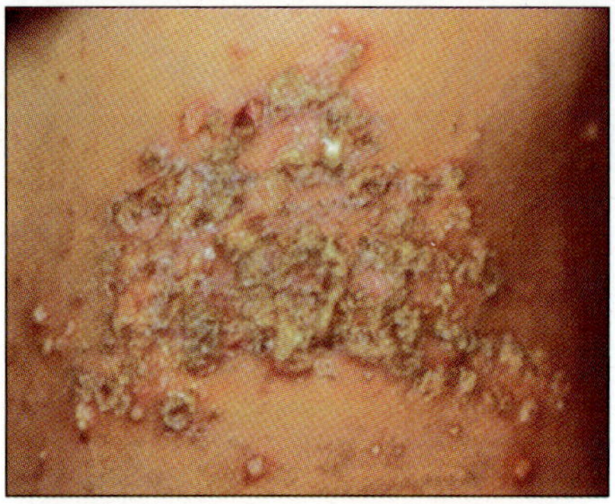

Fig. 2.22 Crust

Scarring

Healing by fibrosis when some part of the dermis is damaged leads to scarring (Fig. 2.23).

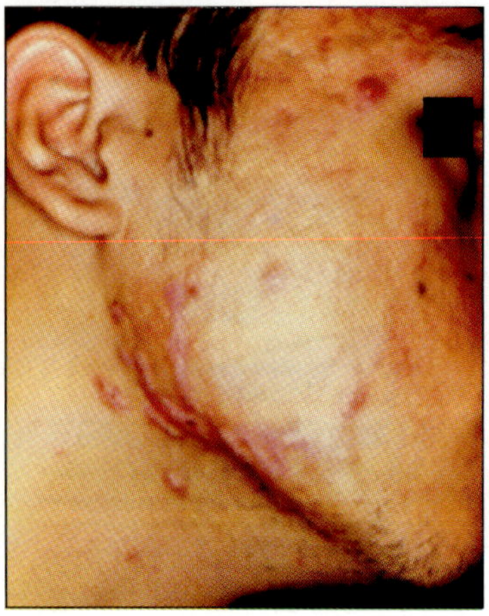

Fig. 2.23 Scarring

Hypertrophic Scar

Is formed when the amount of fibrous tissue formed is more than the tissue destroyed. Such type of scar is raised from the surface but does not grow beyond the original size of the lesion (Fig. 2.24).

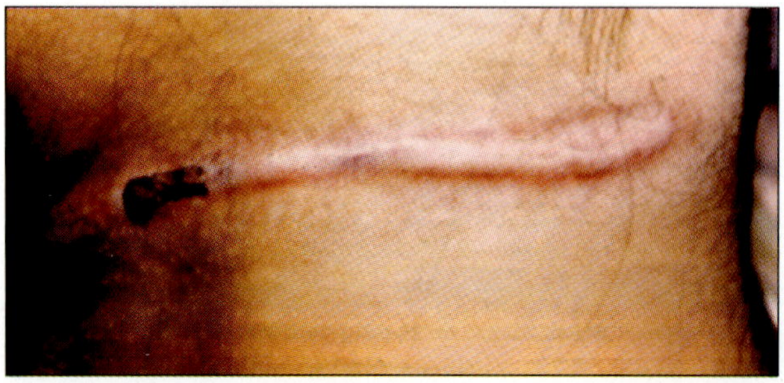

Fig. 2.24 Hypertropic scar

Keloid

When scar continues to grow beyond the limit of the original lesion (Fig. 2.25), it is called **keloid**.

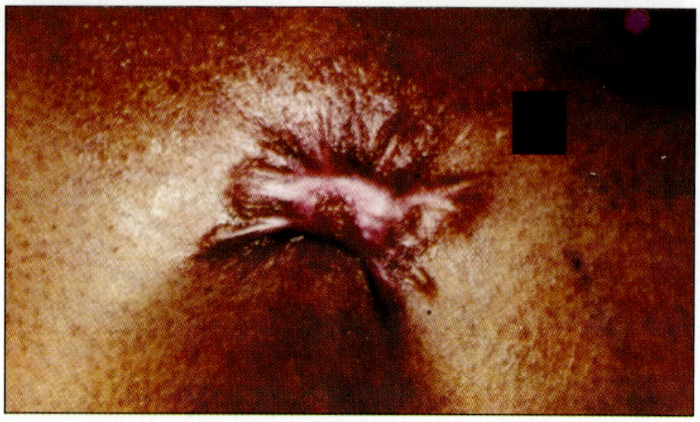

Fig. 2.25 Keloid

Distribution of the Lesions

Lesions Caused by Sunlight

Photodermatitis or the lesions caused by sunlight will be seen on the following exposed parts of the body:

- Extensor of the hands.
- Forearm.
- Upper arms.
- Up to the area covered by sleeves (Fig. 2.26).

Areas such as upper eyelids, upper lip, area behind the pinna and other areas not exposed to sunlight will be spared.

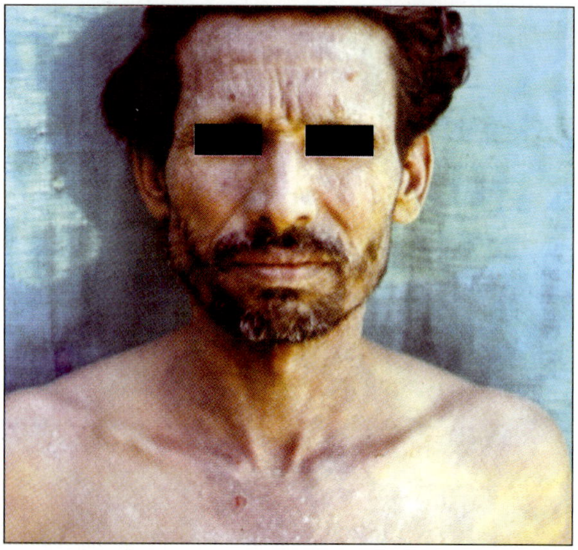

Fig. 2.26 Photodermatitis

Mosquito Bites

Mosquito bites will be seen on the area not covered by clothes (Fig. 2.27).

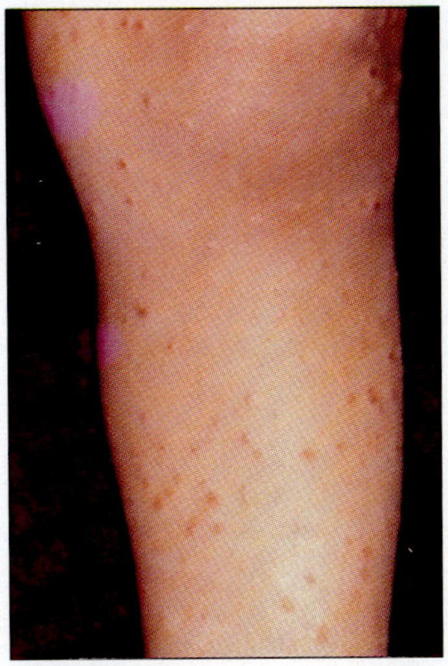

Fig. 2.27 Mosquito bites

Nummular Eczema

Nummular eczema will be present on the extensor surface of extremities (Fig. 2.28).

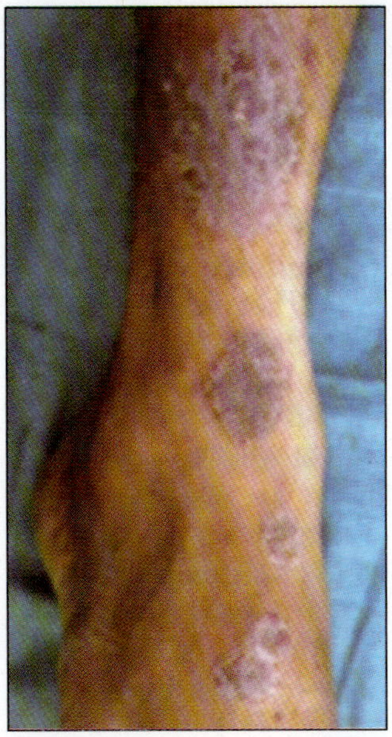

Fig. 2.28 Nummular eczema: extensor surface

Infantile Eczema

Infantile eczema will be seen on the cheeks (Fig. 2.29)

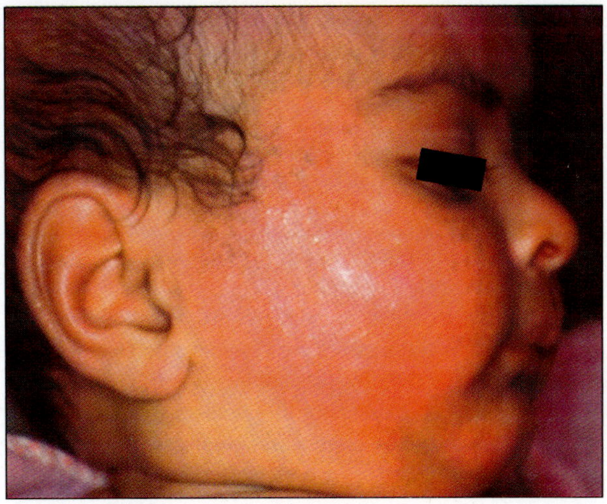

Fig. 2.29 Infantile eczema: cheek

CHAPTER 3

Hereditary Disorders

Hereditary disorders are caused by defective gene(s) which is/are transmitted from one generation to the other.

MODES OF INHERITANCE

- Autosomal dominant.
- Autosomal recessive.
- Sex-linked.

Characteristics of autosomal dominant inheritance

- Manifestation of disease in the heterozygous state through the transmission of even a single abnormal gene allele which is dominant.
- 50% of the children of an affected individual are affected.
- About half of these individuals are new mutants.
- These diseases are associated with a normal life expectancy and physical and mental development.

Characteristics of autosomal recessive gene inheritance

- Manifestation of disease only in the homozygous state as the normal allele is dominant.
- There is a risk of 25% of children getting affected with the disease when the parents are heterozygous; if one of the parents is affected, this risk will increase to 50%.
- These patients have poor life expectancy and grossly retarded mental and physical development.

Characteristics of sex-linked (X-linked recessive) inheritance

- Abnormal gene is transmitted with sex chromosomes.
- Only males are affected.
- Daughters of the affected person will be the carriers.

Different hereditary disorders are given in Table 3.1.

ICHTHYOSIS

Ichthyosis is a disorder of keratinisation that manifests as dry and scaly skin resembling the skin of fish.

Various types of ichthyotic disorders are as follows:

Table 3.1 Different types of hereditary disorders

Ichthyosis
Ichthyosis vulgaris
• Sex-linked ichthyosis
• Lamellar ichthyosis
• Epidermolytic hyperkeratosis
• Non-bullous variety of ichthyosiform erythroderma
Acquired ichthyosis
Neurofibromatosis
Tuberous sclerosis
Xeroderma pigmentosum
Freckles
Palmo-plantar keratoderma
Epidermolysis bullosa

Ichthyosis Vulgaris

Etiology

Inheritance

Inherited as an autosomal dominant gene with high penetration.

Epidemiology

Age

Lesions usually develop between 1 to 4 years of age.

Prevalence

Incidence of 0.3%.

Molecular Defect

Filaggrin deficiency in epidermis.

Clinical Features

- Lesions consist of dirty brown, angulated scales (Figs 3.1, 3.2 and 3.3).
- Present all over the body sparing flexors (Fig. 3.4) like cubital and popliteal fossae, axillae and groins.
- Scales are more prominent on the extensor surfaces of the legs and arms.
- Back is more severely affected than the chest and abdomen (Fig. 3.5).
- Face and scalp are usually clear.
- Lesions are usually asymptomatic.

Associated Features

- Increased marking (Fig. 3.6) and even diffuse **hyperkeratosis** of palms (Fig. 3.7) and soles is seen (Fig. 3.8).

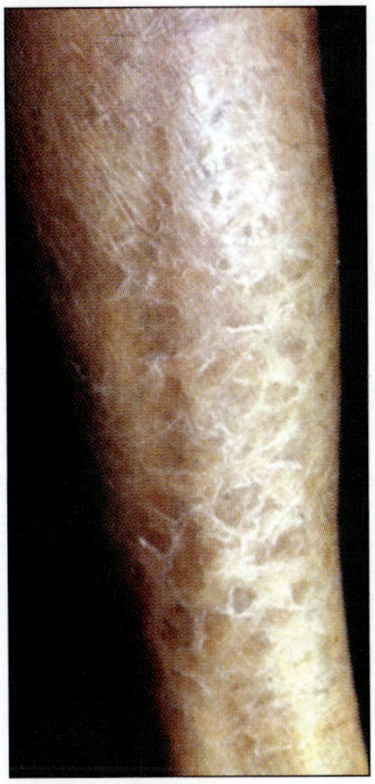

Fig. 3.1 Ichthyosis vulgaris: angulated scales leg

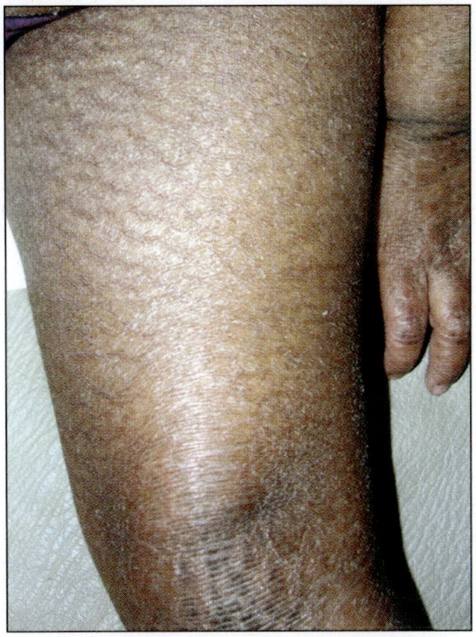

Fig. 3.2 Ichthyosis vulgaris: angulated scales thigh

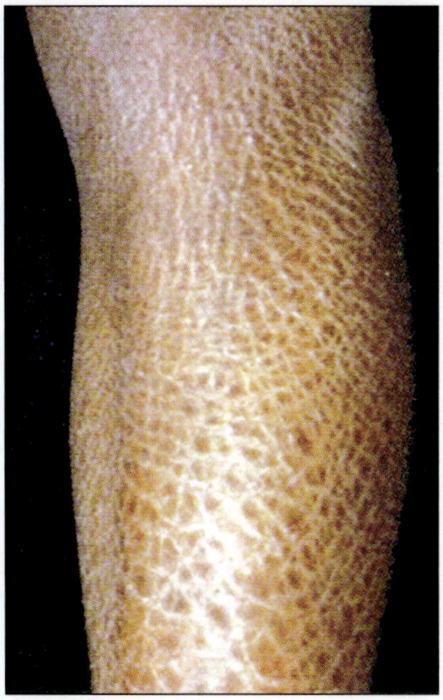

Fig. 3.3 Ichthyosis vulgaris: angulated scales leg

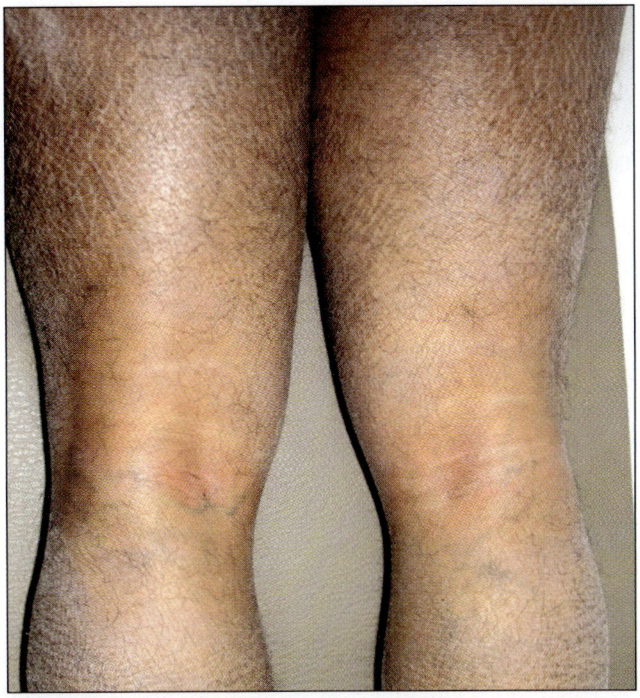

Fig. 3.4 Ichthyosis vulgaris: sparing popliteal fosa

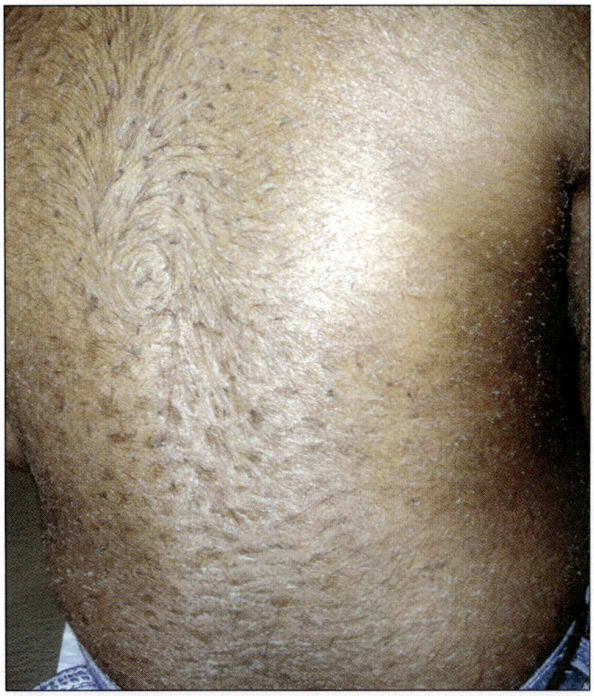

Fig. 3.5 Ichthyosis vulgaris: scales on back

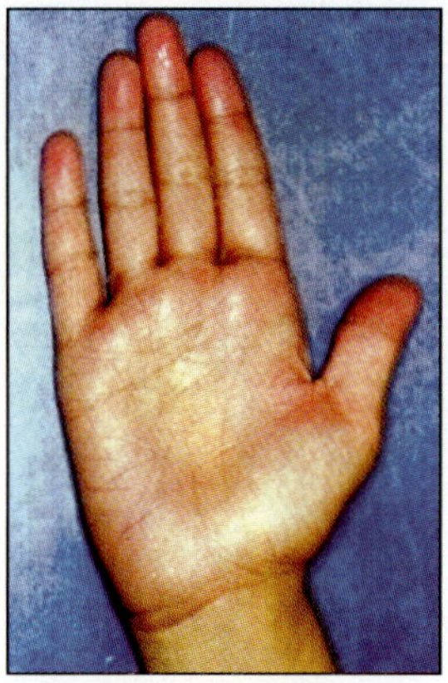

Fig. 3.6 Ichthyosis vulgaris: increased marking palm

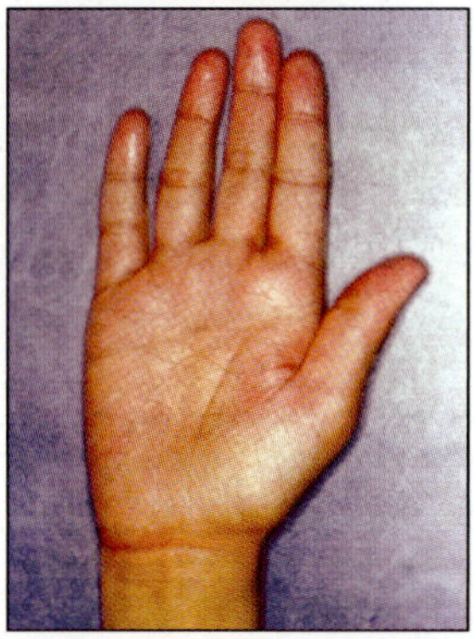

Fig. 3.7 Ichthyosis vulgaris: diffuse hyperkertosis of palm

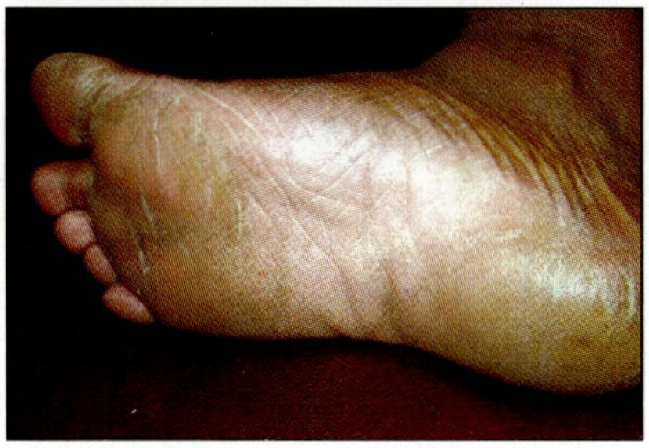

Fig. 3.8 Keratoderma sole: ichthyosis vulgaris

- Presence of **follicular hyperkeratotic papules** (Fig. 3.9) on the shoulders, arms, buttocks and thighs.

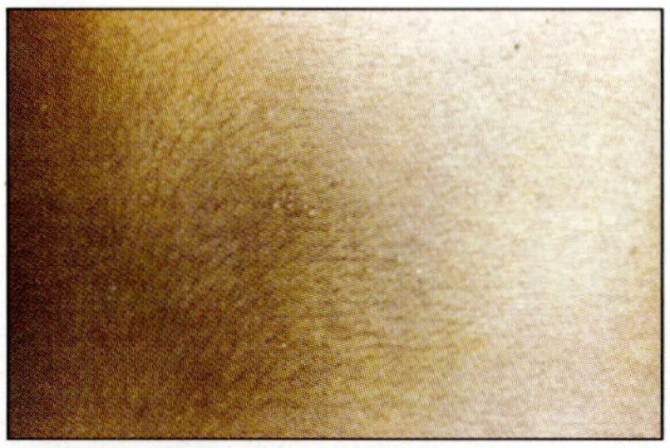

Fig. 3.9 Ichthyosis vulgaris: follicular hyperkeratotic papules

Clinical Course

- The lesions improve during summer months and get aggravated during winter.
- There is some spontaneous improvement at puberty.
- Lesions persist throughout life.

Treatment

- Application of **emollients** like oils, cream and glycerine.
- Glycerine, **a hygroscopic agent**, helps in retaining moisture in the skin; addition of water reduces the stickiness of glycerine.
- Urea 10% in glycerine, **a keratolytic agent**, or cream helps to remove the scales; salicylic acid can be used similarly.

Other Measures

Other measures include:
- Topical retinoic acid.
- Oral vitamin A in a dose of 50,000 IU daily for 2–3 weeks in a month, for 3–4 months.

Sex-Linked Ichthyosis

Etiology

Inheritance

It is transmitted through a recessive gene located on the distal short arm of the X-chromosome.

Molecular Defect

In the cultured fibroblasts, deficiency of an enzyme called steroid sulphatase is seen which may be responsible for the disease.

Epidemiology

Prevalence

1:2000–1:6000 incidence.

Age of Onset

In children.

Sex Predilection

It is transmitted by females but manifests in the males. Maternal uncles might have similar disease.

Clinical Features

- Clinically, the disease is more or less like ichthyosis vulgaris except that it is more widespread and also involves the cubital and popliteal fossae.

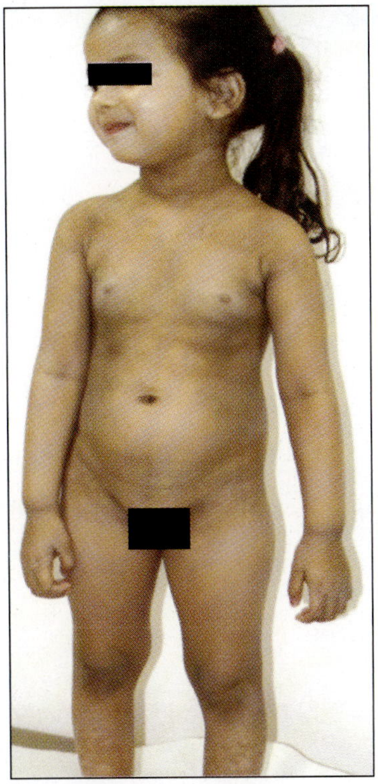

Fig. 3.10 Lamellar ichthyosis

- Scales may be present on the sides of face and even on scalp.
- Follicular hyperkeratotic papules on shoulders, buttocks and thighs are absent.
- Hyperkeratosis and increased marking of palms and soles are also absent.

Associated Features

Following features may be associated with the disease:
- Comma-shaped corneal opacity may develop between 20–30 years of age.
- Cryptorchidism.
- Hypogenitalia.
- Mental retardation.

Clinical Course

Unlike ichthyosis vulgaris, the disease does not improve at puberty.

Treatment

- Genetic counselling.
- Same measures to be taken as ichthyosis vulgaris.
- Patients having cryptorchidism, hypogenitalia and mental retardation may be evaluated by endocrinologist.

Lamellar Ichthyosis

Etiology

Inheritance

- Inherited through autosomal recessive gene of variable expression.
- Consanguineous marriage between close relatives is more likely to result in the manifestation of the disease in offspring.

Molecular Defect

Mutations occur in TGM1 gene that is involved in the synthesis of the enzyme transglutaminase 1.

Epidemiology

Prevalence

Rare disease with an incidence of 1:300000.

Age of Onset

Present at birth or appears during the first few days of life.

Clinical Features

- The features include erythema and hyperkeratosis.
- Erythema is diffuse and generalised with scaling. It is more severe on flexors (Fig. 3.10).
- The skin is smooth, shiny and shows fine wrinkles when pressed between the thumb and the index finger.
- The face and scalp are usually scaly, the scalp may even be crusted.

Associated Features/Diseases

Following diseases are seen associated with the disorder:
- Ectropion.
- Corneal dystrophies.
- Photophobia.
- Small stature.
- Mental retardation.

Clinical Course

- It improves with the advancement of age.
- No relationship with season is seen.

Treatment

Mild cases

Mild cases are treated with the local application of emollient, mild keratolytic and moisturising agents like urea 10% in cream or glycerine.

Severe Cases

Severe cases are treated as follows:
- Corticosteroids in a dose of 10–15 mg prednisolone per day are given for a few months.
- Oral retenoids like etretinate 0.5–1.0 mg/kg/day greatly improve the hyperkeratotic area.
- Oral vitamin A 50,000 IU daily for 2–3 weeks in a month intermittently may help to some extent in adults.
- Candidal infection, if it occurs, should be treated with topical anticandidal medicine.

Non-bullous Variety of Ichthyosiform Erythroderma or Congenital Ichthyosiform Erythroderma

Inheritance

It is inherited as an autosomal recessive gene.

Prevalence

It is a rare skin condition found in 1/300,000 births.

Age of Onset

Early after child birth.

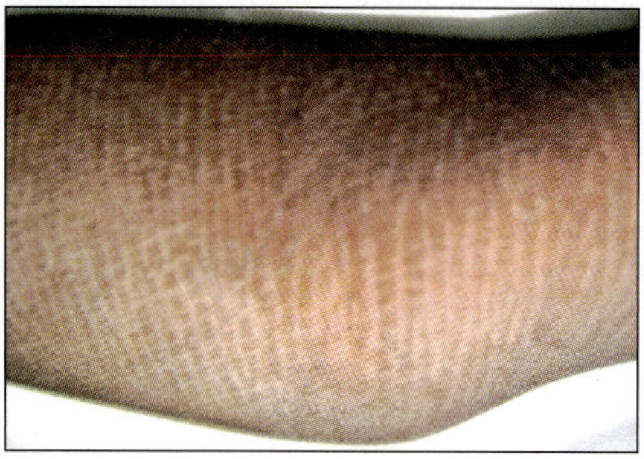

Fig. 3.11 Epidermolytic hyperkeratosis

Most of the affected children are born as **collodion baby**.

Clinical features

- Patient's skin looks erythrodermic, with fine white or flesh colored scales which often involve the entire skin.
- Face may be mildly involved.
- In severe cases, lower eye lids are usually pulled down, giving a red appearance.

Treatment

- Child should be prevented from over exposure to heat.
- Moisturisers containing urea 10% in glycerine or cream is useful.
- Oral retinoid may be used to reduce the scaling but has very little effect on erythema.

Epidermolytic Hyperkeratosis

Synonym

Bullous variety of ichthyosiform erythroderma.

Etiology

Inheritance

- It is transmitted by an autosomal dominant gene.

Molecular defect

Mutations present in keratin genes 1 and 10.

Epidemiology

Prevalence

1 in 200,000–300,000 people are affected.

Age of onset

At birth.

Clinical Features

- Crops of bullae and occasionally erythema and desquamation are seen within a few hours to a week after birth.
- Bullae are followed by hyperkeratotic lesions which start appearing from third month onwards.

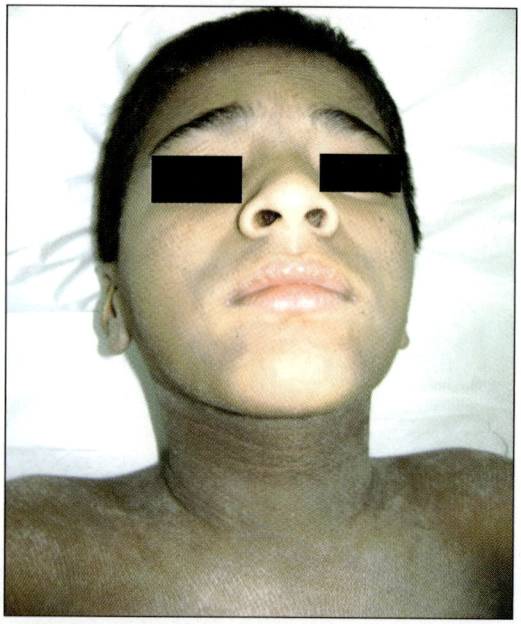

Fig. 3.12 Epidermolytic hyperkeratosis

- Irregular, even linear, warty lesions are seen on flexors like axillae, cubital (Fig. 3.11) and popliteal fossae, groins and sometime even on neck (Fig. 3.12), dorsum of the hands and feet.
- Due to secondary infection, these lesions may emit foul smell.
- Skin is generally dry.
- Palmoplantar keratoderma is seen in some patients.

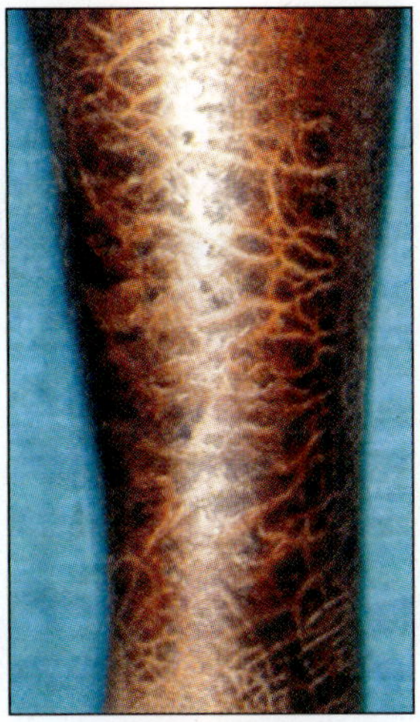

Fig. 3.13 Ichthyosis induced by clofazemine

Treatment

- Infection should be treated with appropriate systemic/topical antibiotics.
- In the later stage, local application of emollient and keratolytic agents such as urea (10% in glycerine) or cream are useful.
- Oral retinoids may be used in severe cases.

Acquired Ichthyosis

When Ichthyosis appears late in life, one should think of the underlying causes (Table 3.2).

Table 3.2 Causes of acquired ichthyosis

Causes
Leprosy, especially on clofazimine treatment (Fig. 3.13).
Hypothyroidism
Sarcoidosis
Malabsorption
Internal malignancy (lymphoma)

NEUROFIBROMATOSIS

Etiology

Inheritance

Inherited through an autosomal dominant gene

Molecular defect

Mutations are seen frequently, NF1 gene located on chromosome 17 is involved.

Clinical Features

- Include soft, sessile, dome-shaped lesions called **neurofibroma**, they can be pedunculated at times.
- Nodules may be present in hundreds, usually on trunk and limbs, ranging from a few millimeters to several centimeters in size (Fig. 3.14).

Plexiform Neurofibroma

Here the fibroma is diffuse, elongated and present along the course of a nerve, specially the trigeminal or upper cervical.

Cafe-au-lait spots

Pigmentation is present in a majority of cases, in the form of sharply defined, light brown, oval patches, 0.5 to 5 cm in diameter.

In about 20% of the cases, a pathognomic feature is the presence of freckle-like pigmented macules in the axillary vaults and in the perineum **(crowe's sign).**

Lisch Nodules

The nodules are melanocytic hamartomas, usually yellow to brown in color and appear as well defined dome-shaped elevations projecting from the surface of the iris.

Buttonhole Sign

The nodules can be invaginated back into the subcutis with the tip of the index finger; they reappear once the pressure is released.

Associated Features

Various associated features are as follows:

- Neurological involvement like intracranial tumour and epilepsy.
- Pheochromocytoma of the adrenal glands.
- Hypertension in childhood.
- Gastrointestinal lesions.
- Recurrent haemorrhage.
- Obstruction and involvement of lower urinary tract resulting in urinary symptoms.
- Enlargement or pain in the neurofibroma suggest the possibility of malignant changes.

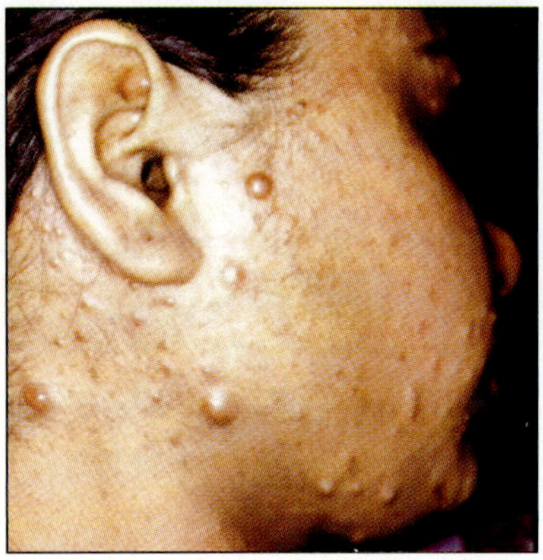

Fig. 3.14 Neurofibroma

Rapid enlargement usually follows haemorrhage in the neurofibroma.

Treatment

- Genetic counselling is important. Fifty per cent of the offspring are at risk of developing neurofibroma.
- Lesions producing pressure symptoms, cosmetic disfigurement or increasing rapidly in size must be excised.
- Epilepsy should be investigated.

Tuberous Sclerosis

Synonym

Epiloia—manifested as a classic triad of **epi**lepsy, **lo**w **i**ntelligence and **a**denoma sebaceum.

Etiology

Inheritance

- Transmitted by an autosomal dominant gene with great variability of expression.
- Nearly half of the cases are due to new mutations.

Molecular Defect

Mutations occur in either the TSC1 or TSC2 genes.

Clinical Features

The clinical features in necrofibroma include a classical triad of the following:

1. Skin lesions such as:
   - Angiofibroma or adenoma sebaceum.
   - Periungual fibromata or Koenen's tumour.
   - Shagreen patch.
   - Ovoid or linear leaf-shaped white macules.
2. Mental retardation.
3. Epilepsy.

Angiofibromas

- Appear between 3 and 10 years of age.
- Become more extensive at puberty.
- Remain unchanged in later life.
- Present as firm, discrete, yellowish or telangiectatic papules, 1–10 mm in diameter.
- Present on naso-labial furrows, cheeks and chin and occasionally in the ears (Fig. 3.15).

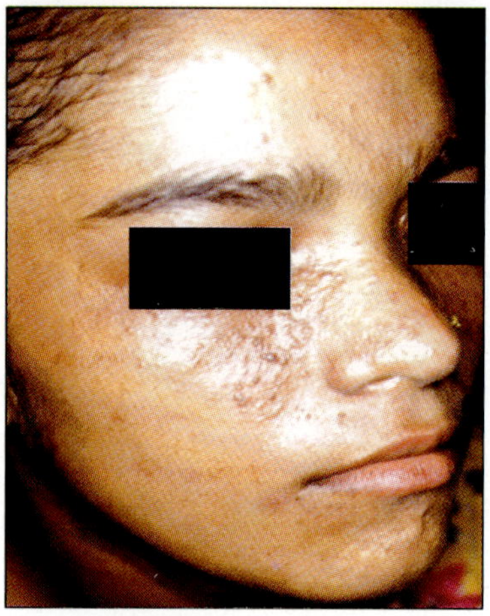

Fig. 3.15 Angiofibroma: face

Periungual Fibromata

- Appear at or after puberty.
- Present as multiple 5–10-mm-long, smooth, firm and fleshy lesion(s) under the nail folds (Fig. 3.16).

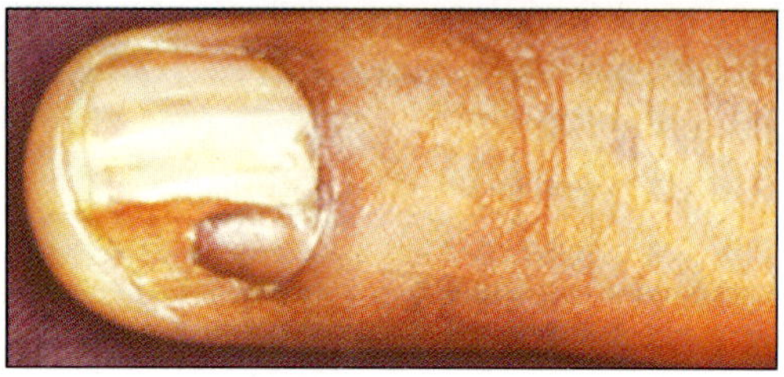

Fig. 3.16 Periungual fibroma

Shagreen Patch

It is an irregularly thickened, slightly raised, soft plaque usually present in the lumbosacral region (Fig. 3.17).

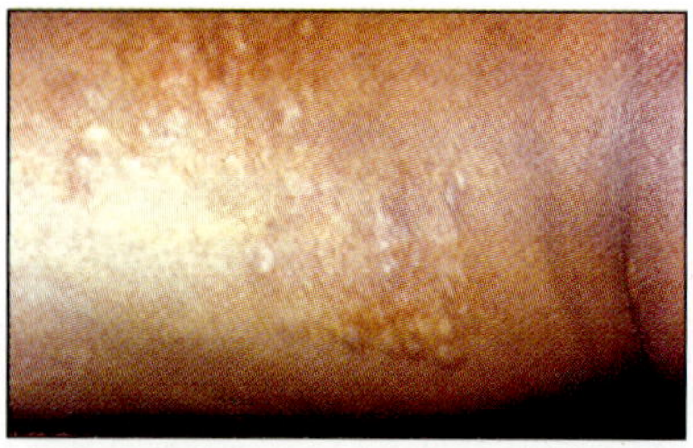

Fig. 3.17 Shagreen patch

Ash Leaf Macules

- May be present at birth or in early infancy.
- Vary from 1 to 3 cm in length (Fig. 3.18).
- Usually present on the trunk or limbs.

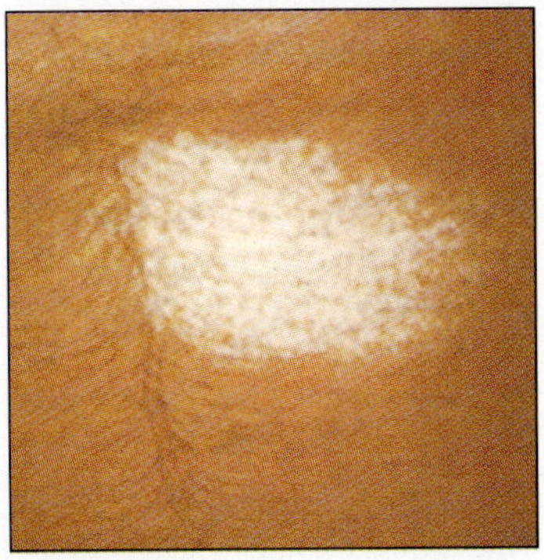

Fig. 3.18 Ash leaf macules

- This is an important **physical marker** as it is present **much before** any other cutaneous lesion.

Mental Retardation

- Seen in 60–70% of cases and is usually progressive.

Epilepsy

Retinal Phacomata

Seen in some of the patients.

Calcified Nodules in the Brain

Seen in the X-ray of the skull, in the region of basal ganglion.

Treatment

- Genetic counselling.
- Destruction of adenoma sebaceums by electro-cautery or lasers may be required.

Xeroderma Pigmentosum

Etiology

Inheritance

Inherited through an autosomal recessive gene.

Molecular Defects

Fibroblasts from most of such patients lack the normal capacity to repair the damaged DNA induced by ultraviolet light.

Clinical Features

- Occurs in infancy.
- Features include photophobia and mild erythema on face.

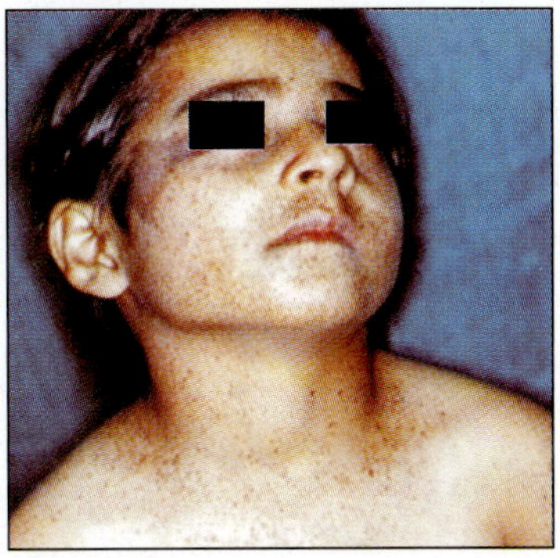

Fig. 3.19 Xeroderma pigmentosum: freckles

- It is followed by increasing dryness and freckling on light-exposed area, which subsequently spreads to unexposed sites as well
- At any time, the freckles are most numerous on the exposed parts (Fig. 3.19).
- Initially these freckles fade in winter but they become permanent later on.
- As the disease progresses, numerous telangiectasia and small angioma appear in between the freckles.
- Small, round or irregular white atrophic macules are also seen in between the freckles.
- At this stage, skin starts showing signs of atrophy as well as hypertrophy.
- Superficial ulcers which heal with difficulty leave disfiguring scars.
- Patients may develop multiple malignant tumours (Table 3.3).

Table 3.3 Malignant tumours in xeroderma pigmentosum

Basal cell epitheliomas.
Squamous cell epitheliomas
Malignant melanomas.
Angiosarcomas.
Fibrosarcomas.

Associated Features

Ocular changes

- Photophobia.
- Ectropion.
- Conjunctivitis.
- Symblepharon.
- Pigmented macules on conjunctiva.
- Vascular pterygium.
- Corneal opacities.
- Ocular neoplasms.

Neurological Defects

- Mental retardation.
- Areflexia.
- Microcephaly.

Clinical Course

Prognosis is variable. Some patients live an almost normal life, while others die in childhood due to an early malignancy.

Treatment

- Protection from sunlight by all available means including local sunscreens.
- Adequate excision of all malignancies. Radiotherapy is contraindicated.
- Oral retenoids as prophylaxis to reduce the occurrence of skin cancer.

Freckles

These are the small brownish spots resulting from the deposition of pigment seen on the skin, especially the face. They darken on exposure to sun.

Etiology

Inheritance

Transmitted through an **autosomal dominant** gene.

Pathogenesis

- Presence of abnormally large, long and rod-shaped melanosomes in the melanocytes is seen in the pigmented macule.
- Melanocytes are normal in number and size.
- The melanosomes form melanin very rapidly after exposure to sunlight.
- Presence of abnormally large quantities of melanin is seen in the epidermis.

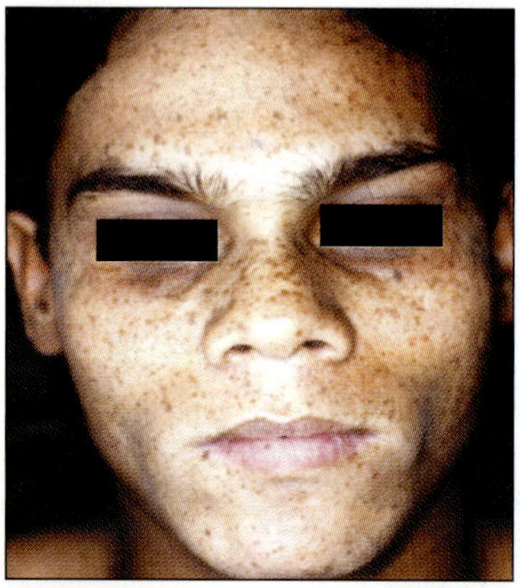

Fig. 3.20 Freckles on face

Clinical Features

- Asymptomatic light brown macules of 2–3 mm size (Fig. 3.20) are seen on the sunlight exposed areas, especially the face, V of neck, dorsal aspects of hands and extensors of forearms.
- The macules increase in number, size and colour in summers; while they become smaller, lighter and fewer in winters.
- Continued exposure to sunlight leads to darkening of the old lesions and appearance of new ones.
- Freckles should be differentiated from lentigenes (Table 3.4).

Table 3.4 Differences between freckles and lentigenes

Freckles	Lentigines
Located on photoexposed parts only	Any part of skin
Each lesion may have variable colour and may be lighter or darker than neighboring lesion	Each lesion has uniform colour
Darken on exposure to sunlight	No change in colour

Treatment

- Protection from exposure to sunlight.
- Use of topical sunscreen.
- Lesions can be treated with a combination of topical retinoic acid 0.025–0.05%, a corticosteroid cream and 2–5% hydroquinone lotion.
- Improvement starts appearing in 4–6 weeks but treatment needs to be continued for prolonged period.
- Freckles can also be removed with electro-cautery, phenol, cryotherapy or lasers.

PALMO-PLANTAR KERATODERMA

These are a group of disorders characterised by hyperkeratosis of palms and soles and may be associated with several diseases and syndromes including ichthyosiform dermatoses.

Diffuse Palmo-plantar Keratoderma or Tylosis

Inheritance

It is transmitted by an autosomal dominant gene.

Clinical Features

- Hyperkeratosis is diffuse and involves the entire surface of palms (Fig. 3.21) and soles.
- May be associated with painful fissures and hyperhidrosis.

- The thickening of palms and soles persists throughout the life with accentuation by trauma.

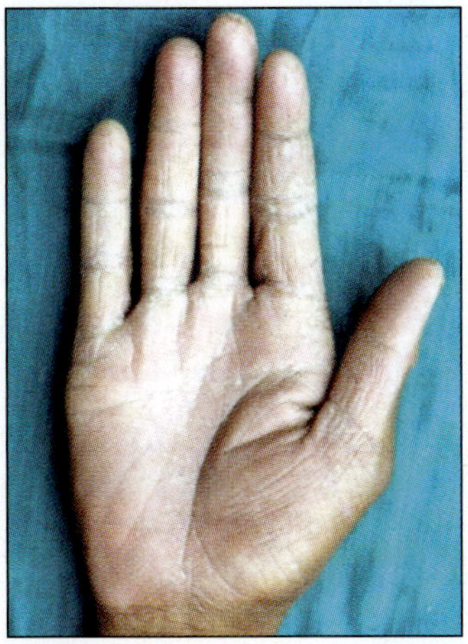

Fig. 3.21 Palmar keratoderma

Mal-de-Meleda

Inheritance

It is transmitted by an autosomal recessive gene.

Clinical Features

- Diffuse palmo-plantar keratoderma extends to the dorsum of hands and feet. It becomes associated with variable degree of erythema (Fig. 3.22).

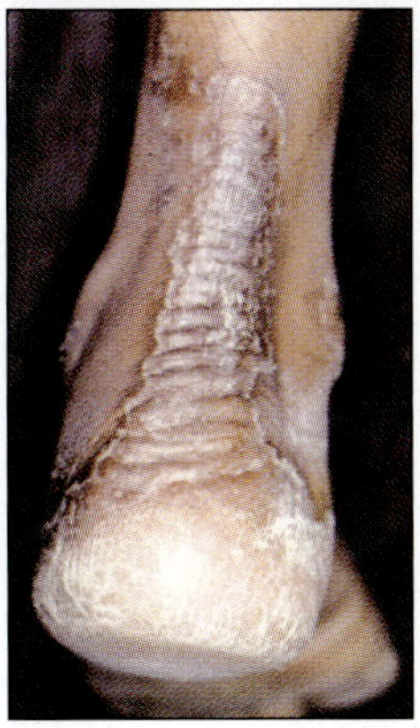

Fig. 3.22 Mal-de-meleda

Associated Features

- Poor physical development.
- Koilonychia.
- Subungual keratosis.

Punctate Keratoderma

Hyperkeratosis is localised to multiple small punctate areas (Fig. 3.23).

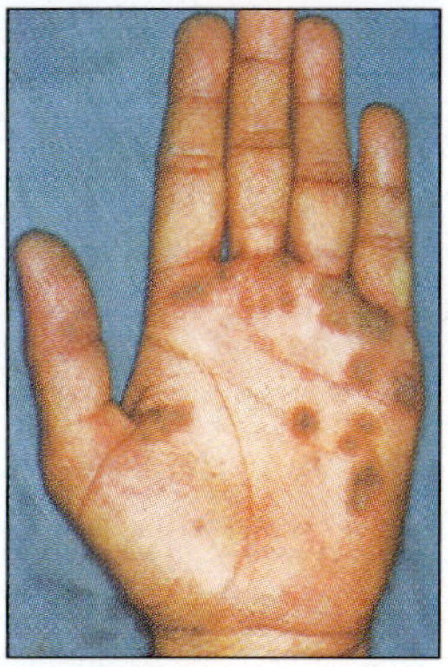

Fig. 3.23 Punctate keratoderma

Localised keratoderma

In this condition, the keratoderma is just localised to certain areas.

Associated Features

Following diseases may be associated with keratoderma:
- Internal malignancy.
- Psoriasis.
- Pityriasis rubra.
- Pilaris keratoderma climactericum.
- Painful fissuring on heal around menopause.

Treatment

- Removal of thick masses of keratoderma to keep the area soft and supple.
- Overnight occlusive dressing by polythene sheet with urea 40% in cream or 10% salicylic acid in vaseline is very helpful in softening and removing the hyperkeratotic masses.
- This may be combined with topical retinoic acid 0.05% and or oral vitamin A 50,000 IU, twice daily.
- Etretinate 0.5–1 mg/kg body weight daily can also be used.

After the initial improvement, treatment with keratolytic agents should be continued to prevent the hyperkeratosis.

EPIDERMOLYSIS BULLOSA

This is a group of genetically inherited diseases (Table 3.5). There is an enhanced tendency to develop blisters on the pressure points and occasionally on mucous membranes.

Table 3.5 Types of Epidermolysis Bullosa

Types
Epidermolytic variety
Junctional variety
Dermolytic variety

Epidermolytic Variety

Inheritance

- Autosomal dominant gene.
- Molecular defect.
- Keratin gene defect.

Clinical Features

- Mild manifestation.
- Blisters are formed due to degeneration of the prickle or basal cell layers.
- Blisters are intraepidermal in location and heal without scar formation.
- Mucous membranes and nails are not involved.

Junctional Variety

Inheritance

Autosomal recessive gene.

Molecular defect.

The anchoring filament protein LAD1 is involved.

Clinical Features

- Manifestations are severe and extensive with the involvement of skin and mucous membranes.
- Involvement of teeth and nails are common and often result in loss of both.
- Blisters are formed within the lamina lucidum.
- Lesions heal without scar or milia formation.

Dermolytic Variety

Inheritance

Some forms are inherited as autosomal dominant, whereas others are inherited as autosomal recessive disorder.

Molecular Defect

Mutations in COL7A1 gene—that codes for anchoring fibril protein—are involved.

Clinical Features

- The blisters are located below the basement membrane.
- Produce scar and milia on healing.
- Binding down of fingers and toes together along with the pseudo-webbing of scar tissues form a club-like fist called **syndactyly.**
- Loss of nails and teeth is very common.

Treatment

General Measures

- Protection from trauma.
- Avoid any activities which are liable to traumatise the skin.
- Shoes should be soft and padded.

After the Occurrence of Blister

- Topical/systemic antibacterial agents for secondary infection.
- Epidermolytic form usually gets benefitted with high dose vitamin E (100 mg twice daily).
- In the dermolytic type, phenytoin 2–4 mg/kg body weight daily is used.

Other drugs

Other drugs used are:
- Cyclosporin
- Minocycline.

CHAPTER 4

Naevi

Naevus is a developmental defect of the skin structure, where there is an overgrowth or (rarely) a lack of one or more components of the skin. Some naevi increase in size for a certain period, but subsequently remain stationary throughout life. Majority of the naevi are present at birth or appear soon after (Table 4.1). Based on the source of origin, naevi can either be epidermal or dermal.

Table 4.1 Various types of naevi

Epidermal Naevi
Verrucous naevus
Inflammatory linear naevus
Naevus sebaceous
Pigmented hairy epidermal naevus
Melanocytic naevi
Halo naevus
Giant melanocytic naevus
Dermal Naevi
Mongolian spot
Naevus of Ota
Naevus achromicus
Vascular Naevi
Capillary haemangioma
Cavernous haemangioma
Naevus vasculosus
Lymphangioma

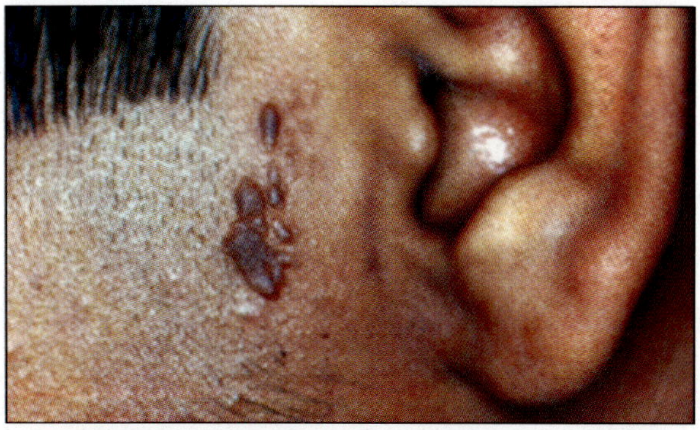

Fig. 4.1 Epidermal naevus

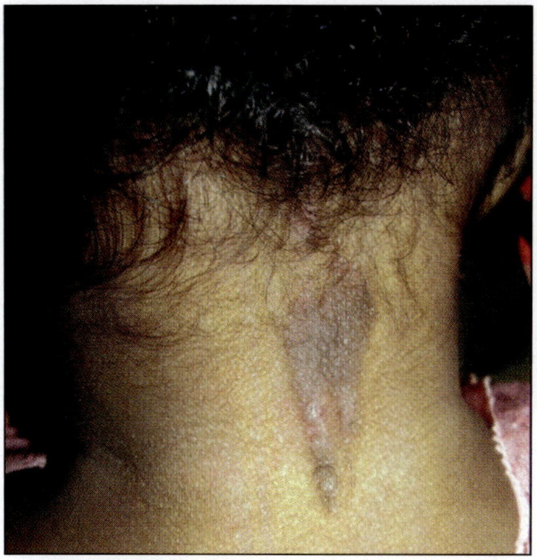

Fig. 4.2 Epidermal naevus: back

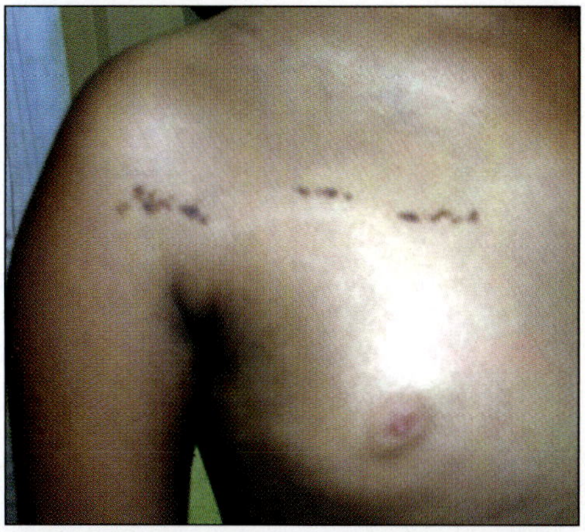

Fig. 4.3 (a) Epidermal naevus: before treatment

EPIDERMAL NAEVI

Verrucous naevus

- It results from the excessive proliferation of the epidermal cells.
- The lesions are usually present at birth or appear in infancy or early childhood.

Clinical Features

- Asymptomatic skin coloured verrucous (Fig. 4.1) lesions are present in a localised area or arranged in a linear or irregular bizarre pattern (Figs 4.2 and 4.3) on different parts of the body.
- Most of the lesions are distributed unilaterally (*naeus unius lateris*).
- The lesions persist throughout life.

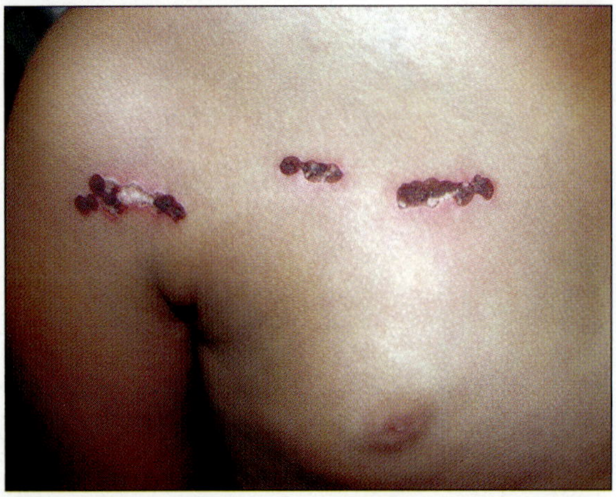

Fig. 4.3 (b) Epidermal naevus: immediately after cryotherapy

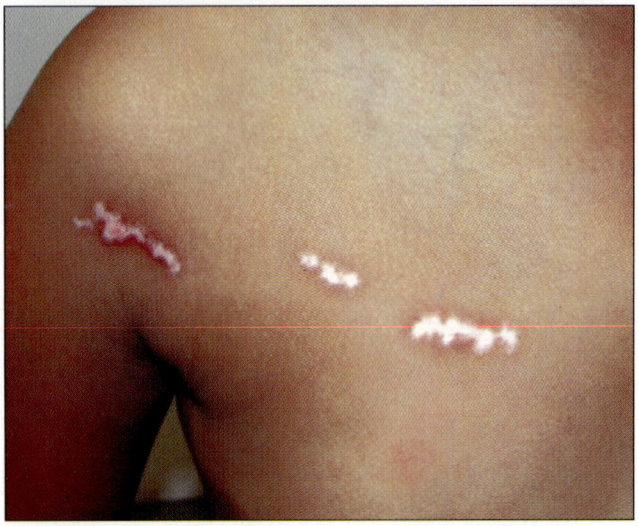

Fig. 4.3 (c) Epidermal naevus: after 1 month of cryotherapy

Treatment

- Excision and repair.
- Electro-coagulation.
- Cryotherapy (Fig. 4.3b and c).
- Lasers.

Inflammatory linear naevus

Synonym

Inflammatory linear verrucous epidermal naevus.

Clinical Features

- Severely itchy, hyper pigmented verrucous papules are seen.
- The lesions are arranged in a linear fashion (Fig. 4.4).
- May extend over an entire extremity.
- Skin biopsy for histopathology reveals an intense perivascular round cell infiltration with acanthosis.

Treatment

- Surgical excision.
- Deep electro-coagulation.
- Intra-lesional corticosteroids.

Melanocytic Naevus

Synonym

Pigmented naevi.

- Usually appears in childhood and adolescence.
- May present at birth.

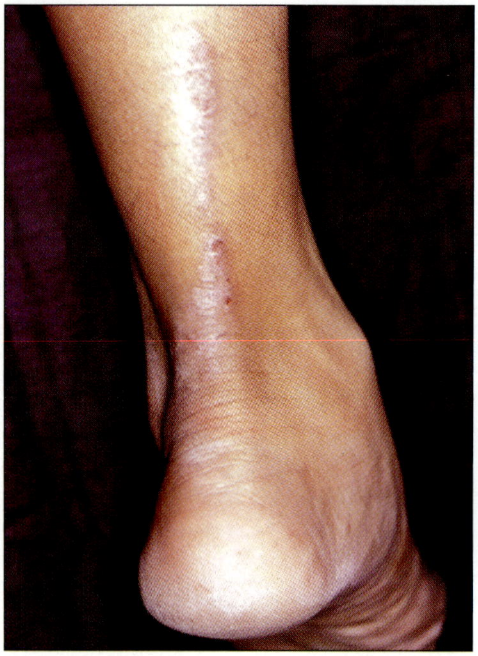

Fig. 4.4 Inflammatory linear naevus

Types

Congenital melanocytic naevus

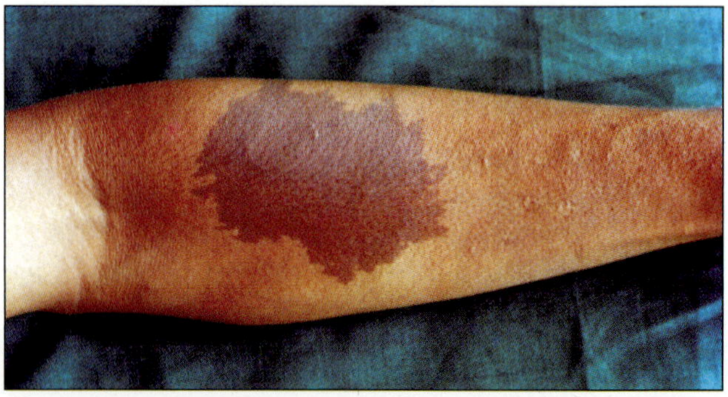

Fig. 4.5 Melanocytic naevus: Hyperpigmented macule

- They are present at birth.
- Naevus cells are located within the epidermis.

Tardive naevus is a congenital variety of naevus similar to the congenital melanocytic variety in the clinical features, but it is not present at birth (rather it appears up to about 2 years of age).

Junctional melanocytic naevus

- Naevus cells located at the dermo-epidermal junction.

Dermal melanocytic naevus

- Naevus cells present in the dermis (Table 4.2).

Compound melanocytic naevus

- Naevus cells are present at the dermo-epidermal junction and within the dermis.

Clinical Features

- They are seen as various morphological forms.
- The most common variety presents as hyperpigmented macules (Figs 4.5 and 4.6) of 1 mm to 1 cm size.
- Located on any area of the body including palms, soles, mucosae of oral cavity and genitalia.
- These naevi remain unchanged throughout life and are usually used as identification marks.

Naevus sebaceous

- The lesion contains hypertrophied deformed structure of epidermis.
- Present at birth or shortly afterwards.

Clinical Features

- Presents as yellow or orange plaques.
- Arranged in linear or irregular pattern.
- May enlarge and become thick.
- Most of the lesions occur on the scalp.

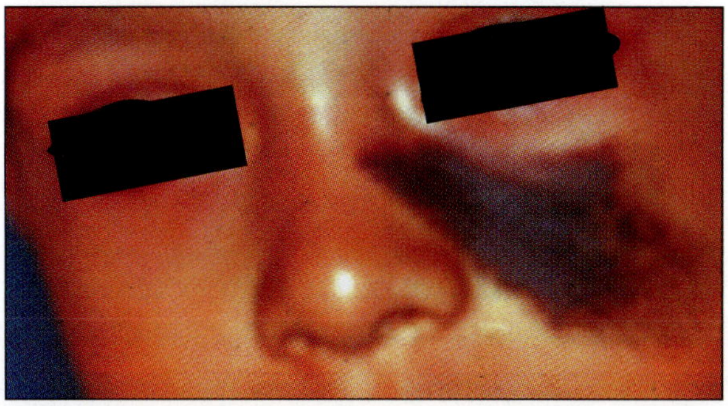

Fig. 4.6 Melanocytic naevus: Pigmented macule

Treatment

- Excision.
- Cryotherapy.
- Cautery.
- Lasers.

Table 4.2 Differences between epidermal and dermal pigmentation

Epidermal pigmentation	Dermal pigmentation
Brown	Slaty grey
Increased by wood's lamp	Not increased by wood's lamp
Due to increased number of melanocytes or synthesis of melanin in the epidermis	Due to presence of melanin in dermis

Pigmented moles

- Dome-shaped pigmented papules or nodules.
- Usually seen on the face (Figs 4.7, 4.8).
- Bunch of coarse hair growing on their surface.
- Majority of these naevi appear by adolescence.

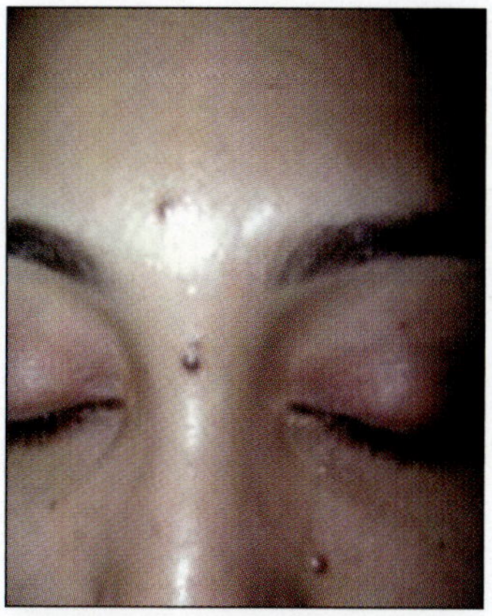

Fig. 4.7 Multiple pigmented moles

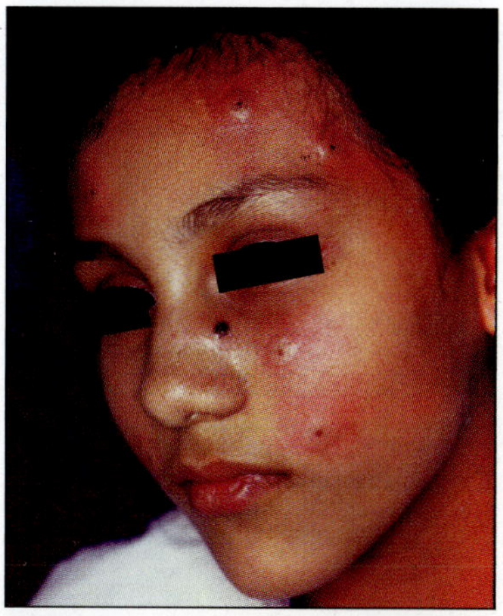

Fig. 4.8 Dome-shaped multiple, pigmented moles: immediately after cryotherapy

Giant Melanocytic Naevus

Synonym

Congenital pigmented naevus (Fig. 4.9).

Clinical Features

- Usually present at birth.
- Dark brown, raised, irregular maxillary projections are seen.
- The lesion develops coarse dark hair at an early stage.
- The lesions can vary from few a millimeters to a large area covering the back of the trunk or whole limb.
- They become thick, dark and warty as the infant grows.

Bathing trunk naevus

When naevus is located on the trunk, it may be associated with other abnormalities, some of which are as follows:

- Spina-bifida.
- Meningocele.

Treatment

Giant melanocytic naevi have a tendency for malignant transformation and thus should be excised at an early age.

Halo Naevus

- It results when pigmented naevus develops a depigmented halo around the lesion.
- The pigmented naevus in the halo naevus ultimately disappears.

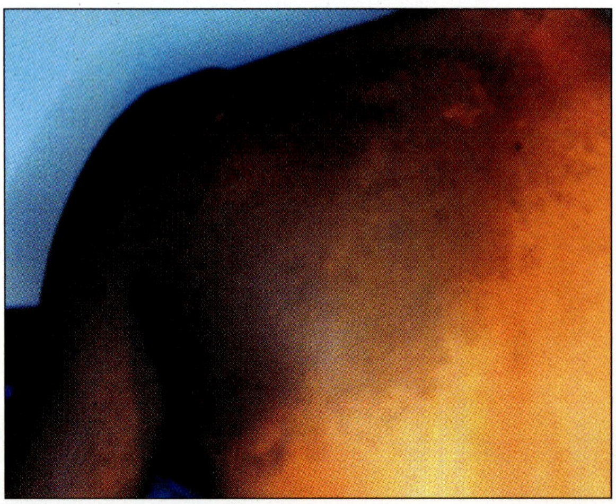

Fig. 4.9 Giant melanocytic naevus

- The depigmented area also vanishes in due course.

Mongolian Spot

- Seen as ill defined bluish macules, most often on the buttocks and back of the newborn.
- Bluish coloration is due to the presence of naevus cells in the upper dermis between the collagen bundles.
- Disappears without any trace during the first year.

Naevus of Ota

- Presents as large coalescing bluish macules.
- Seen on the areas supplied by ophthalmic and/or maxillary branches of the trigeminal nerve.
- Cheek, forehead and eyelids are the commonly affected sites (Fig. 4.10).
- Skin lesions are usually associated with similar lesions in the sclera, conjunctiva (Fig. 4.11) and optic nerve.

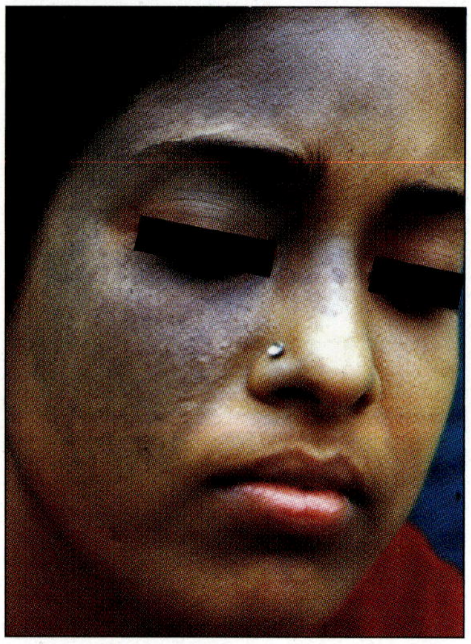

Fig. 4.10 Naevus of Ota on face

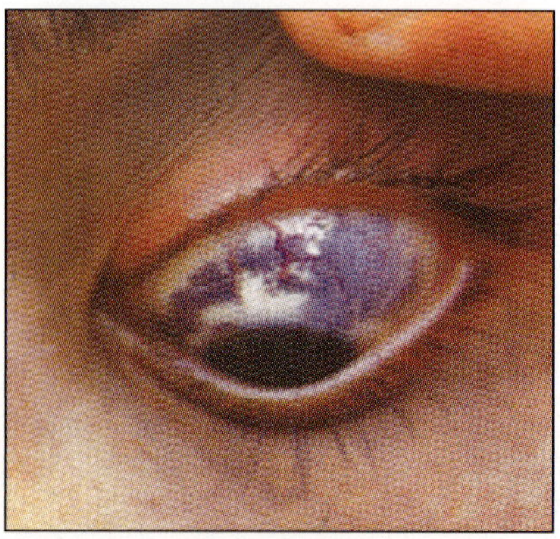

Fig. 4.11 Naevus of Ota on conjunctiva

- Lesions are usually unilateral and more common in females.

Pigmented Hairy Epidermal Naevus

Synonym

Becker's naevus

- It is noticed during adolescence, usually after exposure to sunlight.
- Seen as an irregular, brownish, pigmented macule situated on the shoulders, upper back and chest (Figs. 4.12, 4.14).

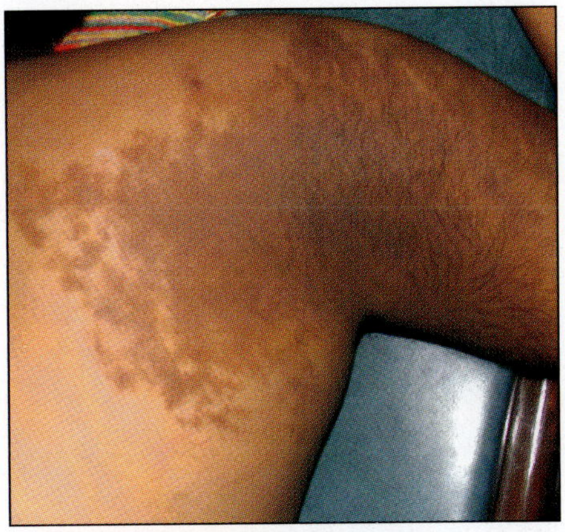

Fig. 4.12 Becker's naevus

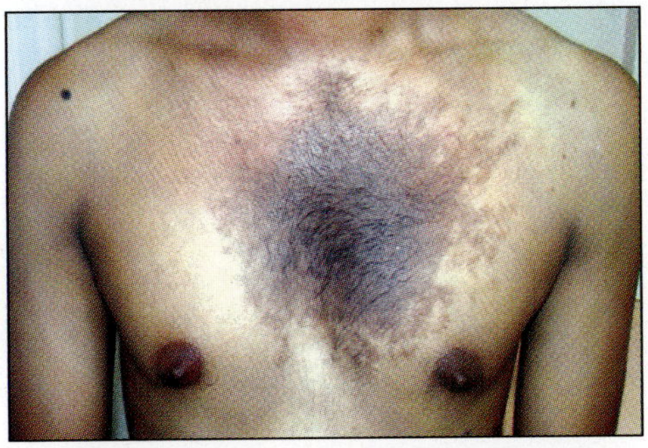

Fig. 4.13 Becker's naevus: before treatment

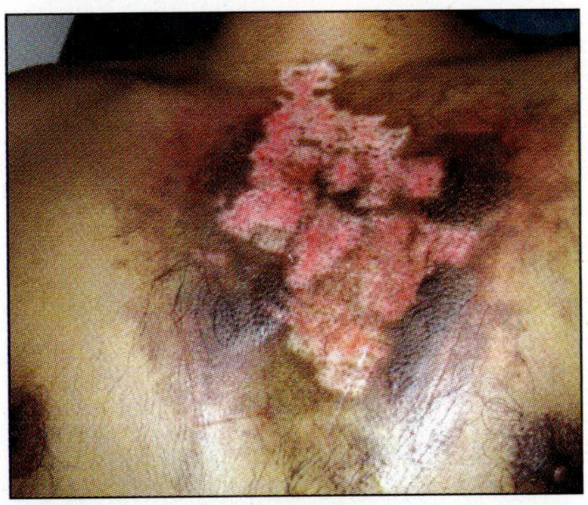

Fig. 4.14 Becker's naevus: after treatment

- Associated with areas of growth of dark coarse hair, which may or may not coincide with pigmented areas.
- It is purely an epidermal condition, no naevus cells are seen at the dermo-epidermal junction or in dermis.

Treatment

- Majority of naevi are harmless.
- A few of them, like small flat pigmented naevi are often used as identification marks.
- Dome-shaped naevi are accepted as beauty spots.
- Unwanted naevi may be excised easily, surgically or with a laser.

Naevus Achromicus

Synonym

Naevus depigmentosus

Clinical Features

- It is present at birth or appears early in life.
- Seen as asymptomatic, depigmented, or occasionally hypo- pigmented macules (Fig. 4.15).

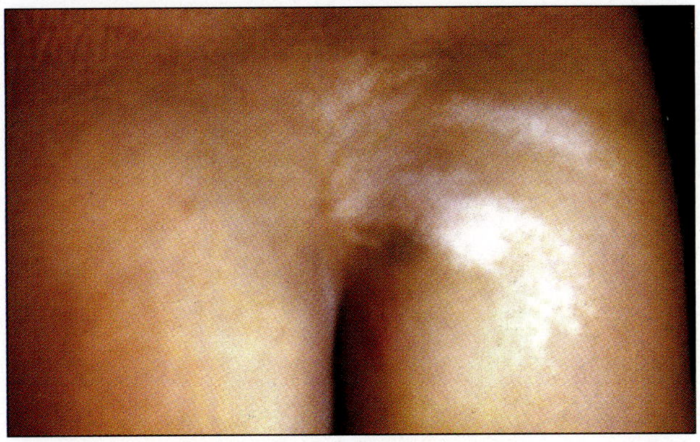

Fig. 4.15 Naevus achromicus on back

- It has a segmental distribution, along the lines of Blaschko.
- There is a functional defect of melanocytes causing decreased melanin synthesis and its transport to the keratinocytes.
- Naevus achromicus needs to be differentiated from vitiligo (Table 4.3).

Treatment

Should best be left alone. If needed, the lesion can be covered with appropriate camouflage or can be serially excised followed by suturing and skin grafting

Table 4.3 Difference between naevus achromicus and vitiligo

Naevus achromicus	Vitiligo
Present at birth	Not present at birth
Segmental/focal	Segmental/focal and generalised
Feathered margins	Scalloped margins
No leucotrichia seen	Leucotrichia on hairy area may be present

Vascular Naevi

The lesion occur due to abnormality seen in the blood vessels.

Types of Vascular Naevus

- Capillary haemangioma.
- Salmon patch.
- Naevus vasculosus.
- Cavernous haemangioma.

Capillary Haemangioma

Synonym

Portwine naevus, naevus flammeus or telangiectatic naevus.

Clinical Features

- Bright red to dark brown macules are seen, varying from a few millimeters to large areas in diameter.
- Comprises small, dilated but mature capillaries of the dermis lined by a single layer of endothelial cells.
- Seen on the face (Figs 4.16 and 4.18), extremities and the trunk.

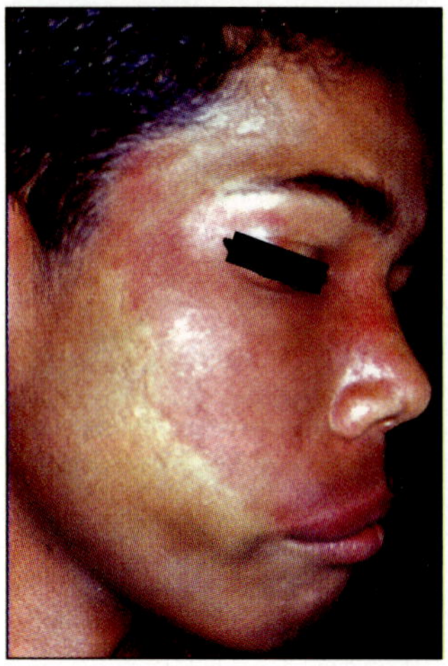

Fig. 4.16 Capillary haemangioma

Sturge-Weber Syndrome

- The lesion is situated in the region of the ophthalmic branch of trigeminal nerve.
- Similar lesions may be present in the eye and leptomeninges which manifest as convulsions and eye problems.
- Intracranial calcification is seen on skiagram of the skull.
- Majority of the lesions are unilateral and present at birth.
- The lesion persists throughout life with thickening and nodule formation.

Treatment

- Excision and grafting of the area.
- Cryotherapy.
- Argon lasers.

Salmon Patch

Clinical Features

- It is a type of very small capillary haemangioma that is present at birth.
- Seen as pale and pink areas with fine telangiectasis.
- Commonly seen on the nape of the neck, centre of the forehead and eyelids.
- These lesions fade rapidly within a year.

Cavernous Haemangioma

Clinical Features

- These lesions are made-up of large, dilated capillaries filled with blood and lined by a single layer of well-differentiated endothelial cells.

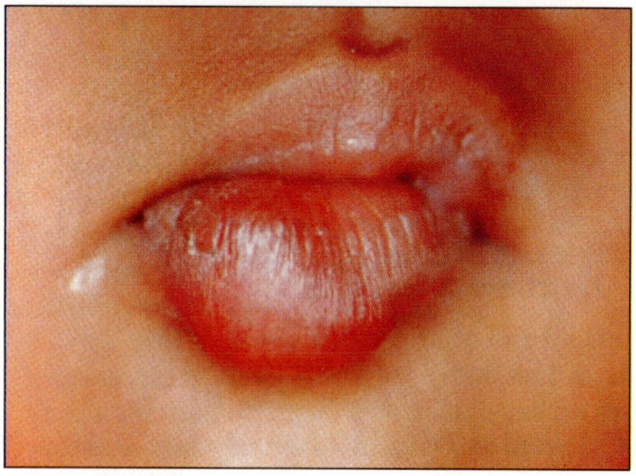

Fig. 4.17 Cavernous haemangioma: lower lip

- They present as red or bluish red, irregular, lobulated masses involving the subcutaneous tissues (Fig. 4.17).
- Usually seen during the first month of life. Lesions do not grow in size and remain constant.
- They can be seen on any part of the body.

- The lesion may produce pressure symptoms, or interfere with the functions of the affected organ when present near vital organs like eye or on the tongue.

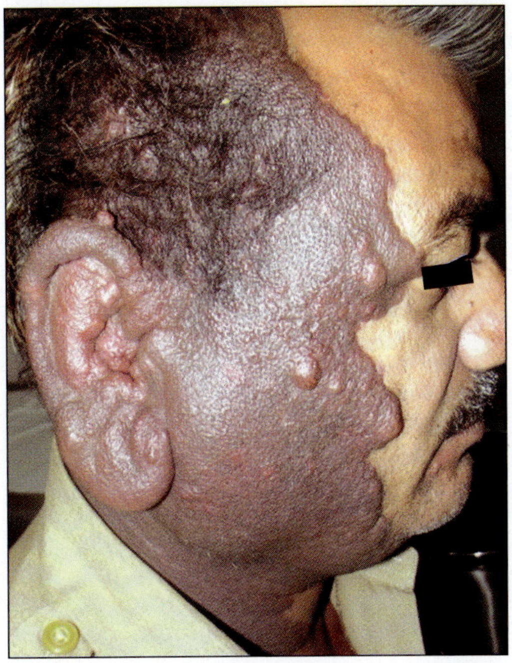

Fig. 4.18 Haemangioma

Treatment

Various methods used in management include:

- Surgical excision including use of diathermy knife.
- Cryotherapy.
- Argon lasers.

Intralesional injection of sclerosing agents like sodium citrate 30%, glucose 30% at fortnightly or monthly interval produces inflammation, fibrosis and scarring leading to occlusion of blood vessels.

Naevus Vasculosus

Synonym

Strawberry naevus/infantile hemangioma.

Clinical Features

- The lesion consists of dilated, immature capillaries lined by several layers of endothelial cells.
- Well circumscribed, dome-shaped, bright red, compressible swelling (Fig. 4.19)
- Commonly seen around eyes, ears, nose or mouth.
- The lesion appears during the first few months of life; initially grows till 2–5 years, then starts regressing spontaneously (Fig. 4.20) and disappears without leaving any mark (Fig. 4.21).

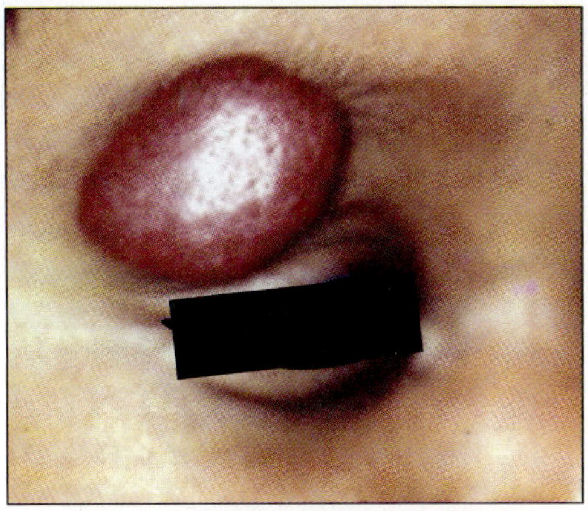

Fig. 4.19 Naevus vasculosus or strawberry naevus

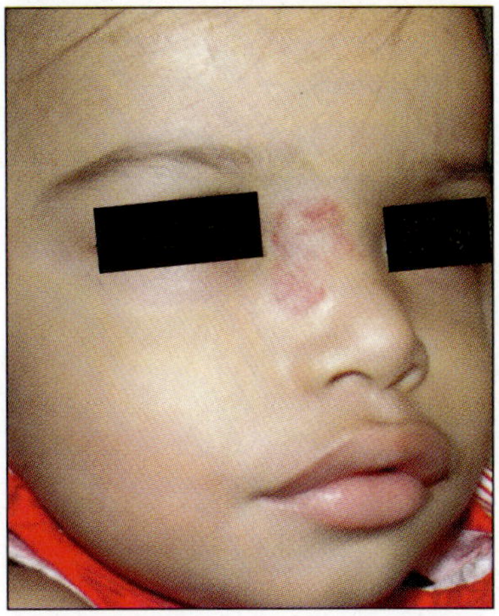

Fig. 4.20 Healing naevus vasculosus

Treatment

- Treatment should be conservative.
- Traumatised bleeding lesion should be treated by pressure on the site of trauma.
- Infection should be treated by topical or oral antibiotics.
- Pressure symptoms on the adjoining structures can be controlled with small dose of oral corticosteroids.

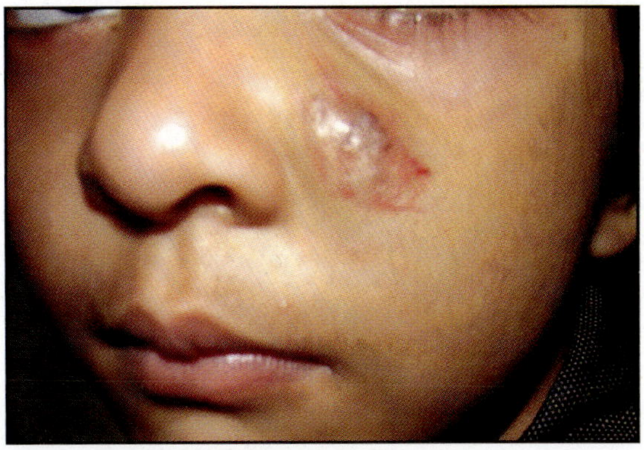

Fig. 4.21 Naevus vasculosus: healed

Lymphangioma

The lesion is seen due to dilatation of lymphatic.

Clinical Features

- It presents as persistent tense vesicles having clear fluid (Fig. 4.22).

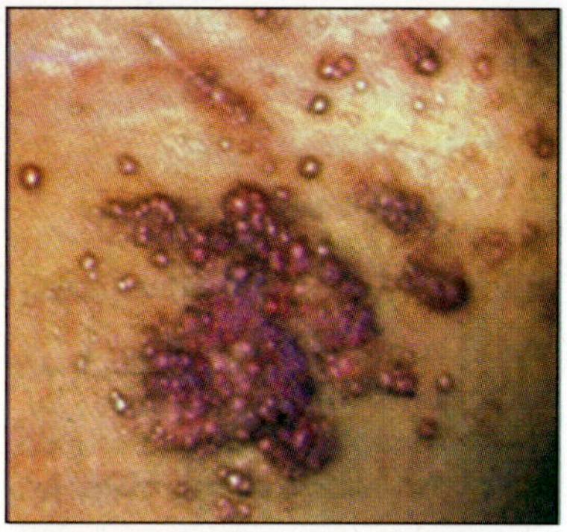

Fig. 4.22 Lymphangioma

- The lesion may present singly or in groups in a localised area.

Treatment

- Protection from trauma to avoid oozing and secondary bacterial infections.
- Oozing can be stopped by pressure on the site.
- Bacterial infection, if present, should be treated with topical/systemic antibiotics,
- Surgical excision,
- Cryotherapy.
- Lasers.

Chapter 5

Nutritional Deficiencies

Nutritional deficiencies usually occur due to insufficient intake of food due to poverty, lack of appetite, malabsorption from the gastrointestinal tract and increased demands due to chronic illness or presence of gastrointestinal parasites in the gut (Table 5.1). Nutritional deficiencies may predispose the individual to certain diseases like infection etc. (Table 5.2).

Table 5.2 Common diseases due to nutritional Deficiencies

Diseases	Deficiencies
Phrynoderma	Vitamin A and/essential fatty acids
Pellagra	Nicotinic Acid
Angular stomatitis	Vitamin B2 or Riboflavin
Scurvy	Vitamin C
Acrodermatitis enteropathica	Zinc

PHRYNODERMA

Etiology

Occurs due to deficiency of vitamin A and/or essential fatty acids

Clinical Features

- Frequently seen in children.
- Present as asymptomatic, hard, acuminate, rough, follicular papules.
- Usually seen on the extensors (Fig. 5.1) of the knees, elbows and buttocks (Fig. 5.2).

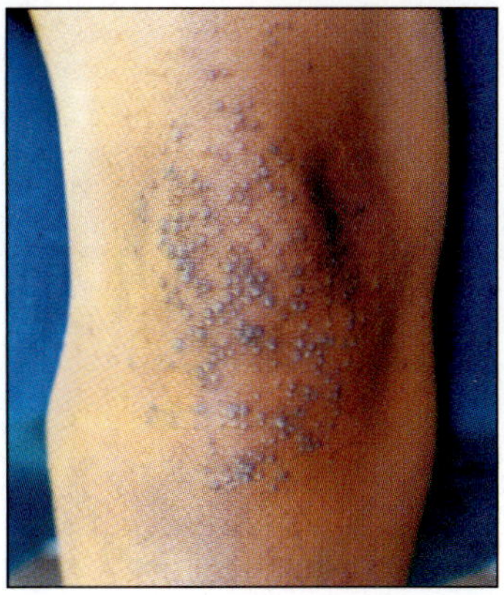

Fig 5.1 Phrynoderma: Hard, acuminate, follicular papules

Table 5.1 Causes of nutritional deficiencies

1. Poor intake of food.
2. Lack of appetite or eating selected items of food.
3. Malabsorption due to gastrointestinal tract diseases.
4. Increased demands in the following conditions:
   - Chronic illnesses
   - Treatment with certain drugs, e.g., isonicotinic acid hydrazide (INH) etc.
5. Presence of gastrointestinal parasites

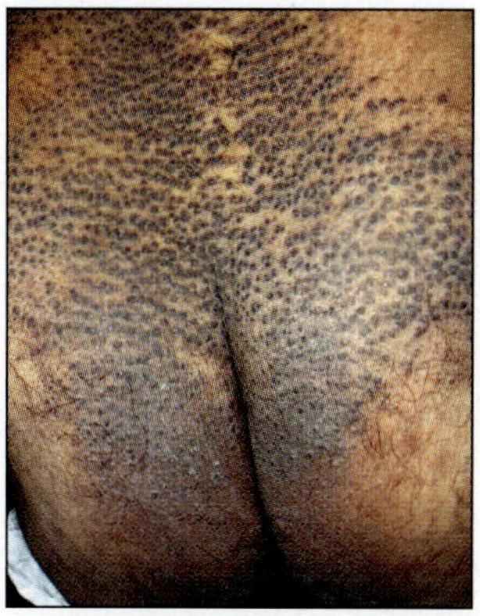

Fig. 5.2 Phrynoderma: Buttocks

Other signs associated with vitamin A deficiency may be as follows:

- Dry skin with ichthyotic scales.
- Small, triangular, white patches on the inner sides of the cornea called Bitot's spots.

Treatment

- Investigate and treat for gastrointestinal parasitic infestation.
- Local treatment with keratolytic agents like 10–40% urea cream along with oral 50,000 IU vitamin A daily for about 2–3 months

PELLAGRA

Etiology

- The disease occurs due to deficiency of nicotinic acid; deficiency of nicotinic acid is due to inadequate intake in the diet (in chronic alcoholism) or gastrointestinal disorders which impede its absorption.

Occasionally, the deficiency occurs in tuberculosis patients who are on isonicotinic acid hydrazide, a chemical closely related to nicotinic acid which competes with it

- Deficiency can also be seen in patients on 6-mercaptopurine or 5-fluorouracil or carcinoid tumor
- In Hartsnups disease, there is a defective absorption of tryptophan that in turn affects the niacin formation.

Clinical Features

Deficiency of nicotinic acid makes the individual more sensitive to sunlight. Erythematous macules covered with large dark brown scales (Fig. 5.3) present in areas exposed to:

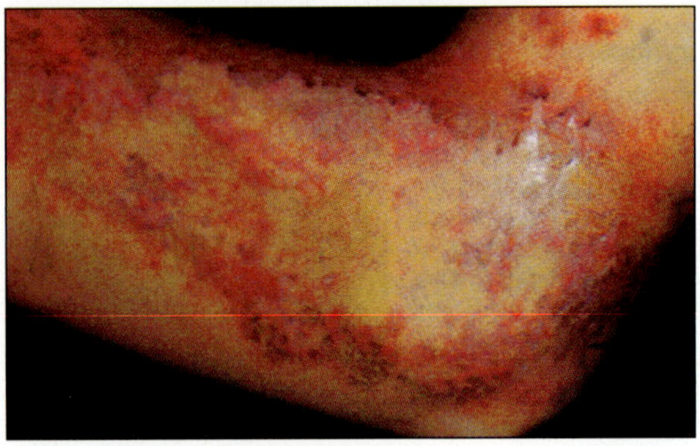

Fig. 5.3 Pellagra-erythematous macules with brown scales

- Sunlight like face, V of neck (Casals's necklace), dorsa of hands or extensor aspect of arms and feet.
- Heat.
- Friction or pressure.
- Lesions are well-marginated and get exacerbated on exposure to sunlight.

Other Associated Features

- Atrophic, red, beefy tongue.
- Diarrhea: Bloody diarrhoea due to hyperemia of intestine.
- Diarrhoea: impairment of memory, depression and psychosis.
- Occasionally, peripheral neuritis.

Treatment

- Nicotinic acid or nicotinamide 200 mg thrice daily clears the lesions in 7–10 days.
- Skin should be protected from sunlight.

DEFICIENCY OF VITAMIN B2 OR RIBOFLAVIN

Etiology

- Dietary shortage like consuming diet devoid of dairy products, animal products and leafy vegetables.
- Acute illness:
  i) Nausea and vomiting.
  ii) Amoebic and bacillary dysentery.
- Chronic illness
  (i) Bypass surgery in GI tract.
  (ii) Cirrhosis of liver.

Clinical Features

The deficiency presents as follows:

Cheilitis

Lips become dry, cracked and at times crusted and ulcerated

Angular Stomatitis

There may be maceration, fissuring and proliferative growth at the angle of mouth (Fig. 5.4).

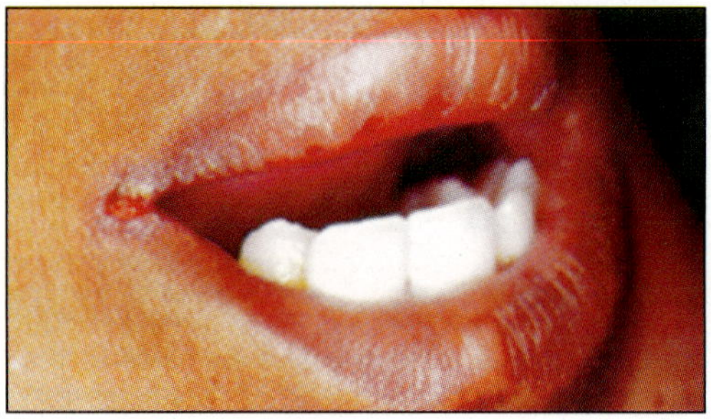

Fig. 5.4 Angular stomatitis: maceration on angle of mouth

Seborrhoeic Dermatitis like Lesions

Seen as scaly lesions around nose, eyes and ears which may also involve scrotum and vulva.

Treatment

Vitamin B complex, specifically riboflavin, 5–15 mg is given 2–3 times daily till the clearance of lesions.

SCURVY

Etiology

Scurvy is caused by the deficiency of vitamin C or ascorbic acid, most often due to scarcity of fresh fruits and vegetables in the diet.

Clinical Features

- Loss of appetite and listlessness are the early signs.
- Depression, resentfulness and non-cooperativeness.
- Swollen gums which bleed easily.
- Perifollicular purpuric spots on the leg.
- In infants, dental development may be impaired.
- Occasionally, tender subperiosteal haematomas are seen.

Treatment

Oral dose of 300–500 mg of vitamin C daily.

ACRODERMATITIS ENTEROPATHICA

Etiology

Occurs due to deficiency of zinc in the body.

Three types of deficiencies are seen:

Type I

Resulting from the inability to absorb zinc from the gastrointestinal tract.

Type II

Due to deficiency of zinc in mother's milk.

Type III

Deficiency due to artificial feed.

The deficiency may occur in infants during feeding (type II), after weaning (type I) or in adults after gastrointestinal bypass operations (type III).

Clinical Features

- Presents as vesiculation and ulceration around the nose, mouth, anal opening (Figs 5.5 and 5.6) and genitalia.
- Acral areas like hands and feet are also involved.
- Diarrhoea may precede or follow the skin manifestations.

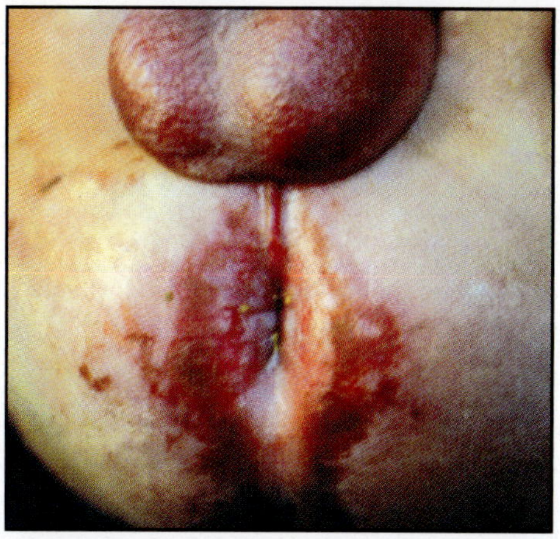

Fig. 5.5 Acrodermatitis enteropathica: erythema on anal opening and scrotum

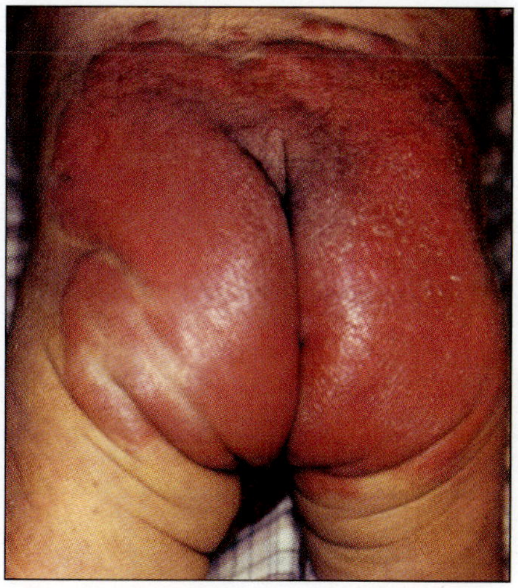

Fig. 5.6 Acrodermatitis enteropathica: erythema on anal opening and buttock

Treatment

- Zinc in a dose of 2 mg/kg body weight orally for 7–10 days.
- Treatment should be continued for a prolonged period to prevent relapse.

CHAPTER 6

Metabolic Disorders

Metabolic disorders of the skin, e.g., amyloidosis, xanthelasma or porphyria, result due to the deposition of causative substance in the skin. Sometimes, these lesions are so characteristic that they provide clues to the correct diagnosis. Sometimes defects in enzyme regulation have been found responsible for the metabolic disorders. Common metabolic disorders are listed in Table 6.1.

ETIOLOGY

Defects in enzyme regulation that can be either of the following:

- Acquired.
- Genetically transmitted.

Table 6.1 Common metabolic disorders involving the skin

Porphyrias.
Xanthelasma palpebrarum.
Cutaneous amyloidosis:
• Macular amyloidosis.
• Lichen amyloidosis.

Porphyrias

It is a group of disorders characterised by an excessive production of porphyrins and their precursors causing an elevation of these chemicals in:

- Blood.
- Urine.
- Faeces.

Porphyrias are usually inherited except a few which are acquired.

Etiology

The porphyrins are important intermediates in the biosynthesis of haem from glycine and succinyl-CoA. Each step in the pathway is controlled by specific enzymes. Deficiency (inherited or acquired) of these enzymes leads to the accumulation of intermediary porphyrins, many of which cause photosensitivity induced by light of wave length 400 nm.

Classification

Classification of porphyrias is presented in Table 6.2.

Table 6.2 Classification of porphyrias

• Congenital erythropoietic porphyria
• Erythropoietic protoporphyria
• Porphyria cutanea tarda
• Acute intermittent porphyria
• Variegate porphyria

Congenital Erythropoietic Porphyria

It is a rarely occurring variety of porphyria.

Inheritance

Autosomal recessive.

Clinical Features

- Severe photosensitivity is seen soon after birth.
- Manifests as blistering and scarring on sun exposure, which eventually deforms.
- Hypertrichosis seen on sun-exposed parts.
- History of passing red coloured urine which shows fluorescence under Wood's lamp.
- Brown discoloration of teeth seen, which show flourescence under Wood's lamp.
- Red cells show stable fluorescence.
- Haemolytic anemia may be present.

Treatment

- The results of treatment are usually unsatisfactory.
- Photo protection.
- Gene therapy may be tried.

Erythropoietic Protoporphyria

This is a rarely occurring variant of porphyria.

Inheritance

Autosomal dominant.

Clinical Features

- Photosensitivity develops in infancy or early childhood.
- Manifests as burning, erythema and urticaria on sun exposed parts.
- Thickening of the skin and superficial scarring (Fig. 6.1) develop over a period of time.
- History of passing red-coloured urine is absent.
- Liver disease like hepatitis C and gallstones may be present.

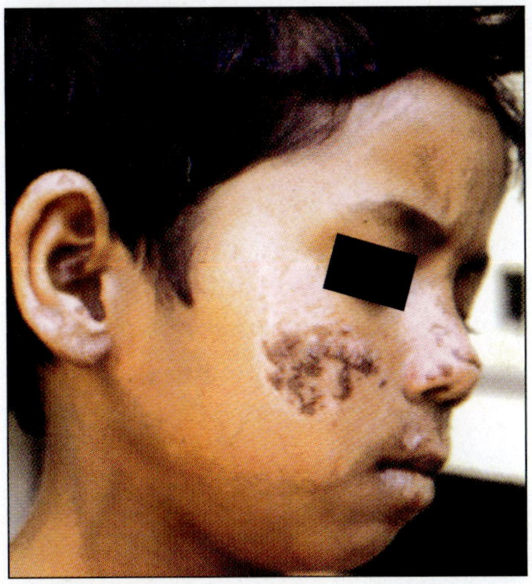

Fig. 6.1 Erythropoietic protoporphyria

Treatment
- Excessive exposure to sunlight should be avoided.
- Skin should be protected from light with clothes and sunscreen creams.
- β-carotene, a free radical scavenger, 60–180 mg/day orally.

Porphyria Cutanea Tarda

Porphyria cutanea tarda (PCT) is the most commonly occurring form of porphyrias. The two main recognised variety of this disease are—sporadic form and familial variety.

Sporadic Form
It is the common variety. It occurs in adulthood against a background of liver damage (due to alcoholism, hepatitis C virus infection).

Familial Variety
Occurring at an earlier age, it is an autosomal dominant disorder.

Clinical Features
- Blisters occur on the photo-exposed parts on exposure to sun and in response to minor trauma.
- Over a period of time, the skin becomes thickened, sclerodermoid and scarred.
- In addition, these parts develop hypertrichosis.
- Urine is pink and shows a bright coral pink fluorescence under the Wood's light.

Treatment
- Photo protection.
- Avoidance of 'triggering' factors like alcohol.
- Venesection till haemoglobin falls below 12 g/dl. This reduces the serum ferritin levels to the lower limit of the reference range and has a protective effect by limiting haem synthesis.
- Low dose therapy with hydroxychloroquin (100 mg, twice a week); it increases the excretion rate of excessively formed porphyrins.

Variegate Porphyria

This variety of porphyria presents after puberty.

Clinical Features
- Cutaneous lesions present as blisters over the photo exposed parts on sun exposure.
- Sclerodermoid changes are seen.
- The lesions are precipitated by drugs (Table 6.3).
- Sometimes presents as acute intermittent porphyria with the following symptoms:
  i) Abdominal pain.
  ii) Neuropsychiatric symptoms.
  iii) Passage of red-coloured urine.

Table 6.3 Drugs precipitating variegate porphyria

- Barbiturates
- Griseofulvin
- Sulphonamides
- Estrogens

Xanthelasma Palpebrarum

Etiology

- The disease is marked by the local collection of lipid-containing cells (xanthoma cells) in the dermis and on, and around the eyelids.
- This is usually a localised condition.
- Sometimes, it is the manifestation of hyperlipoproteinaemia with abnormal serum lipids.

Clinical Features

The lesion is seen as soft, yellow papules and plaques on the upper and lower eyelids (Fig. 6.2), and around the inner canthus.

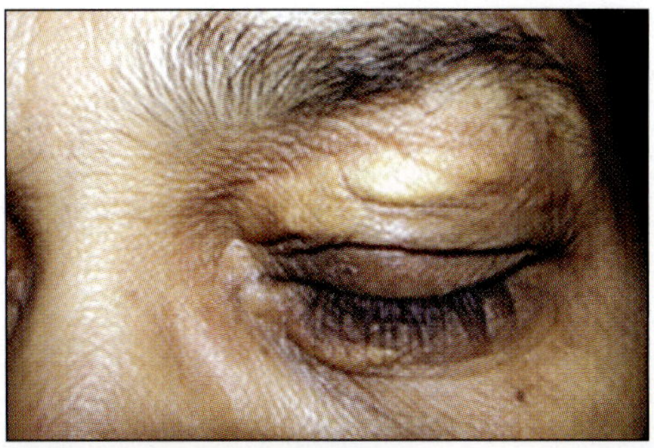

Fig. 6.2 Xanthelasma palpebrarum

Treatment

- Destruction of the lesions with one of the following:
  i) Chemical cautery.
  ii) Electric cautery.
  iii) Cryotherapy.
  iv) Lasers.
- Patients with high cholesterol should be treated with anticholesteraemic drugs.

Cutaneous Amyloidosis

It is seen as a local deposit of amyloid confined to the skin. It is due to some interference in the local protein metabolism. There are of two types of cutaneous amyloidosis—macular amyloidosis and lichen amyloidosis.

Macular Amyloidosis

Clinical Features

- Presents as pigmentation usually at the interscapular region.
- Pigmentation is arranged in a rippled pattern (Fig. 6.3).

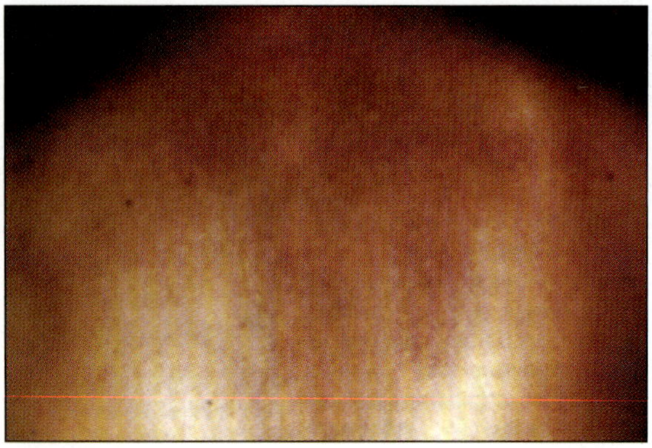

Fig. 6.3 Macular amyloidosis: ripple pattern pigmentation

Treatment

- Results of treatment are unsatisfactory.
- Local massage with retinoic acid 0.025–0.05% and hydroquinone lotion 2–5% into the skin one after another at night.
- Oral dose of cyclophosphamide 50 mg daily may be used.

Lichen Amyloidosis

Clinical Features

- Seen as discrete, firm, brown or yellow, smooth, shiny and sometimes scaly papules (Figs. 6.4 and 6.5) and nodules.
- Lesions are commonly seen on legs, lumbar region and the extensor surface of the arms.
- Old lesions become hyperkeratotic and pigmented.
- Itching is usually severe in most of the cases.

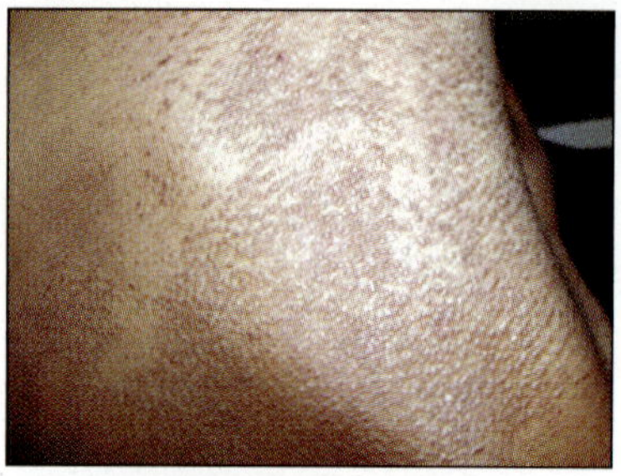

Fig. 6.4 Lichen amyloidosis: early lesions

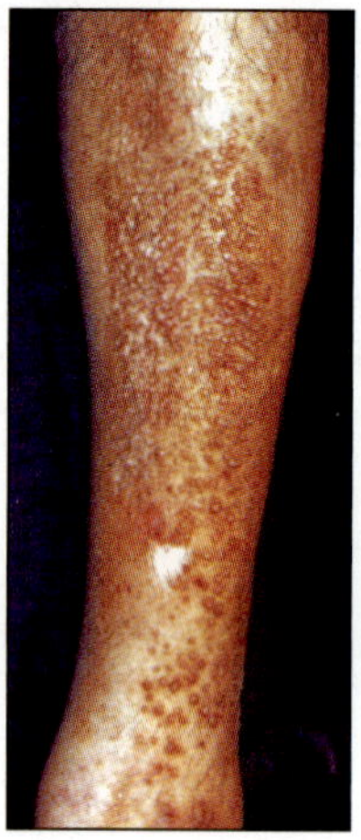

Fig. 6.5 Lichen amyloidosus: firm brown papules on the leg

Treatment

- Massage of potent corticosteroids like clobetasol propionate.
- Oral cyclophosphamide 50–100 mg daily clears the lesions in 6–12 months.
- Oral retinoids, especially, etretinate.
- Lesion may improve with intralesional steroids, dermabrasion and cryotherapy.
- Recently, **dexamethasone cyclophosphamide pulse** (DCP) therapy has been found curative.

CHAPTER 7

Diseases Due to Physical Agents

Skin normally protects itself from environmental assault of trauma, friction, heat, cold and radiations (Table 7.1). However, when environmental factors become too strong, they may produce a variety of skin lesions (Table 7.2).

Table 7.1 Common environmental agents that cause skin lesions

• Friction. • Heat. • Light.	• Trauma. • Cold. • Radiations.

Table 7.2 Common dermatoses produced due to different environmental agents

• Friction blisters. • Callosities. • Corns. • Burns. • Erythema ab igne. • Frost bite. • Chilblains or perniosis.

DISEASES CAUSED DUE TO FRICTION

Friction Blister

Etiopathogenesis

When a pressure of high intensity—as produced by wearing tight shoes—acts against the epidermis, it results in the formation of a blister.

Pathogenesis

Degeneration and necrosis of pickle cells results in the formation of intra-epidermal blisters.

Sites

Blisters are located on areas which have been subjected to friction. Some such areas are:

- Back of heels.
- Dorsum of toes especially little and big toes in case of shoes.
- Palmer skin against head of metacarpal bones in case of hard manual labour.

Treatment

- Main focus of the treatment lies in preventing it from further trauma, further friction can be prevented by putting a piece of cotton between the skin and shoes.
- Blisters, as a rule, dry up and start healing in 2–3 days.
- Local cream containing corticosteroids and antibiotics are effective in the early stage.

Callosities

Etiopathogenesis

Callosities are produced by repeated friction of low intensity that results in circumscribed areas of hyperkeratosis.

Clinical Features

- Hands (Fig. 7.1) of labourers, industrial workers and farmers are commonly affected.
- Seen on the soles (Fig. 7.2) beneath the metatarsal heads due to abnormalities of the foot, abnormal gait and unsuitable footwear.

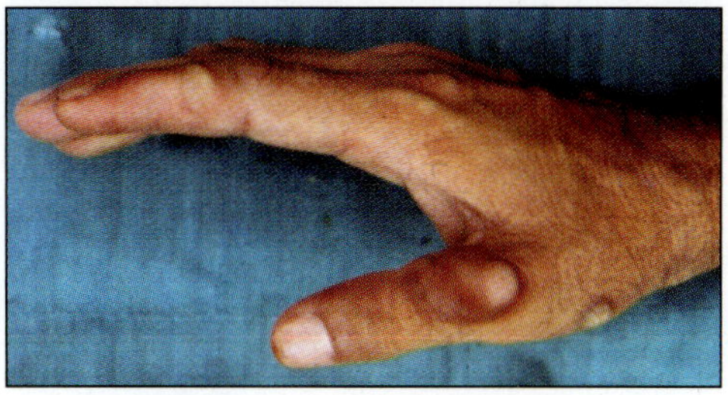

Fig. 7.1 Callosities: hand

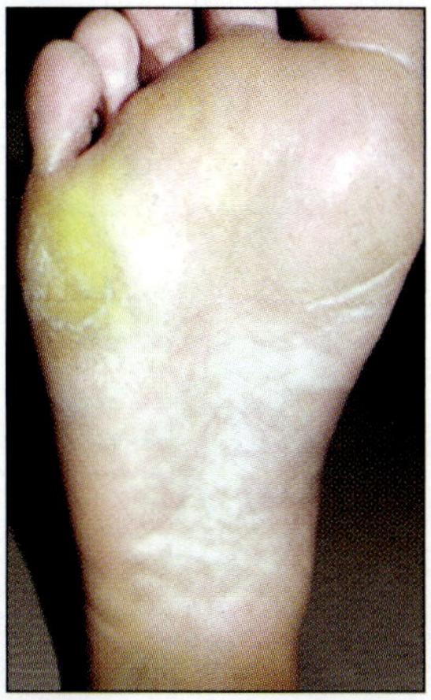

Fig. 7.2 Callosities: foot

Treatment

- Further friction must be prevented.
- Thickened area of the lesion is treated by local application of keratolytic agents like urea 40% or salicylic acid 10–40% in cream or vaseline with occlusive dressing.
- Paring of the lesions.

Corns

Etiopathogenesis

These are the localised, smaller callosities produced by friction and pressure caused by ill-fitting shoes or the projecting ends of the shoe nails. The lesion consists of a central hyperkeratotic spike projecting downward towards the dermis.

Clinical Features

- Due to continuous pressure on the surface, the deeper end of the corn may start pressing on the underlying epidermis resulting in thinning of the stratum malpighii.
- If the corn presses upon an underlying nerve twig, it causes acute pain. Otherwise the lesions are painless.

Treatment

- Prevention of further friction.
- Treatment as described for callosities.

DISEASES CAUSED BY HEAT

Burns

Etiology

- If an object with a temperature of more than 60°C remains in contact with the skin for some time, it is likely to produce burns.
- The type of the burns depends upon the temperature of the object and the duration of contact with the skin.

Clinical Features

Burns due to very High Temperature

- It may cause charring of the tissue with deep ulcer formation and even causing the exposure of the underlying bone.
- Pain may be absent if nerve endings are destroyed.

Burns due to Moderately High Temperature or Brief Duration of Contact

There is pain, erythema and mild oedema.

Burns due to Mildly High Temperature or Prolonged Duration of Contact

It may cause separation of epidermis from dermis leading to formation of tense blister(s).

Treatment

Superficial burns of limited area can be treated by the dermatologist.

During the First Few Minutes after Burn

- Counter the heat by cooling the area with plain tap water.
- Corticosteroids topically and orally will prevent the blister and scar formation.
- Formed blisters should not be ruptured.
- Ruptured lesions are susceptible to secondary infection.
- Topical antibiotics are given to prevent secondary infection.

For Extensive Infection

- Appropriate oral antibiotic.
- Analgesics are given to relieve pain.

Erythema Ab Igne

Prolonged and repeated exposure to low temperature heat which is insufficient to produce a burn such as from oven, room heater or other similar device, can produce persistent dilatation of arterioles leading to erythema and hyperpigmentation in reticular distribution.

It commonly affects the front of both legs, but may involve the area chronically exposed to the heat.

Treatment

- Avoid further exposure to heat.
- Skin gradually returns to its normal colour.
- Hydroquinone 2–5% application twice daily improves the color of lesions fast.

DISEASES DUE TO COLD

Frost Bite

Etiology

Freezing induced by extreme cold causes frost bite. Exposure of a few seconds may be sufficient to produce a frost bite, especially in the presence of strong wind in high altitudes during climbing or military duties.

Clinical Features

- The affected area becomes numb and white; the discomfort of feeling cold disappears on rewarming.
- Commonly affected areas are the exposed parts, e.g., toes, feet, fingers, ears, tip of nose and cheek.
- In **mild cases**, the skin in these areas develops erythema and discomfort which returns to normal in few hours.
- In **severe cases**, blisters, ulcers and gangrene may occur along with severe pain.

Treatment

- Immediate removal of the patient from the cold environment to normal atmosphere.
- Local heating should be avoided as the part may develop excessive oedema.
- Systemic corticosteroids, antibiotics and vasodilators should be started immediately to reduce the inflammation and prevent secondary infection.
- Topical application of corticosteroids and antibiotic creams is also helpful.
- Low molecular weight dextran infusion is given.
- Gangrenous area may be amputated.
- Oral vasodilators should be continued.

Chilblains

Synonym

Perniosis.

Etiology

It is an abnormal reaction to cold and develops when the skin is exposed to cold followed by warmth.

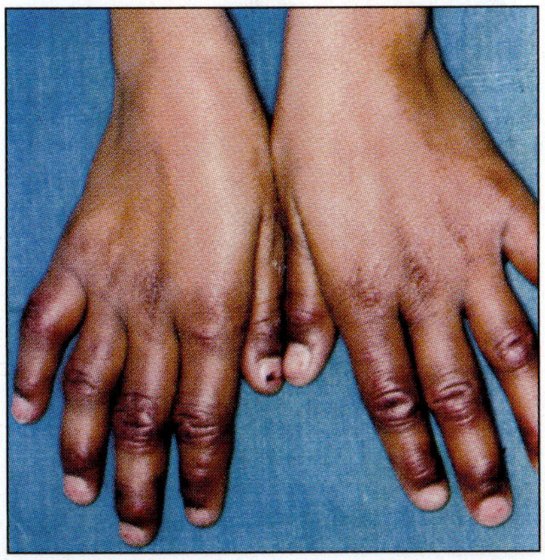

Fig. 7.3 Chilblain: fingers

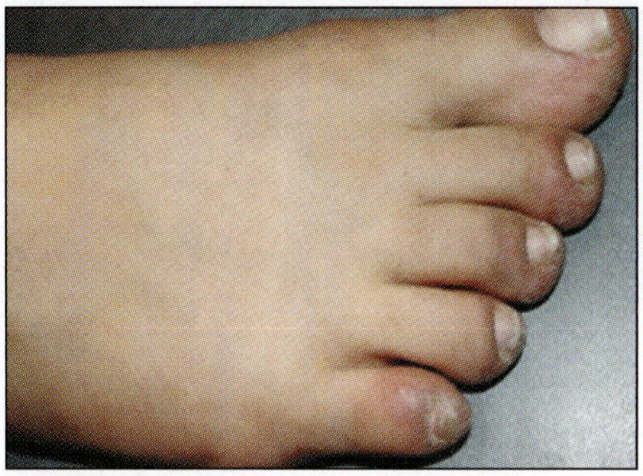

Fig. 7.4 Chilblain: tip of toes

Clinical Features

- The fingers and toes of these patients are cold to touch.
- Painful or itchy, erythematous and oedematous areas are seen on the dorsa of the fingers (Fig. 7.3), toes (Figs 7.4–7.6), nose and ears.
- From erythematous, the lesions usually change to dark brown in colour.
- In severe cases, blisters and ulceration may occur.
- The lesions heal spontaneously in 7–14 days.

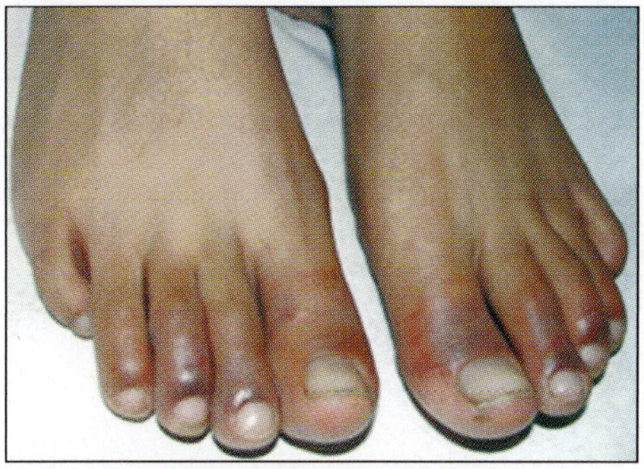

Fig. 7.5 Chilblain: dorsum of feet and toes

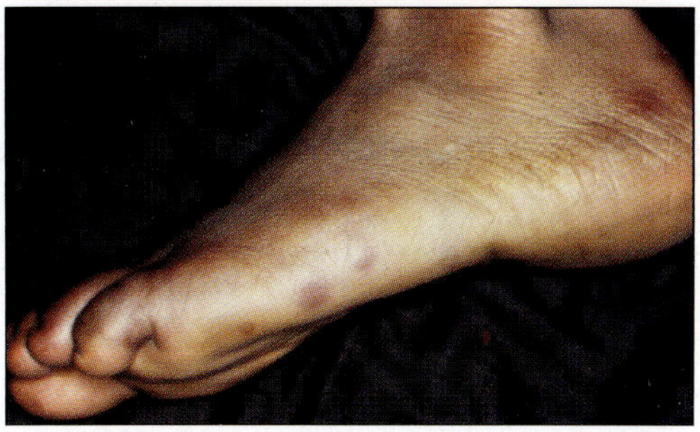

Fig. 7.6 Chilblain: sole

Recurrences are common. Chilblains continue to recur every winter for a few years.

Treatment

- Should protect from cold by using warm water and wearing woolen clothes during winter.

- Vasodilators may be given orally.
- Once the chilblain has appeared, topical corticosteroids with antibiotic cream can be applied.

DISEASES CAUSED BY SUNLIGHT AND RADIATION

The spectrum of solar radiation that reaches the surface of earth is presented in Table 7.3.

Table 7.3 Solar radiation reaching the surface of earth

Spectrum (nm)	Name
200–290	Ultra-violet C or UVC.
290–320	Ultra-violet B or UVB.
320–400	Ultra-violet A or UVA (also called long wave or UVR).
400–700	Visible spectrum.
above 700	Infra-red (also called the heat spectrum).

Skin is protected from the harmful effects of the sunlight by the following factors:

- The epidermis, especially stratum corneum, that absorbs the UVC and to a certain extent, the UVB bands.
- The melanin pigment in the basal cell layer of epidermis.

Diseases Caused by Sunlight

Diseases caused by sunlight (Table 7.4) may be caused under the following conditions:

- When a normal person is subjected to excessive exposure to sunlight. When a person reacts abnormally to even normal exposure to sunlight.
- When a normal person temporarily becomes susceptible to sunlight due to the presence of some photosensitiser in the body.

Table 7.4 Diseases caused by sunlight

Photosensitivity.
Acute solar dermatitis or sunburn.
Chronic solar dermatitis.
Polymorphous light eruption.
Actinic lichenoid grouped papular eruption.

Photosensitivity or Photodermatitis

Etiology

When a large number of chemicals found in plants or synthetic compounds are present in the system (Table 7.5), they make a human more sensitive to sunlight.

Table 7.5 Common photosensitisers

Drugs	• Demethylchlortetracycline.
	• Sulphonamides.
	• Griseofulvin.
	• Psoralens.
	• Chlorpromazine.
Dyes	• Eosins present in some cosmetics and perfumes.
	• Tar products.
	• Psoralens and other chemicals present in plants.

If an individual gets exposed to sunlight when such substances are present in his/her system, s/he is likely to develop dermatitis on the exposed parts of the body.

Clinical Features

- The skin lesions seen are erythema, scaling and even vesiculation, along with itching in the areas exposed to sunlight (Fig. 7.7).
- Hyperpigmentation, with or without itching, is also seen.
- When the photosensitiser is a local applicant on the skin, the pattern of the lesion will correspond to the areas coming in contact with the photosensitiser.
- The area not exposed to sunlight (Fig. 7.8) and/ or to the photosensitiser, will not develop any skin lesions

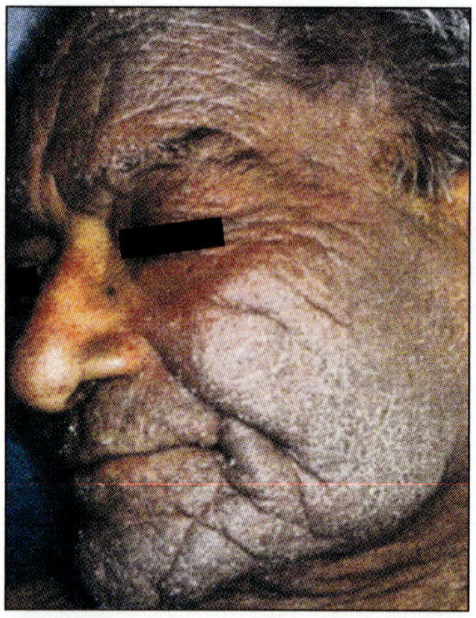

Fig. 7.7 Photodermatitis

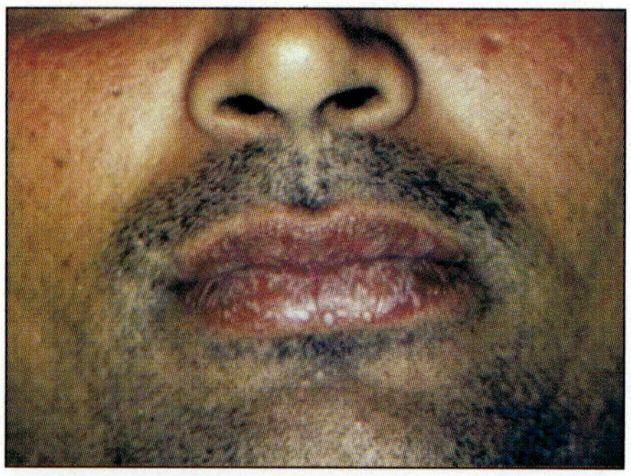

Fig. 7.8 Area spared in photodermatitis

Treatment

- Pinpoint the substance responsible for the reaction and avoid further exposure.
- Protect from sunlight by using sunscreens.
- Cover the body by full sleeves, high-neck clothes and cap.
- During the acute phase of dermatitis use the following:
  i) Saline compresses twice daily may show some effect.
  ii) Local or systemic corticosteroids.

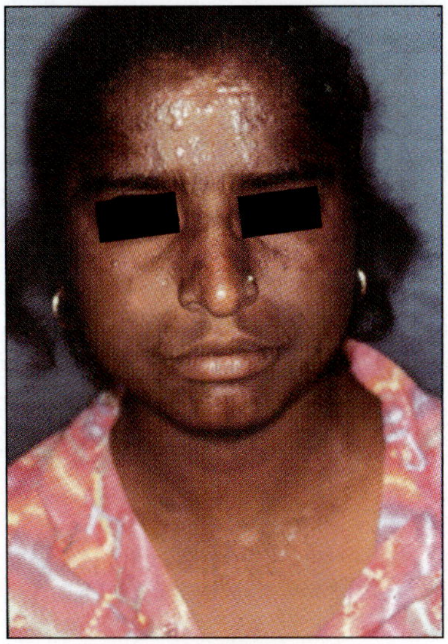

Fig. 7.10 Polymorphous light eruption

Acute Solar Dermatitis

Synonym

Sunburn.

Etiology

It is observed in normal individuals, when they are exposed to excessive sunlight for a prolonged period. For example, in one of the following situations:

- Outdoor picnic.
- A trip to a hill-station, especially if the area is covered with snow.
- Visit to a sea-side resort.
- Prolonged stay in the desert areas.

Clinical Features

- Itching and erythema occur within a few hours in the area exposed to sunlight (Fig. 7.9).
- If the exposure is too much, the person may develop papulovesicles; skin peeling and hyperpigmentation may follow.
- Most commonly affected areas are the face—especially the forehead, cheeks and bridge of the nose, pinna, V of the neck, extensor surface of forearm and arms up to the edge of sleeves and the dorsum of hands (sparing fingers).

Treatment

- Normal saline compresses, applied 2–3 times daily, may help.

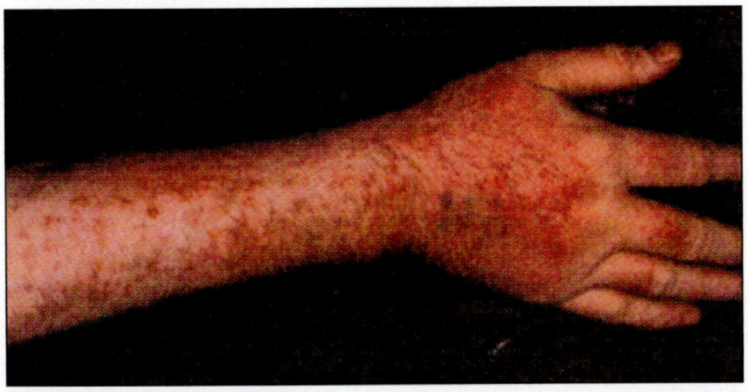

Fig. 7.9 Solar dermatitis

- Local gentle massage with corticosteroid creams, 2–3 times daily, may be effective when used early.
- The skin should be protected from further exposure to sunlight by covering as much areas of the skin as possible with clothes.
- Over the areas that cannot be covered with clothes like face and hands, a local sunscreen should be applied in the day, which should be repeated every 3–4 hours or whenever the area is washed.
- Sunscreen should be used prophylactically during excessive exposure to sunlight.

Chronic Solar Dermatitis

Etiology

The condition is seen in people like farmers, sailors, labourers and others who are engaged in professions that expose them to sunlight for prolonged periods.

Clinical Features

- Skin is wrinkled with irregular atrophy.
- Hypertrophy and hyperpigmentation seen on the affected parts.
- Depigmentation is also seen on the area of the skin exposed to sunlight.
- The condition becomes prominent when the individual grows old.

Treatment

- Hardly any treatment can change the lesion once it is fully developed.
- To prevent this condition, the individuals engaged in professions that expose them to prolonged sunlight should use local sunscreens throughout their professional lives.

Polymorphous Light Eruption

Etiology

This is an abnormal reaction to normal exposure of sunlight. It usually occurs in women under 30 years of age.

Clinical Features

The clinical features include a mixture of lesions (polymorphism) like papules, erythematous and scaly plaques (Fig. 7.10), vesicles, etc. Patients may even present a picture of acute dermatitis. Commonly affected parts are the ones exposed to sun.

Treatment

In Acute Stage

- Short course of systemic steroids.
- Saline compresses 2–3 times daily might help.
- Topical application of corticosteroid creams.

In Chronic Stage

- Broad spectrum sunscreens locally during the day.
- Chloroquine/hydroxychloroquine in a dose of 200 mg daily to children; and 400 mg daily to adults, 15 days in a month for 2–3 months acts, as a systemic sunscreen.
- Protect the skin from sunlight throughout life by using suitable clothes, umbrella and local sunscreens.

Prophylaxis

Gradual increase of low dose UVB or PUVA therapy, 2–3 times/week for several weeks.

Actinic Lichenoid Grouped Papular Eruption

This condition is commonly seen in children and young adults due to exposure to sunlight.

Clinical Features

Asymptomatic small, skin-coloured, grouped micro-papules on the extensor surface of one or both forearms that increase in sunlight.

Treatment

- Corticosteroid creams clear the lesions.
- The area should be protected by wearing full-sleeved clothes to prevent the recurrence.

Sunscreens

These are creams or lotions which filter or reflect the damaging UVR. Initially, the sunscreens contained only substances which were able to absorb or filter out only 290 nm UVB of the UVR. These substances included para-aminobenzoic acid (PABA), salicylates, benzo-phenone and cinnamates.

Subsequently, sunscreens were developed which were able to protect skin from UVA also by reflecting the rays. These included titanium dioxide and zinc oxide. They protect skin from both UVA and UVB.

Sun Protection Factor

Efficiency of sunscreens is measured by their ability to inhibit UVB-induced sunburn. **Sun protection factor (SPF)** is a number that expresses the relationship between the numbers of times of exposure to UVB that causes skin burning with and without the sunscreen protection.

Chapter 8

Bacterial Infections

PYODERMA

Infections of the skin caused by bacteria are called **pyoderma**. Pyogenic infection of normal skin is called **primary pyoderma,** while infection caused over a pre-existing skin disease is called **secondary pyoderma**. Most of the bacterial infections of the skin are caused by *staphylococcus aureus* or *streptococcus pyogenes*. There are different types of bacteria found on the skin surface (Table 8.1).

Table 8.1 Bacterial flora of the skin

Resident flora of the skin
This is the group of bacteria which is regularly found on the skin surface of normal individuals and cannot be removed easily by scrubbing.

They include:

- *Staphylococcus albus*
- *Streptococcus viridians*
- *Streptococcus faecalis*
- Several aerobic diphtheroids
- Anaerobic cutaneous diphtheroids
- *Corynebacterium acnes*
- *Corynebacterium*
- *Propionibacterium granulosum*

Majority of these bacteria do not produce any disease.

Transient flora
This group consists of organisms which come on the skin surface from the environment, i.e., from infected individual or healthy carrier of similar bacteria and are rapidly removed by a few minutes' scrubbing.These bacteria stay on the skin for a variable period.

This group includes:

- *Staphylococcus aureus*
- *Streptococcus pyogenes*
- *Pseudomonas aerugenosa*

Majority of these strains produce diseases.

Temporary resident flora of the skin
Group of bacteria like *Mima herellea* group and *Escherichia coli,* are found in small numbers at certain areas on a few people. These are present only on some occasions.

Skin Barrier

Skin acts as a barrier to the bacterial infections through constant desquamation of its outer layer and the active chemical agents produced by splitting of the esters in sebum by its flora.

Common pyodermas are listed in Table 8.2.

Table 8.2 Common pyodermas

- Impetigo.
- Ecthyma.
- Cellulitis.
- Erysipelas.
- Boils or furuncles.
- Carbuncles.
- Superficial folliculitis.
- Deep folliculitis.
- Pseudo folliculitis.
- Acute paronychia.
- Acute intertrigo.
- Secondary pyodermas.
- Infectious eczematoid dermatitis.

Impetigo

This is the infection of the superficial layers of the skin caused by *Streptococci* or *Staphylococci* or both the organisms.

Clinically, impetigo is seen in two forms (Table 8.3):

- Impetigo contagiosa.
- Bullous impetigo.

Table 8.3 Difference between Impetigo contagiosum and Bullous impetigo

Impetigo contagiosa	Bullous impetigo
Caused by *staph. aureus* or *strep. pyogenes* or both.	Caused by *staph. Aureus.*
Usually affects children.	Usually infants are affected.
Bullae are thin walled and transient.	Bullae are thick walled persistent and may become large.
Erythematous halo common.	Erythematous halo absent.
Bright yellow and thick crusts.	Brownish thin crusts.
Central clearing—not seen.	Central clearing—seen.
Lymphadenopathy—frequent.	Lymphadenopathy—rare.
Involvement of mucous membrane—rare.	Mucous membranes may be involved.
Lesions—predominantly on face.	Lesions—on face and other parts.

Impetigo Contagiosum

Epidemiology

Prevalence

A frequent infection.

Age
Commonly affects the small children.

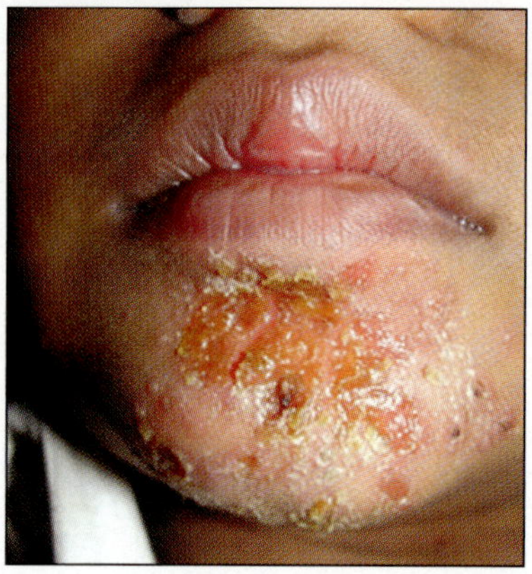

Fig. 8.1 Impetigo contagiosum: yellow crust and pus-face

Clinical Features

Usually affecting the face of small children, it presents the following features:

- Very thin walled vesicles are seen. They rupture rapidly, leaving behind superficial ulcers covered with bright yellow crusts (Figs 8.1, 8.2, 8.3) and pus.
- They extend irregularly to the periphery without central healing.
- Crusts eventually get dry and separate without scarring.
- Regional lymph nodes may be involved with fever and other constitutional symptoms.

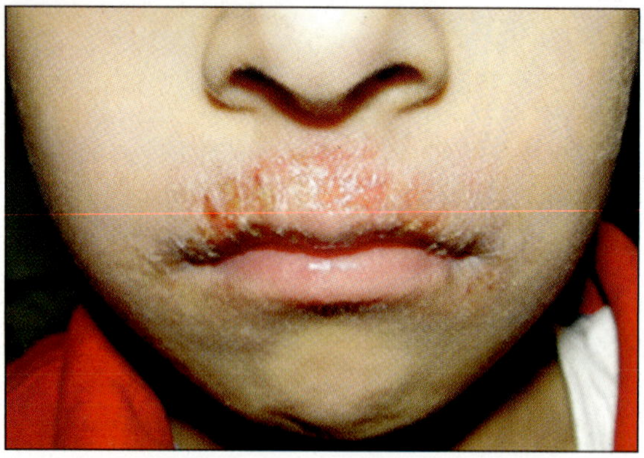

Fig. 8.2 Impetigo contagiosum: upper lip

Bullous Impetigo

Epidemiology

Prevalence
Sporadic.

Age
Commonly affects the newborn and young children.

Clinical Features

- Diffusely scattered, asymptomatic, tense bullae of 1–2 cm size are seen. They persist for 2–3 days.
- Blisters are filled with clear fluid.
- After rupture, thin flat brownish crusts are formed.
- Central healing with peripheral extensions results in circinate lesions (Fig. 8.4).
- Regional adenitis and constitutional symptoms are usually absent.

Sites

Can affect any part of the body including palms and soles.

Diagnosis

Gram stain will show intra- and extracellular gram positive cocci in chains (*streptococci*) or clusters (*staphylococci*). Pus culture will identify the organism.

Ecthyma

It is often seen as a complication of impetigo contagiosa.

Precipitating Factors

- Poor hygiene.
- Malnutrition.

Age

Commonly seen in older children.

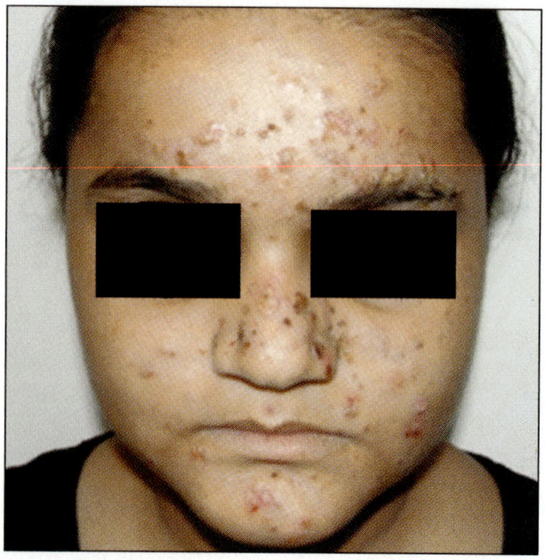

Fig. 8.3 Impetigo contagiosum in older child

Clinical Features

- The lesion extends deep into the dermis.

- The pus is usually stained with blood.
- The crusts are dark brown or black, hard and adherent to the skin (Fig. 8.5).

Crusts are removed with difficulty and leave behind purulent irregular ulcers (Fig. 8.6) which heal in a few weeks with scarring.

Sites

Determined by minor injuries or any predisposing skin conditions.

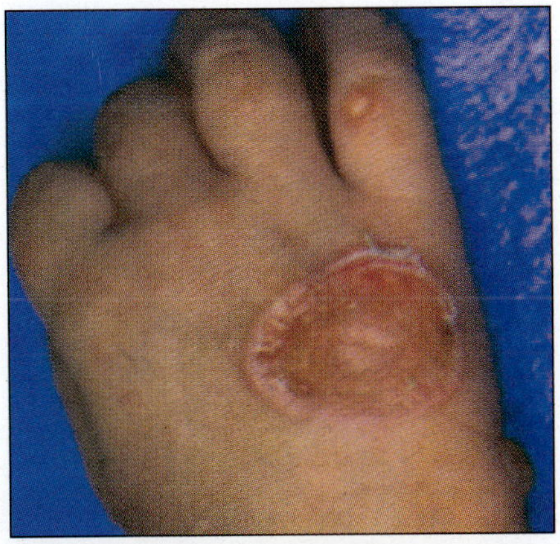

Fig. 8.4 Bullous impetigo: circinate lesions

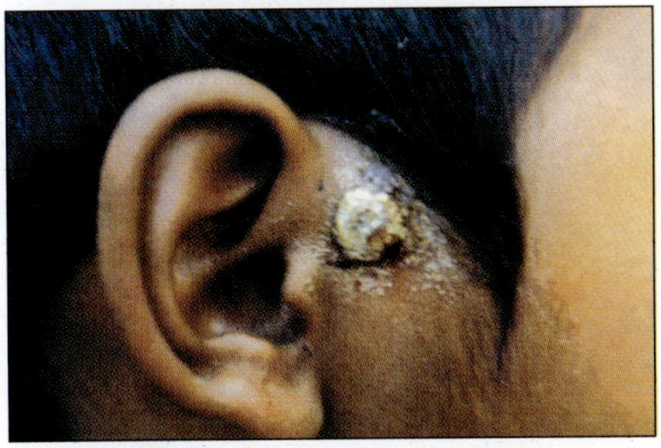

Fig. 8.5 Ecthyma: dark brown hard crust

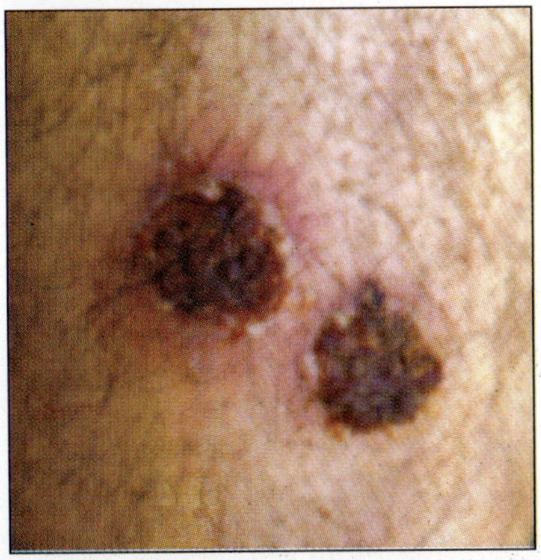

Fig. 8.6 Ecthyma: irregular deep ulcers

Cellulitis

This is an infection of the deep dermis and subcutaneous tissue.

Etiology

The most common causative organism is *Streptococus pyogenes.* The infection arises as a complication of one of the following conditions:

- Wound.
- Ulcer.
- Other skin conditions.

Predisposing Factors

Lymphoedema or venous stasis predispose to the development of cellulitis. It may develop suddenly even in previously normal skin.

Clinical Features

- Seen as an erythematous, tender swelling, which is deep and has an ill-defined border (Figs 8.7 and 8.8). It can be seen on any part of the body.
- Usually associated with fever and malaise.

Erysipelas

Etiology

This is the infection of the upper layer of the dermis caused by *Streptococci.*

Clinical Features

Seen as a sharply-defined, slightly elevated, tender, erythematous area (Figs 8.9 and 8.10) associated with high fever and malaise.

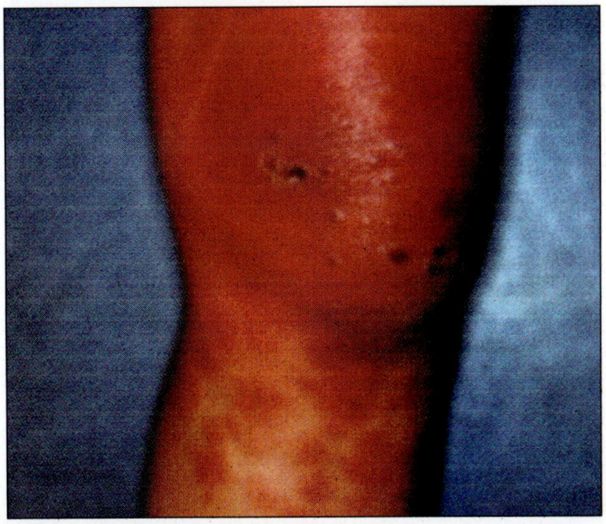

Fig. 8.7 Cellulitis: ill-defined border

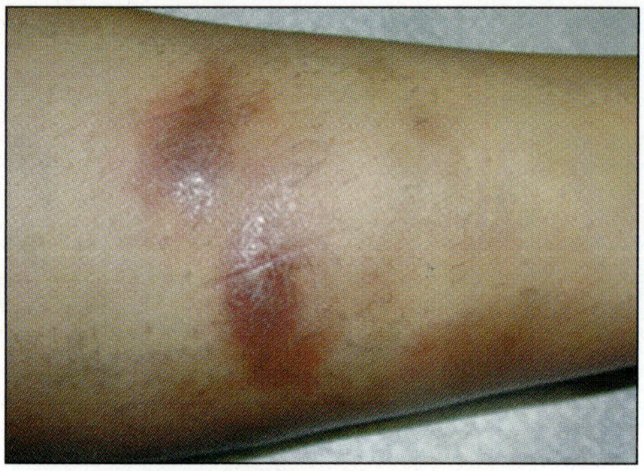

Fig. 8.8 Cellulitis due to boils

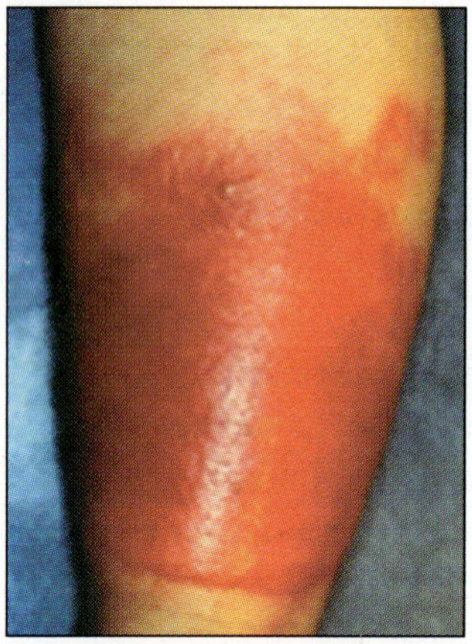

Fig. 8.9 Erysipelas: bright red, well defined

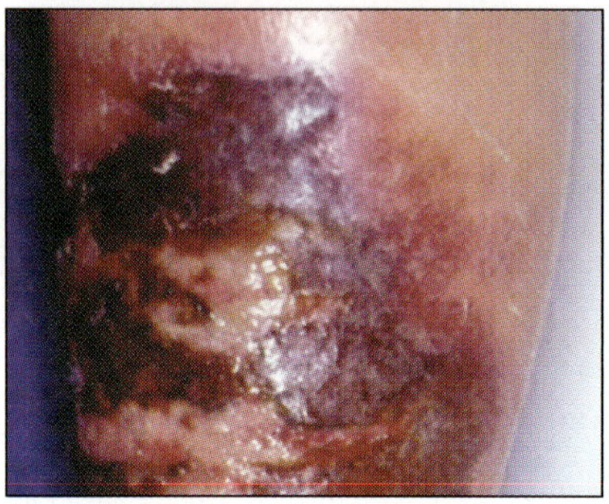

Fig. 8.10 Erysipelas: healing

Boils or Furuncles

Etiology

This is an acute infection of the hair follicles and the surrounding tissue most commonly caused by *Staph. aureus*.

Predisposing Factors

The predisposing factors for recurrent boils are as follows:

- Diabetes.
- Malnutrition.

Clinical Features

- It starts as a small, deep-seated, tender and inflammatory follicular nodule that turns to a pustule (Figs 8.11 – 8.13) in a few days.
- The hair is shed during the early stage of the disease.
- Lesion is usually single and can be seen on any part of the body.
- When it is present on upper lip and cheek, possibility of cavernous sinus thrombosis is there, a rare and dangerous complication seen commonly in children and diabetics.

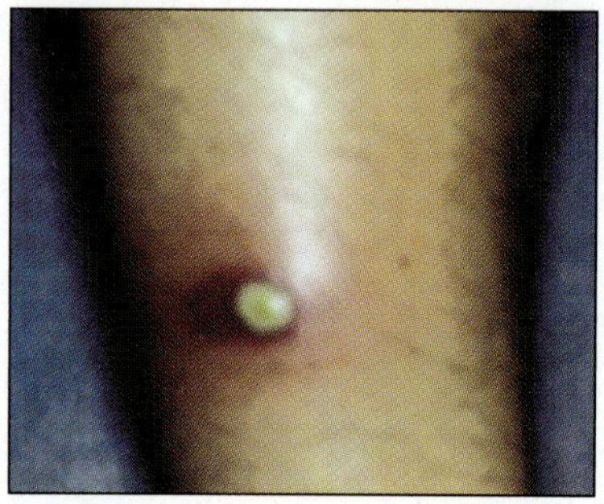

Fig. 8.11 Boil on leg

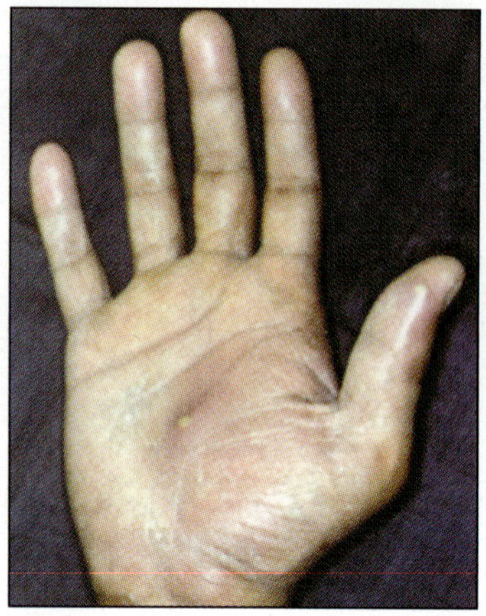

Fig. 8.12 Boil on palm

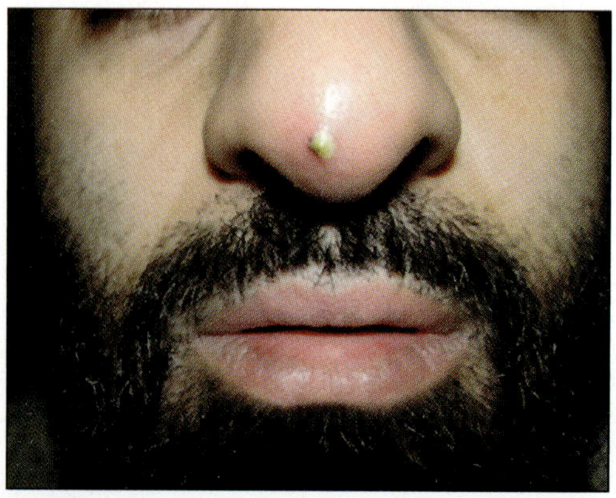

Fig. 8.13 Boils on nose

Carbuncles

Etiology

This is the deep infection of a group of contiguous follicles associated with an intense inflammatory reaction in the surrounding and underlying tissues including subcutaneous fat (Fig. 8.14). The most common causative organism is *Staph. aureus*.

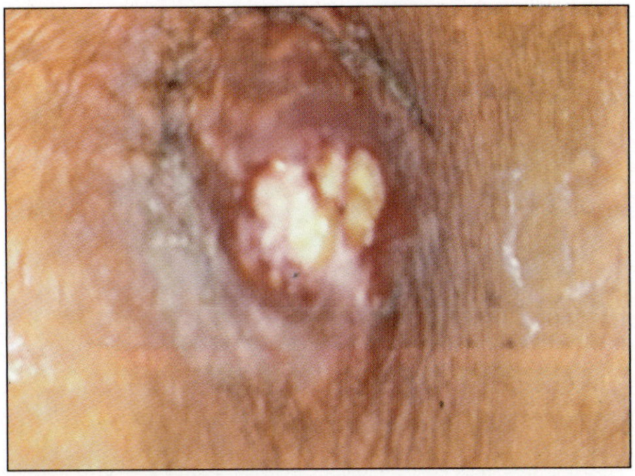

Fig. 8.14 Carbuncles

Precipitating Factors

- Uncontrolled diabetes.
- Malnutrition.
- Prolonged steroid therapy.

Clinical Features

Huge painful swelling is seen in a localised area discharging pus from multiple follicular openings. The lesions are extremely painful and associated with constitutional symptoms.

Sites

- Nape of the neck.
- Shoulders.
- Hips.
- Thighs.

Superficial Folliculitis

Etiology

Infection of the opening of hair follicles, it can also be caused by chemicals such as oils and petrolatum.

Clinical Features

Pustules are present around the coarse hair (Fig. 8.15).

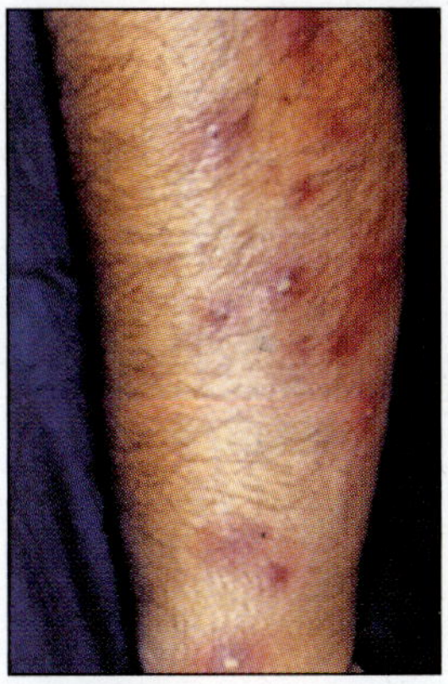

Fig. 8.15 Superficial folliculitis

Bockhart's Impetigo

- It is a common form of superficial folliculitis.
- Dome-shaped yellow pustules are seen surrounded by red areola (Fig 8.16).
- Seen commonly on legs and thighs.

Age

Common in adults.

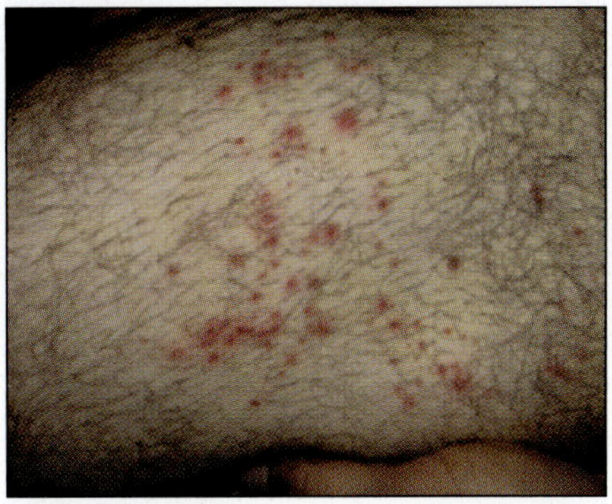

Fig. 8.16 Folliculitis: thigh

Chronic superficial folliculitis of legs

Superficial folliculitis is seen mainly in Indian adult males (Fig. 8.17).

Clinical Features

- Itchy superficial and occasionally deep follicular pustules are seen on the legs and thighs.
- The lesions are resistant to treatment.

Deep Folliculitis

Etiology

This is a subacute or chronic infection of the deeper parts of the hair follicles, commonly caused by *Staph. aureus*.

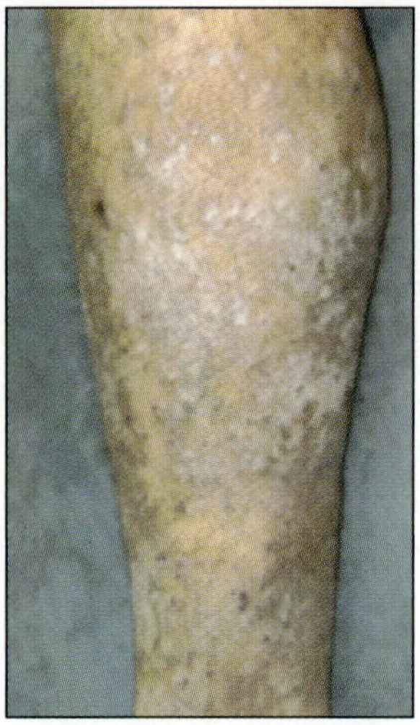

Fig. 8.17 Chronic superficial folliculitis of leg

Age and Sex

Seen only in males after puberty.

Clinical Features

- Erythematous, oedematous, discrete papules and pustules are seen around coarse hair.
- If neighbouring follicles are involved, perifollicular oedema may coalesce and form raised plaques, studded with pustules, often with some crusting (Fig. 8.18) but the hair is usually retained.

Sites

It most commonly affects the regions which have coarse hair.

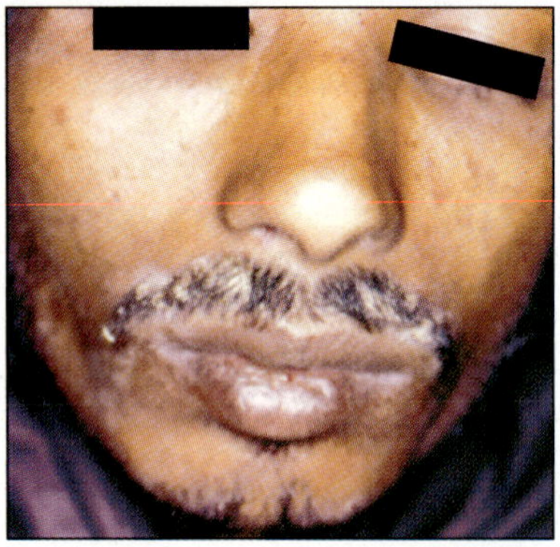

Fig. 8.18 Deep folliculitis: moustache (*Sycosis barbae*)

Sycosis barbae

In this condition, the lesions occur in bearded areas.

Sycosis nuchae

In this condition, the lesions are present on back of the neck.

Pseudo-folliculitis

Etiology

This is an inflammatory disorder of hair follicles of the beard region that occurs due to the sharp tips of shaved hair which penetrate the walls of the follicles or curve backwards to reenter the skin.

Predisposing Factors

People of any race with curly hair can develop it, if they shave frequently.

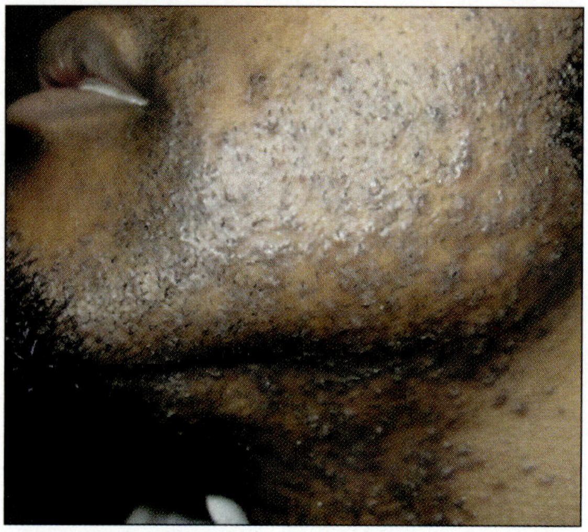

Fig. 8.19 Pseudofolliculitis

Clinical Features

Follicular and non-follicular papules are seen over the beard region.

Treatment

- Stop shaving.
- Local application of steroid antibiotic cream.

Acute Paronychia

Etiology

Infection of the nail-fold caused commonly by *Staph. aureus*. It occurs due to local injuries such as:

- Nail bites.
- Ingrowing nails.
- Splits and splinters.
- Complication of chronic paronychia.
- Spontaneously without any cause.

Clinical Features

- Painful, red swelling of the nail fold (Fig. 8.20). It may be associated with lymphadenopathy and constitutional symptoms.

- May be associated with constitutional symptoms like fever and malaise.

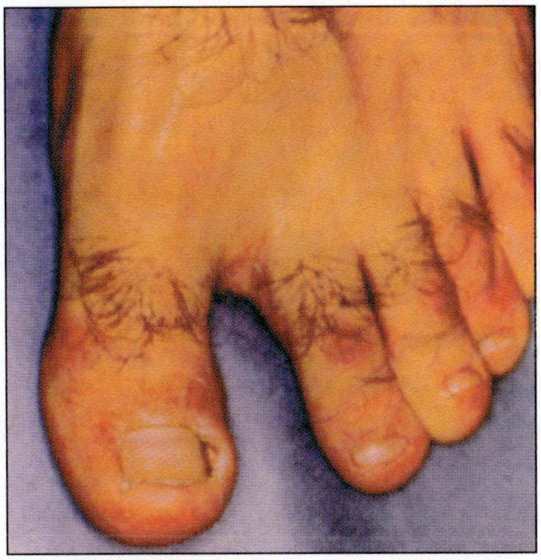

Fig. 8.20 Acute paronychia

Acute Intertrigo

- This is the painful crusting and fissuring seen in the depth of the skinfold (Fig. 8.21), associated with oedema and inflammation.
- Recurrence is very common.

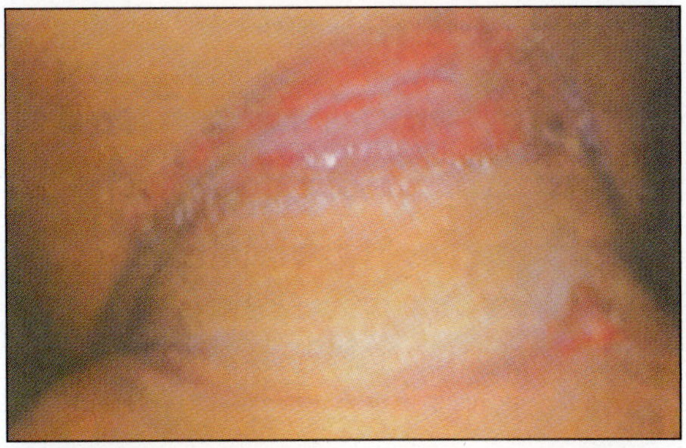

Fig. 8.21 Acute intertrigo: neck

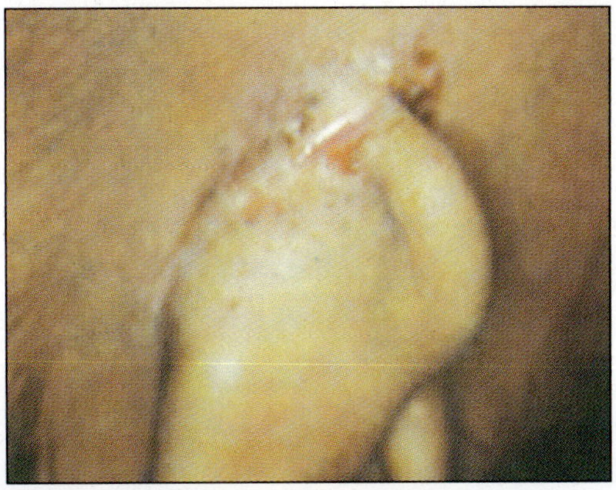

Fig. 8.22 Acute intertrigo: post auricular area

Sites

Retro-auricular folds (Fig. 8.22) and interdigital areas.

Secondary Pyodermas

Many primary diseases like scabies, pediculosis, contact dermatitis, insect bites, etc. may also get secondarily infected with pyogenic organisms producing pyodermic lesions which are called secondary pyodermas.

Clinical Features

- The existing primary lesions of the disease start discharging pus and even develop pustules and crusts.
- May be associated with constitutional symptoms like fever and malaise.

Infectious Eczematoid Dermatitis

Synonym

Infective eczema.

Etiology

This occurs due to hypersensitivity to the infecting pyogenic organisms or their antigenic products.

Clinical Features

Eczematisation around the original lesions of pyoderma occurs presenting as itchy, diffuse, papulo-vesicular or scaly lesions (Figs 8.23–8.25)

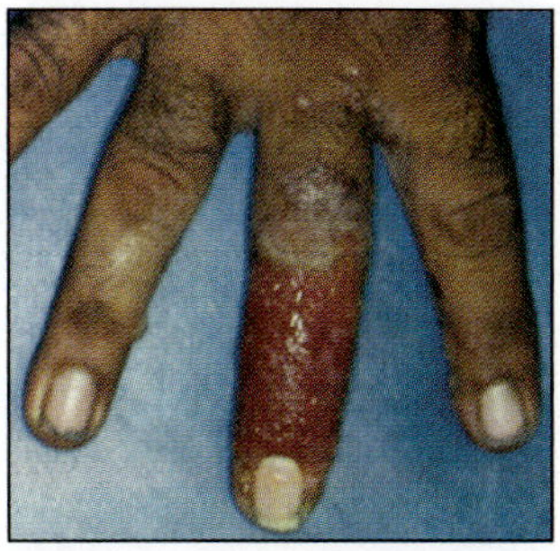

Fig. 8.23 Infectious eczemoid dermatitis: finger

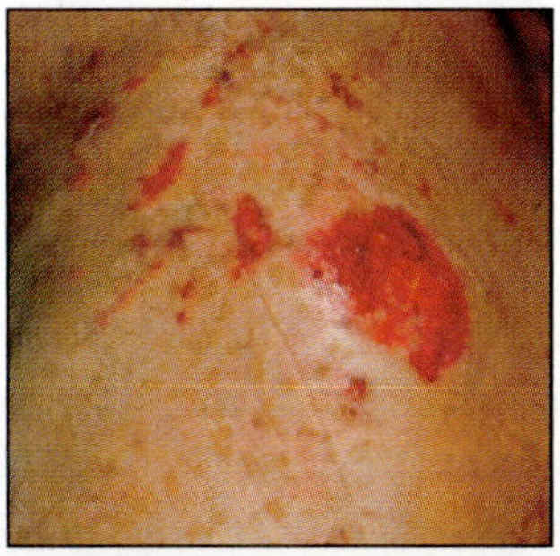

Fig. 8.24 Infectious eczematoid dermatitis: hand

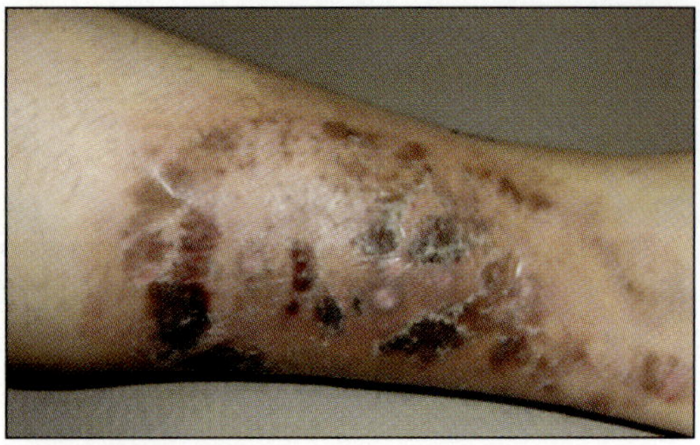

Fig. 8.25 Infectious eczematoid dermatitis: healing

Staphylococcus Scalded Skin Syndrome

Synonym

Also known as pemphigus neonatorum or Ritter's disease.

Etiology

It is caused by *Staphylococcus aureus* and induced by exotoxins or exfoliatin A and B, which is released by *Staph. aureus*.

Predisposing Factors

Children under five-years-of-age are at high risk. However, week immune system and long term kidney disease also increase the risk.

Clinical Features

- It causes detachment in the epidermal layers by breaking desmosomes.
- It presents with widespread fluid filled blisters which are thin-walled and rupture easily or there is positive Nikolsky's sign.
- Staphylococcal scalded skin syndrome spares the mucous membrane.

Diagnosis

- Confirmed by isolating *staph. aureus* from blood.
- Skin biopsy may show separation of superficial layer of the epidermis, i.e., intra-epidermal separation.
- Where as in toxic epidermal necrolysis, separation occurs at the dermo-epidermal level.

Treatment

- Mainstay of treatment is supportive therapy along with the eradication of primary infection.
- Thus rehydration, antipyretic drug and antibiotics to cover *Staph. aureus* is the mainstay of treatment.
- If treated properly, the prognosis is excellent.

Erythrasma

Etiology

It is a superficial infection of the skin caused by *Corynebacterium minutissimum*—a gram positive bacterium which is a normal skin flora.

Predisposing Factors

It occurs most commonly in diabetic, elderly and immune compromised patients. Hyperhidrosis, obesity,moisture and occlusion also increase the risk.

Clinical Features

The infection presents as macerated, scaly plaques between the toes or erythematous to brown patches with thin plaques in intertriginous areas.

Treatment of Pyodermas

Tables 8.4 and 8.5 present the course of treatment for pyodermas.

Table 8.4 General management of pyodermas

- Clean with ordinary soap and water.
- Clean the hairy areas with shampoo.
- Use of oil should be avoided.

Recurrent infections

Causes of recurrent infections may be:

- Poor hygiene.
- Malnutrition.
- Immune deficiency.
- Concomitant diseases like diabetes mellitus.
- Lymphomas

Treatment with immunosuppressants or corticosteriods.

Table 8.5 Medical management of pyodermas

Limited lesions
Topical antibiotic like the following: Gentian violet and brilliant green. Bacitracin, mupirocin and sodium fucidate.
Indications for systemic antibiotics
The lesions are extensive. Regional lymph glands are enlarged and tender. There is fever and malaise. The infection is deep as in deep folliculitis, erysipelas, cellulitis and carbuncles. Pus discharge for culture and susceptibility to various antibiotics is done and specific antibiotics given adequately.

Pitted Keratolysis

Synonym: Keratoderma salcatum

First reported by castellani in 1910 in a Ceylonese patient.

Etiology

- Caused by bacteria.
- Due to wearing tight shoes and excessive sweating.

Symptoms

- Marked thickening of horny layer of the soles (Fig. 8.26).

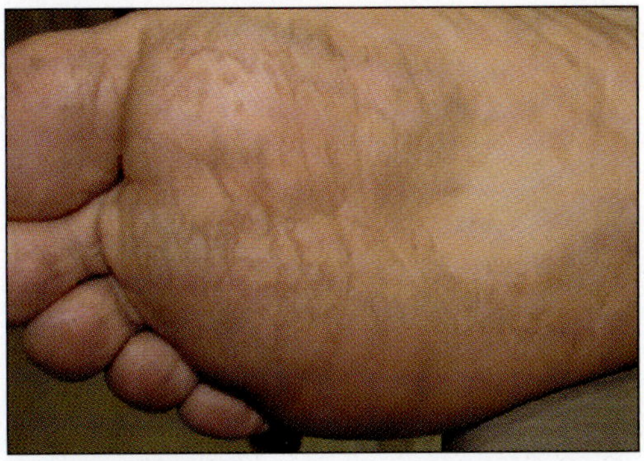

Fig. 8.26 Pitted keratolysis

- Crater like pits.
- Surface of feet and toe, especially on weight bearing areas, are involved.
- Due to dirt in holes and fissures, lesions stand-out sharply against yellowish-brown back ground.

Treatment

- Topical antibiotics.
- Wearing tight shoes and excessive sweating to be avoided.

CHAPTER 9

Tuberculosis

TUBERCULOSIS OF THE SKIN

Tuberculosis of the skin is caused by *Mycobacterium tuberculosis* found in the sputum, faeces, urine or pus of the infected cases. Infection with atypical mycobacteria can clinically resemble the *M. tuberculosis* infection.

Mode of infection

- Tubercular infection of the skin occurs by direct inoculation of the organisms into the skin.
- The pathogen may also enter the body via the respiratory system or gastrointestinal tract and reach the skin through the blood stream.
- Alternatively, there may be contiguous spread from an underlying focus.

Predisposing Factors

- Poverty.
- Overcrowding.
- Lack of hygiene.
- Malnutrition.

The clinical picture depends upon the mode of infection of the skin and the state of specific hypersensitivity (Table 9.1).

Table 9.1 Various presentations of tuberculosis of the skin

- Tubercular chancre.
- Lupus vulgaris.
- Tuberculosis verrucosa cutis.
- Scrofuloderma.
- Tuberculosis cutis orificialis or orificial tuberculosis.
- Tuberculides
  - Papulo-necrotic tuberculides.
  - Lichen scrofulosorum.

Tubercular Chancre

Incidence

Very rare.

Etiology

- When *Mycobacterium tuberculosis* gets inoculated into the skin of a person who has never been exposed to *Mycobacterium tuberculosis*.
- No hypersensitivity to *Mycobacterium tuberculosis*.

Clinical Features

- Nondescript, brownish, painless nodule.
- Breaks down within a week into a ragged ulcer having undermined edges with a hemorrhagic base.
- Regional lymph nodes are invariably enlarged.
- Heals spontaneously in many months.

Sites

Exposed parts of the body are affected

Lupus Vulgaris

Incidence

Commonest form.

Etiology

It occurs in a person with a moderate to high degree of immunity to *Mycobacterium tuberculosis* (Figs 9.1—9.3).

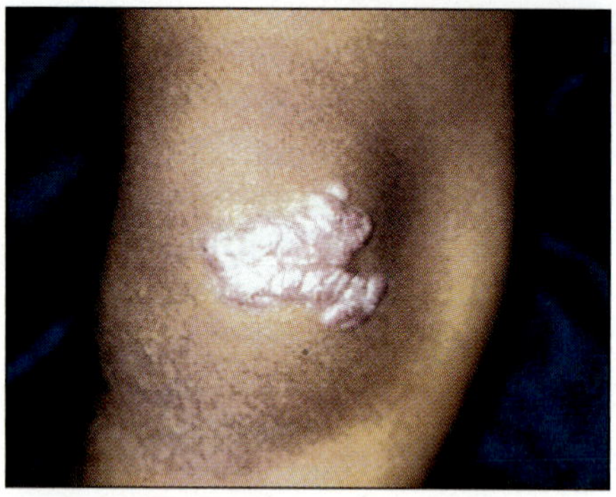

Fig. 9.1 Lupus vulgaris: knee

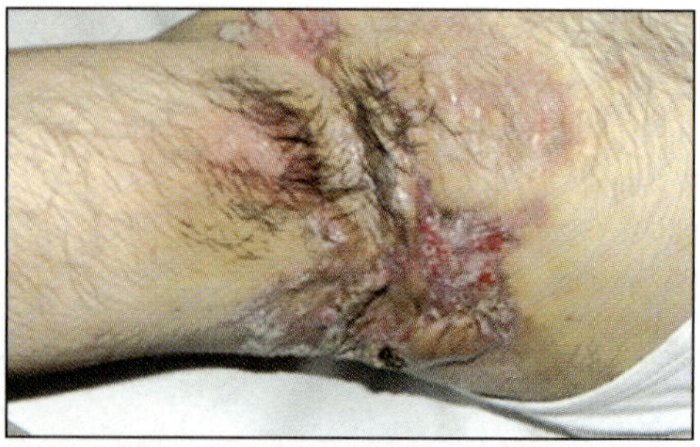

Fig. 9.2 Lupus vulgaris on chronic ulcer

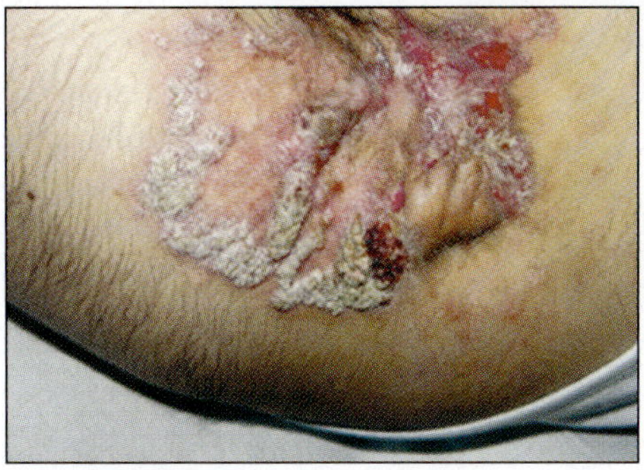

Fig. 9.3 Lupus vulgaris

Clinical Features

- Single, occasionally multiple, erythematous, irregular, indurated plaque(s) (Figs 9.1–9.3).
- The lesion is ulcerated in some areas while healing with scar formation is seen in other areas.
- Scars are usually thin, white and smooth, but unstable.
- Lesion slowly extends irregularly at the periphery.
- Lesion is more verrucous and dry.
- Apple jelly nodules comprise several large and soft nodules arranged in an annular fashion.
- Lesions present on the face may destroy the adjoining area like nose, eyelid and pinna.
- Carcinoma may develop in a long-standing lesion.

Sites

- Situated on the exposed parts of the body like face, arms and legs.
- Face is the most favoured site.
- In India, buttocks and trunk are very frequently involved.
- Occasionally present on the groins, shoulders and even on the glans penis.

Tuberculosis Verrucosa Cutis

Synonym Warty tuberculosis.

Clinical Features

- Lesions are similar to lupus vulgaris, except that they are more verrucous (Fig. 9.4).
- It is differentiated from common wart by the presence of erythema around it.

Sites

- The lesion is usually situated on the dorsum of the hand or feet.
- Sometimes may be seen on knees, ankles and buttocks.

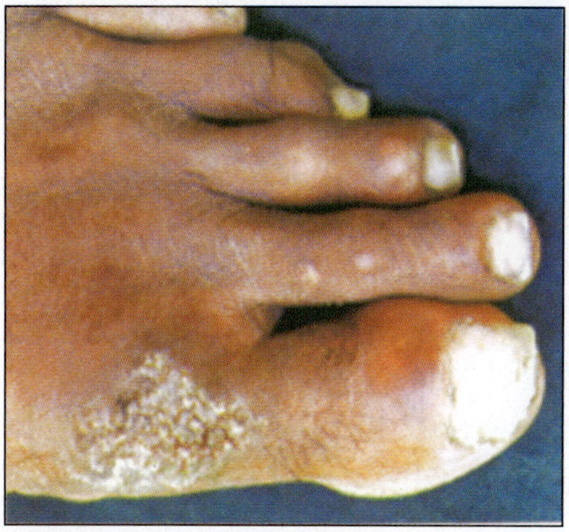

Fig. 9.4 Tuberculosis verrucosa cutis

Scrofuloderma

Etiology

This occurs due to the rupture of skin caused by the extension of infection from underlying tubercular foci in the following areas:

- Lymph glands.
- Bone or joints.

It occurs in an individual with poor to moderate immunity.

Clinical Features

- Single or multiple sinuses with undermined edges are seen which discharge thin, yellow pus and are located at the site of lymph nodes (Fig. 9.5), bone or joint.
- Sometimes lupus vulgaris develops around the sinus due to the implantation of *Mycobacterium tuberculosis* in the adjoining area.
- Scarring of the lesion produces an irregular mass adherent to the underlying structure.
- Pus discharge from the sinuses contains abundant *Mycobacterium tuberculosis*.

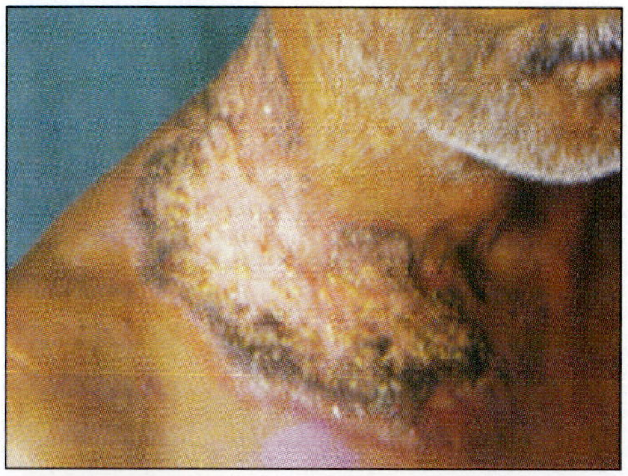

Fig. 9.5 Scrofuloderma

Tuberculosis Cutis Orificialis

Synonym

Orificial tuberculosis.

Incidence

The occurrence of tuberculosis cutis orificialis is very rare.

Etiology

It occurs due to the direct inoculation of *Mycobacterium tuberculosis* into the oral, anal or urogenital mucosa.

It occurs in patients with advanced tuberculosis.

Clinical Features

The skin adjacent to the orifice (in the mouth, around anus and on the genitalia) develops multiple painful shallow ulcers with undermined edges.

Tuberculides

A group of eruptions arise in response to internal foci of tuberculosis. This clears with anti-tubercular treatment.

Types

- Papulo-necrotic tuberculides.
- Lichen scrofulosorum.

Papulo-necrotic Tuberculides

Etiology

- It is a hypersensitivity reaction and occurs in an individual with moderate to high degree of immunity.
- Usually the primary tubercular focus is not clinically active at the time of eruption.

Clinical Features

- There is a sudden appearance of erythematous papules which become necrotic at the centre within a few days.
- The necrotic papules become crusted and heal leaving behind hyperpigmented and pitted scars over 2–3 weeks.
- New crops may keep on recurring for a few months to years.
- Tuberculous granuloma is seen on histology with the absence of bacilli in skin biopsy specimens.

Sites

The lesions are more or less symmetrically scattered all over the body, more so, on the extremities.

Lichen Scrofulosorum

This affects young children and occurs due to haematogenous spread of *Mycobacterium tuberculosis* from a tubercular focus.

Clinical Features

- Multiple asymptomatic groups of small, skin-coloured papules are seen (Fig. 9.6).
- Occasionally, mild scales are present.
- The lesions persist for variable periods and heal without scarring.

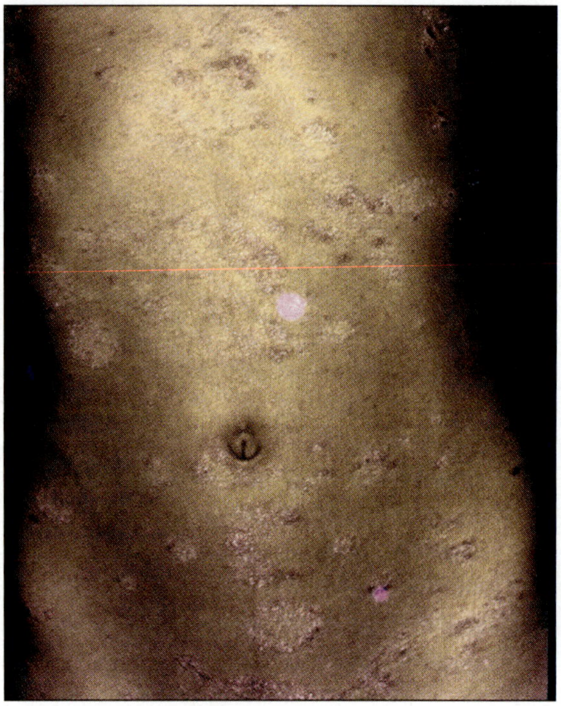

Fig. 9.6 Lichen scrofulosorum

Diagnosis of Cutaneous Tuberculosis

- Biopsy from the lesion demonstrating a classical caseating tubercular granuloma.
- Smear made from the lesion or pus discharge are usually negative for acid fast bacilli stained with Ziehl–Nielsen stain.
- Culture of pus from the lesions are also usually negative, except in some cases of scrofuloderma.
- **Polymerase chain reaction** (PCR) for identification of *M. Tuberculosis* from skin is also doubtful.
- Mantoux test is positive in tuberculosis verrucosa cutis and tuberculides.
- Still, the diagnosis is based on the characteristic morphological features of the lesions.

Treatment

Like treating tuberculosis of any other organ, the initial treatment consists of giving at least three drugs to avoid the development of resistance. Most commonly used drugs are:

- Isonicotinic acid hydrazide (INH): 300 mg daily.
- Rifampicin: 600 mg daily.
- Ethambutol: 800 mg daily.
- Pyrazinamide: 750 mg twice daily can be given in place of any of the above drugs.

The initial phase and long term treatments are presented in Table 9.2.

Table 9.2 Treatment of skin tuberculosis: Present regime

Initial Phase
At least three drugs to reduce the number of viable bacilli as quickly as possible, for 8–12 weeks.

Continuation Phase
In this phase, the standard 6-months regimen for an adult is as follows:

- Pyrazinamide: 1.5–2 gm daily for the first 2 months.
- Ethambutol: 800 mg (15 mg/kg body weight) daily for the first 2 months.
- Isonicotinic acid hydrazide: 300 mg daily for 6 months.
- Rifampicin: 450–600 mg daily for six months.

Other Drugs

Vitamin D2 (calciferol), given in the treatment of lupus vulgaris, acts on the tissue and not on bacilli. It promotes fibroblast proliferation leading to strangling of the tubercles. Dose is 150,000 units daily given for 5 days a week.

Sarcoidosis

Etiology

It may be due to an unusual reaction to *mycobacterium tuberculosis.*

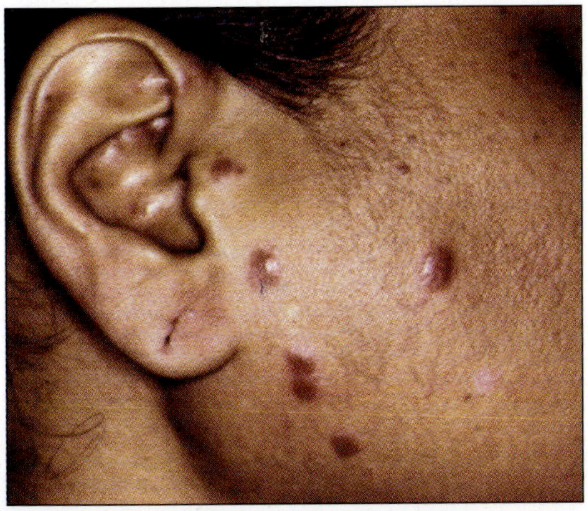

Fig. 9.7 Sarcoidosis: reddish purple juicy papules

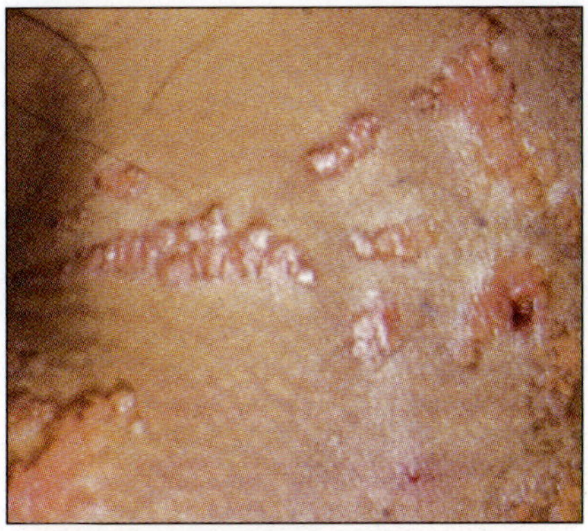

Fig. 9.8 Sarcoidosis: juicy papules

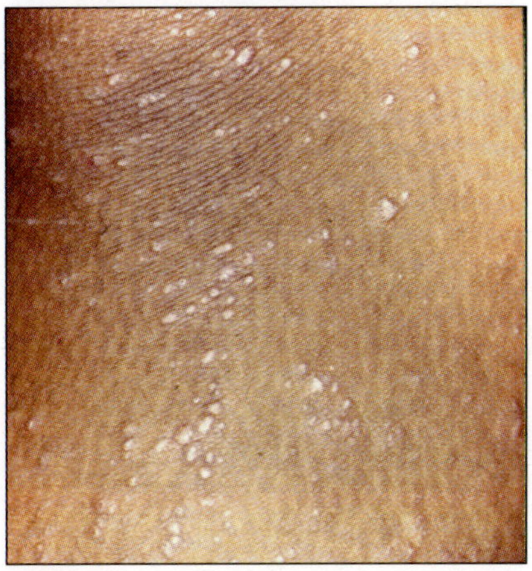

Fig. 9.9 Sarcoidosis: micropapule

Clinical Features

- It is a multisystem disease involving the following:
  - i) Respiratory system.
  - ii) Reticuloendothelial system.
  - iii) Skin.
  - iv) Skeletal system.
  - v) Cardiovascular system.
- Multiple reddish, purple, juicy papules (Figs 9.7–9.10) and deeper nodules and plaques are present.
- Bluish swelling of the following:
  - i) Fingers.
  - ii) Nose.
  - iii) Ears.

Erythema Nodosum

Clinical Features

- Presents as painful, erythematous, raised, tender nodules mostly on the shin.
- May be associated with malaise, fever and arthralgia of ankles and knees.
- The lesions heal without ulcerating.

Diagnosis

Biopsy shows naked tubercle containing foci of macrophages and giant cells without surrounding lymphocytes.

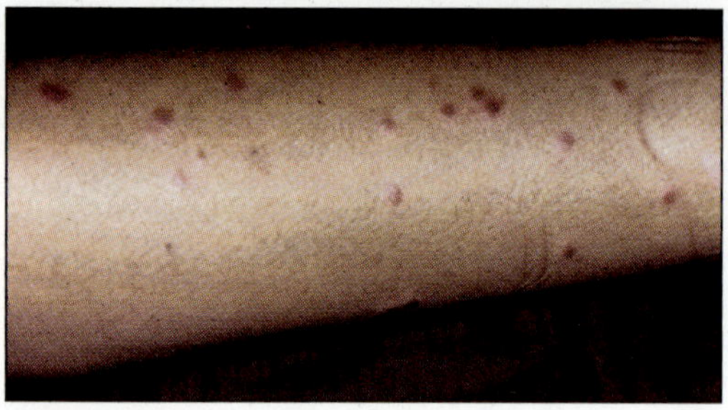

Fig. 9.10 Sarcoidosis: reddish papules on arm

Table 9.3. Causes of erythema nodosum

• Sarcoidosis.	• Crohn's disease.
• Leprosy.	• Streptococcal infection.
• Brucellosis.	• Drugs.
• Ulcerative colitis.	• Malignancy.

Treatment

- Large lesions leave scars and require treatment.
- Systemic corticosteroid.
- Dexamethasone pulse—where dexamethasone 100 mg dissolved in 500 ml 5% glucose is transfused over 1–2 hours on 3 consecutive days, every month, till the clearance of all lesions.
- Underlying disease should be treated.

Chapter 10

Leprosy

Leprosy is a chronic infectious disease that probably originated in India and is caused by *Mycobacterium leprae*. It generally occurs only in human beings. India has the greatest number of leprosy sufferers.

Etiology

- Leprosy is caused by *Mycobacterium leprae* which was discovered in 1873 by G.H.A. Hansen at Bergen in Norway.
- It closely resembles the bacillus which causes the tuberculosis on staining with Ziehl–Nielsen stain; but it is less acid-fast than *Mycobacterium tuberculosis*.
- *Mycobacterium leprae* is pleomorphic, straight or slightly curved, rod-like or ovoid. It may be fragmented or granular.

Incidence

- Occurs only in humans and is prevalent in the tropical countries.
- In 2015, the prevalence of the disease globally was 176,176 cases (0.2 cases per 10,000 people). Number of new cases reported globally in 2015 was 211,973 (2.9 new cases per 100000 people)
- It is not a hereditary disease.
- Children born of infectious leprosy parents—if separated soon after birth and protected from exposure—will escape from the disease.
- Incidence of conjugal transmission of leprosy (from one spouse to another) is very low, i.e., between 2 to 5 per cent.

Source of Infection

Infected human beings, especially the untreated multibacillary patients of leprosy, are the only source of infection.

Transmission of Infection

Transmission of leprosy depends primarily on the following factors:

- Direct implantation of bacilli laden droplets from nasal secretions or skin ulcers of infected individuals onto the mucous membranes or skin of healthy individuals.
- It may also be transmitted by one of the following:
  i) Scratch.
  ii) Abrasion.
  iii) Insect bite.
- The role of biting insects like mosquitoes, cockroaches, flies and bugs in transferring the bacilli from an untreated patient to the susceptible individuals is also quite possible.
- People living in areas where leprosy is highly prevalent, are susceptible to infection, especially if there is an infected individual living in the same house.
- All the patients are not infectious.

The transmission of infection also depends on the following factors:

- Infectiousness of the infected person.
- Susceptibility of the contact person.
- Closeness.
- Frequency of contact.
- Duration of contact.

Pathogenesis

- Principally, it affects the peripheral nerves and the skin.
- Organisms from the droplets deposit into the dermis through the epidermis.
- The clinical features of the disease depend on the immunity status of the individual; resulting in the localised form of disease when the cell mediated response is good. The disseminated form of disease is caused when the immunity status is poor.

Clinical Forms

Depending on the status of the infected individual's resistance to leprosy bacilli, i.e., cell-mediated immunity, clinical presentation, pathological and bacteriological features, the disease is classified as per Ridley–Jopling classification (Table 10.1),

Table 10.1 Classification of leprosy

- Tuberculoid leprosy (TT).
- Borderline tuberculoid leprosy (BT).
- Mid borderline (BB).
- Borderline lepromatous (BL).
- Lepromatous leprosy (LL).

Tuberculoid and lepromatous leprosy are the stable variants, whereas the other three are unstable variants of the disease.

Four other clinical types are seen. These are as follows:

- Indeterminate leprosy.
- Histoid leprosy.
- Neuritic leprosy.
- Maculo-anesthetic leprosy.

Indeterminate Leprosy (I)

An early stage of leprosy that presents as an asymptomatic ill-defined, hypopigmented macule(s) (Fig. 10.1) with the following symptoms:

- There may/may not be a loss of sensation.
- Nerve supplying the macule is not enlarged.
- Slit-smear from macule is mostly negative.
- Lepromin test may be positive or negative.
- Careful examination of the well-stained serial sections usually reveals acid-fast bacilli in dermal nerve fibrils infiltrated with lymphocytes.

Course

- Many of the lesions disappear spontaneously without any treatment.
- Quite a few progress to other forms of leprosy.
- Patient should be examined at 3 to 6 months interval to assess the progress of the disease.

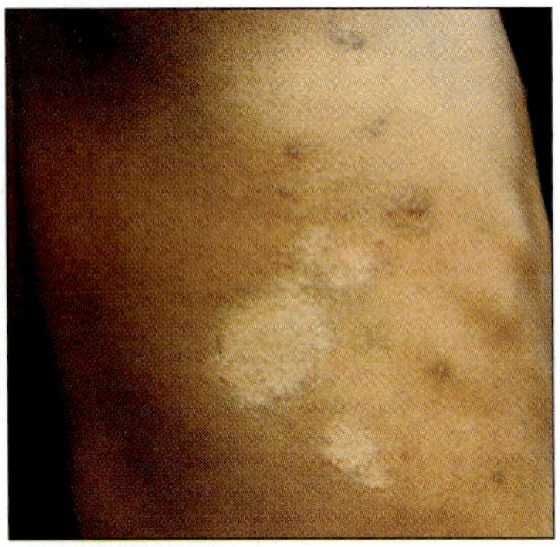

Fig. 10.1 Indeterminate leprosy

Tuberculoid Leprosy (TT)

Occurs in individuals who have good immunity against the leprosy bacilli, but are not strong enough to eradicate infection altogether

Clinical Features

- The disease remains confined to a localised area of the skin; the lesion can be seen on any part of the body.
- Lesion is usually single, but there may be two or three oval or rounded plaques with well-defined distinct margins (Fig. 10.2–10.4). Actively dividing bacilli are seen at the margins of the lesions.
- Total loss or impairment of the superficial sensations, i.e., of pain, touch and temperature occurs; it is difficult to detect the loss of sensation in a lesion situated on the face because of a rich supply of sensory nerves to the facial skin
- The patch is usually rough, hairless or with sparse hair.
- Sweating is markedly impaired on the affected area.
- An enlarged cutaneous nerve may be seen entering the lesion (Fig. 10.5) at one end and emerging from the other end.
- Slit and smear examination for acid-fast bacilli is negative from the patch.
- Tuberculoid leprosy patients are usually non-infectious.

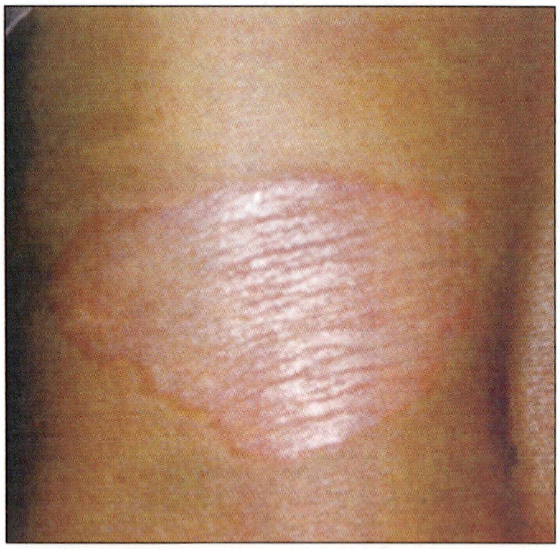

Fig. 10.2 Tuberculoid leprosy

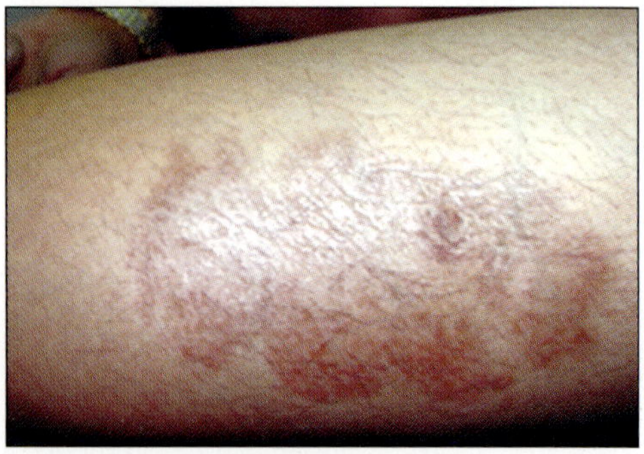

Fig. 10.3 Treated tuberculoid leprosy

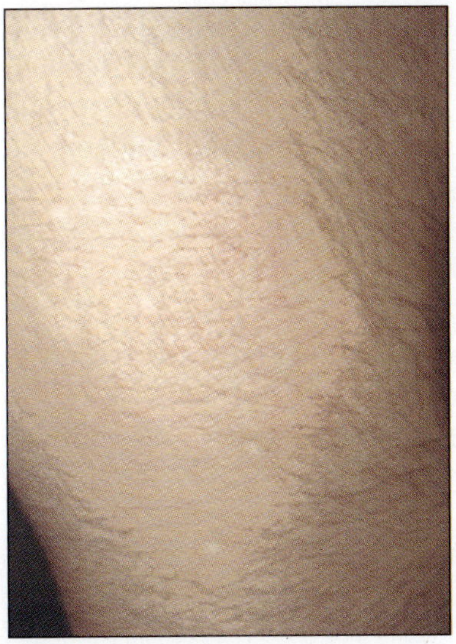

Fig. 10.4 BT leprosy

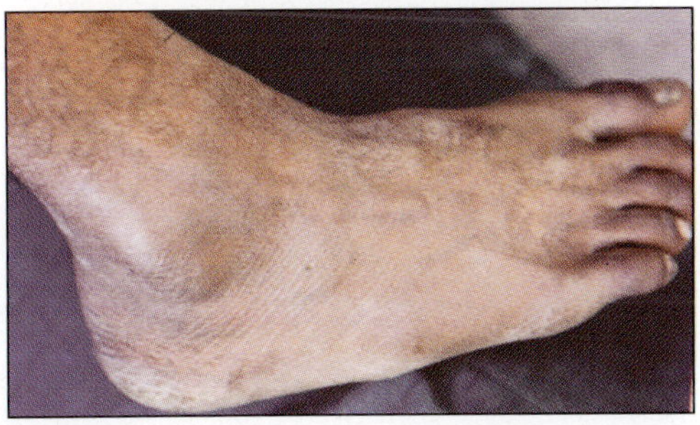

Fig. 10.5 Thickened masculo-cutaneous nerve

Maculo-anaesthetic Leprosy

It is largely seen in Indians.

Clinical Features

- Consists of single or a few hypopigmented macules with well-defined borders (Fig. 10.6) and the loss of superficial sensation.
- Regional nerve may be enlarged.
- Slit and smear examination is negative for acid-fast bacilli.

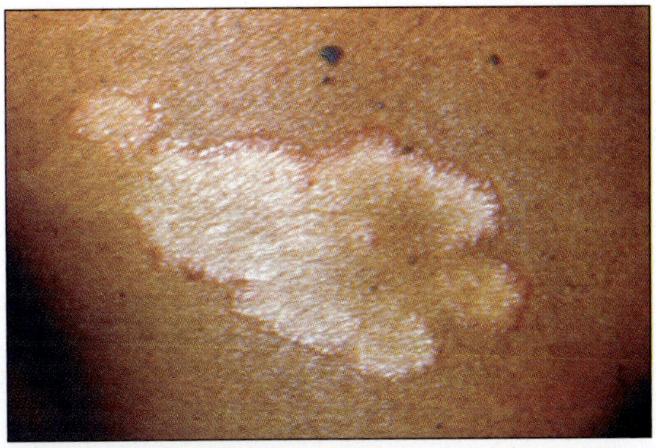

Fig. 10.6 Maculo-anaesthetic leprosy

Neuritic Leprosy

It occurs due to the involvement of one, or at times, several peripheral nerve trunks by leprosy bacilli. Ulnar nerve is very commonly involved.

Clinical Features

- Enlarged, and sometimes, tender cutaneous nerve(s) with a loss of sensation in the corresponding area of skin which otherwise looks completely normal.
- Patient may present with heaviness, tingling and numbness.
- Severe pain is present if acute inflammation occurs in the affected nerve.
- This may cause paralysis and atrophy of the muscles (Fig. 10.7), particularly of the hands and the feet causing deformities (Table 10.2).

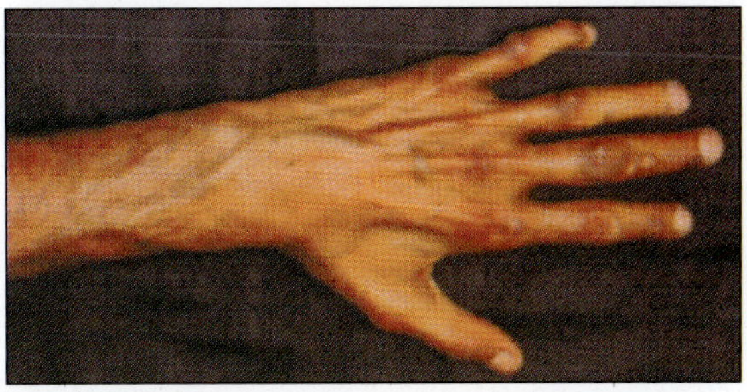

Fig. 10.7 Claw hand

Table 10.2 Deformities occurring due to involvement of nerve in neuritic leprosy

- Claw hand
- Claw toes
- Wrist drop
- Foot drop

Borderline Leprosy

Synonym

Dimorphous leprosy

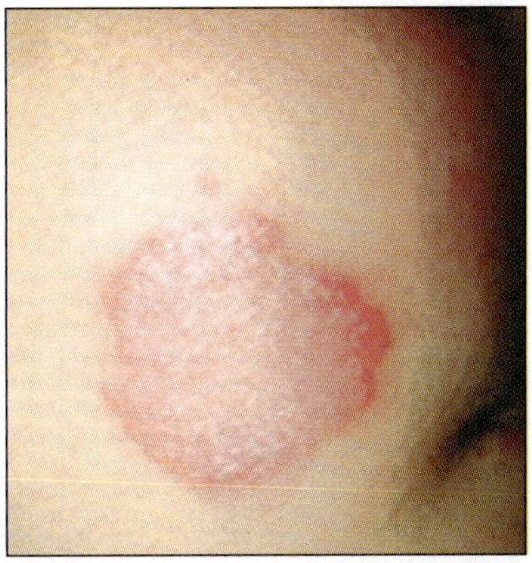

Fig. 10.8 BT Leprosy

- It is the most common variety of the leprosy.
- The degree of impairment of immunity against leprosy bacilli is variable.
- It has been subdivided into the following categories:
  i) **Borderline-tuberculoid** (BT) (Figs 10.4 and 10.8).
  ii) **Borderline** (BB) (Figs 10.9–10.11).
  iii) **Borderline lepromatous** (BL) leprosy.

Clinical Features

- Lesions of the borderline leprosy may be erythematous, having different shapes, such as, raised centre and sloping at the periphery, i.e., dome shaped, inverted saucer or annular appearance.

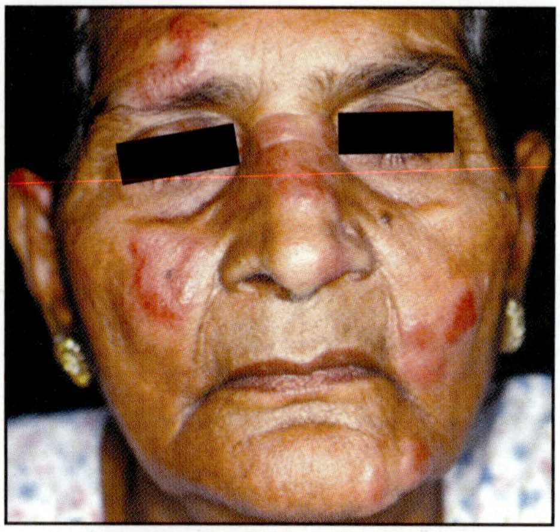

Fig. 10.9 Borderline lepromatous leprosy: active lesion

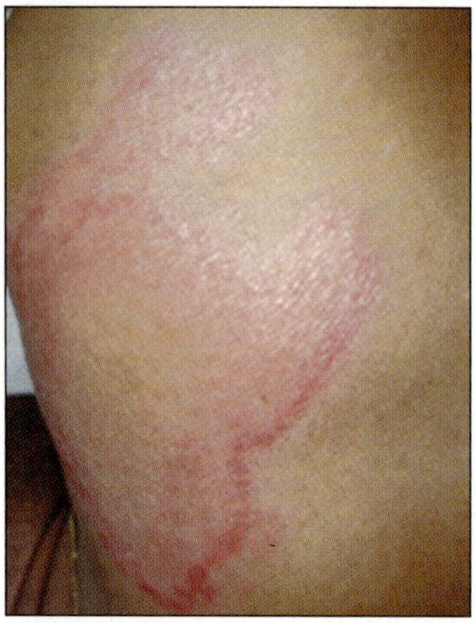

Fig. 10.10 Borderline lepromatous leprosy: active lession

- Depending on the position on the borderline spectrum, macular or other lesions vary greatly in number, size and shape; nearer to the **lepromatous end**—the lesions are more numerous, shiny, less defined, symmetrical and anaesthetic. The opposite occurs nearer to the **tuberculoid end**.
- However, in a single patient, some lesions may be typically BL, while the others may suggest BB or BT. This indicating that the exact typing of leprosy is not possible.
- Slit and smear examination for acid-fast bacilli from the lesions are usually positive.
- Concentrations of bacilli increase from very few in BT to a large number in BL.

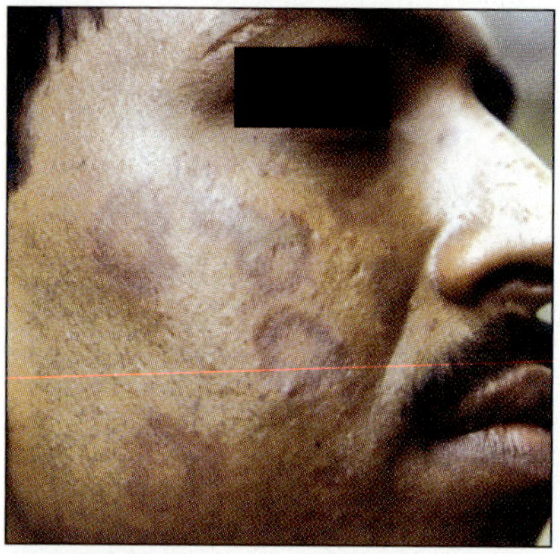

Fig. 10.11 B.B. leprosy: subsiding lesion

Lepromatous Leprosy

Occurs in individuals who have very little or no resistance to leprosy bacilli.

Clinical Features

- Lepromatous leprosy is a systemic disease that may involve any part of the body.
- Leprosy bacilli multiply rapidly leading to extensive spread to the skin, mucous membranes, bones, eyes, liver, lungs, etc.
- Nasal stuffiness and discharge, with or without blood, may be the earliest manifestation.
- Ulceration of the nasal mucosa is common. Antero-inferior aspect of the nasal septum is the site of predilection.
- Some skin areas, like the ear lobules (Fig. 10.12) and lateral part of the eyebrows, may show diffuse infiltration with loss of hair (supraciliary madarosis).
- The skin lesions consist of multiple erythematous and indurated plaques, nodules and even diffuse infiltrated area present on any part of the body. Later on, scarring may occur (Fig. 10.15).
- The margins of the plaques are ill-defined.

- There is no loss of sensation.
- Sometimes the skin may look completely normal.
- Cutaneous nerves may be enlarged in some cases.
- Presence of multiple infiltrated nodules on the face (Fig. 10.13) produce 'leonine-facies' (lion-like appearance).
- In the advanced stage of the disease, the involvement of nerve and bones may cause 'glove and stocking anaesthesia' and the terminal portion of fingers and toes might get absorbed leading to shortening of the digits.

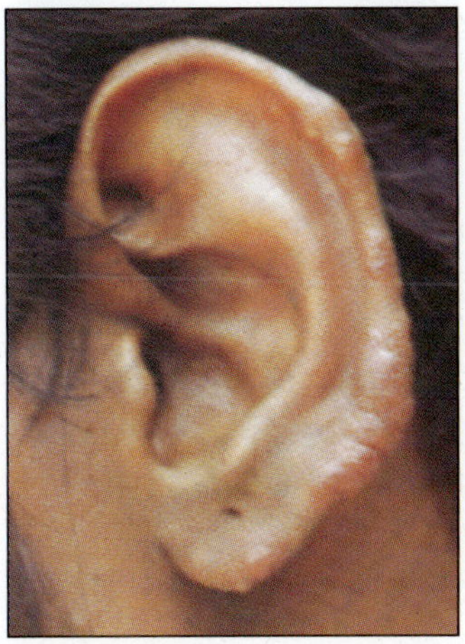

Fig. 10.12 L.L. leprosy: pinna

- At the site of trauma, patient may develop painless non-healing ulcers (Fig. 10.14).
- Slit and smear examination from the lesions, nasal mucosa or even from normal looking skin shows acid fast bacilli.

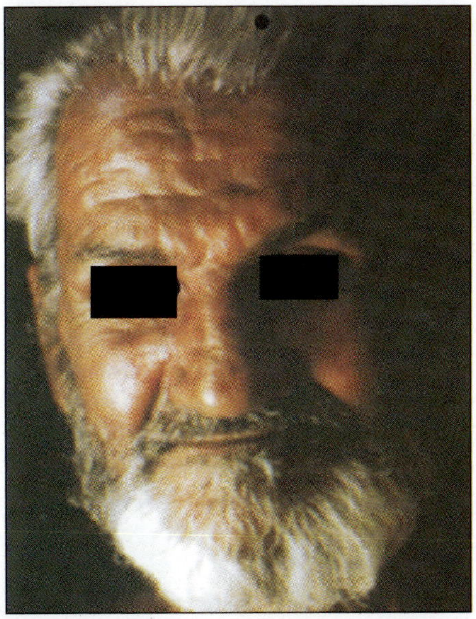

Fig. 10.13 L.L. leprosy: face

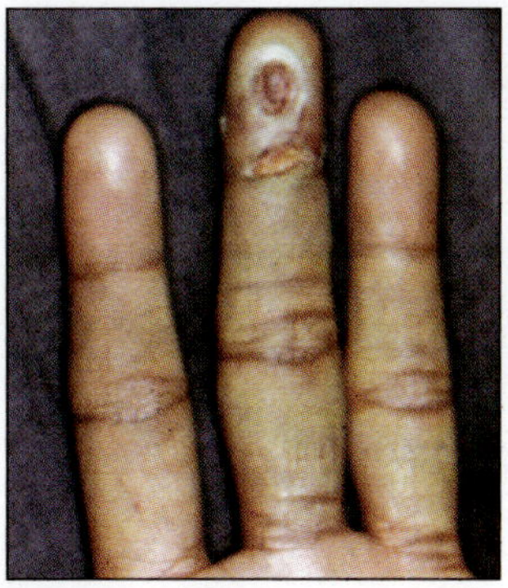

Fig. 10.14 Trophic ulcer in finger

Histoid Leprosy

Wade in 1963 described a special type of leprosy characterised by the presence of firm, erythematous, glistening or juicy nodules in the skin (Fig. 10.16).

These patients usually belong to multibacillary type of leprosy.

It is called **histoid** because biopsy shows elongated or spindle-shaped histiocytes containing bacilli.

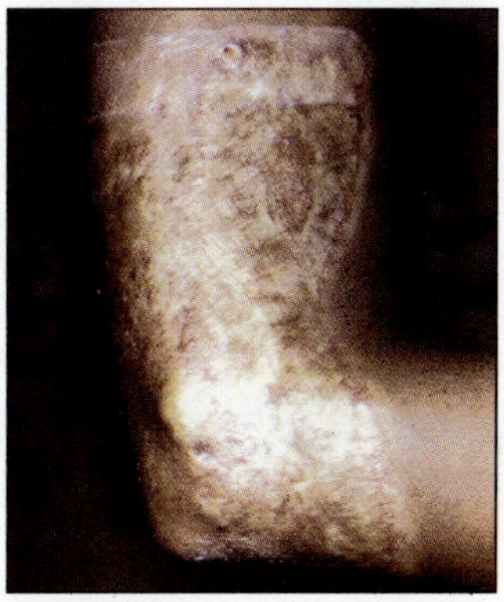

Fig. 10.15 Scar leprosy: elbow

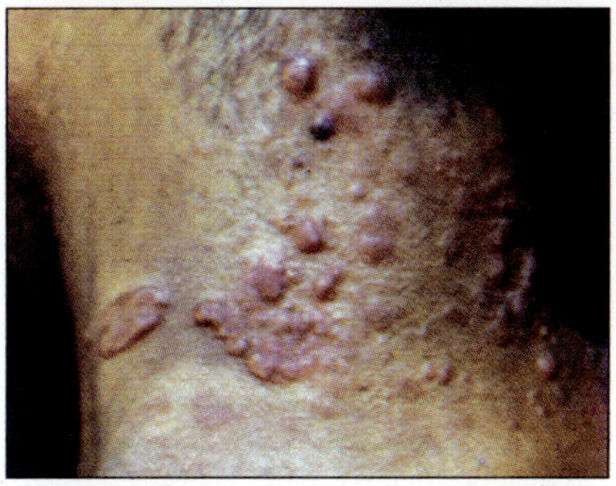

Fig. 10.16 Histoid leprosy

Reactions in Leprosy

These reactions are the sudden exacerbations of leprosy, following effective treatment and reduction in the bacillary load. These occur due to immunological changes.

Sometimes they are spontaneous, or they may be due to other various causes (Table 10.3).

Table 10.3 Causes that precipitate the lepra reactions

- Intercurrent infections like malaria, virus etc.
- Mental and/or physical stress.
- Anaemia.
- Pregnancy.
- Parturition.
- Surgical interventions.

Types of Lepra Reactions

Type I Reaction

- This is a Type IV hypersensitivity reaction and involves the cell-mediated immunity.
- Seen in the entire spectrum of leprosy, except the lepromatous type.
- Type I reaction can be classified into upgrading and downgrading reactions, based on the improvement or deterioration of the cell-mediated immunity.

Upgrading Reaction

- It is due to an increase in the cell-mediated immunity.
- Commonly occurs during treatment.

Downgrading reaction

- When the reaction is associated with a decrease in the cell-mediated immunity.
- Seen in a patient who is not receiving treatment.
- It is impossible to clinically differentiate between the upgrading and downgrading reactions.

Clinical Features

- It manifests as a local aggravation of the lesions which may suddenly become more erythematous and indurated with an increased loss of sensation (Fig. 10.17).

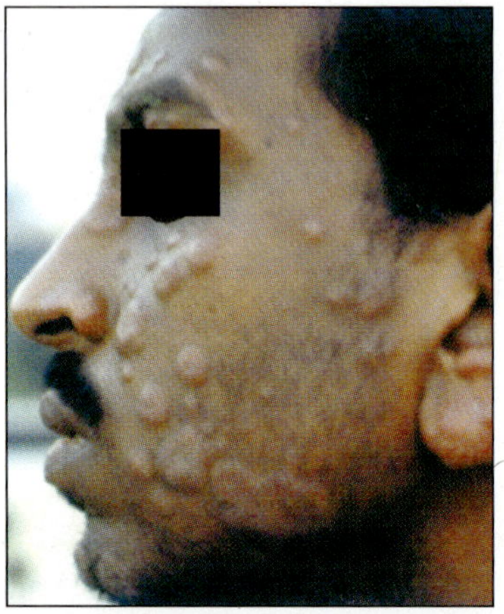

Fig. 10.17 B.B. leprosy with type I reaction

- Lesion becomes painful and may develop paraesthesia.
- The nerve may become extremely painful and tender.
- Acute neuritis may cripple the patient overnight.

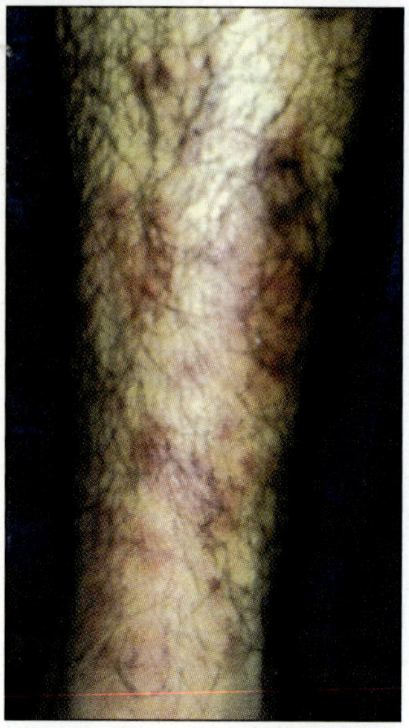

Fig. 10.18 Erythema nodosum leprosum (ENL)

Type II Reaction

Synonym

Erythema nodosum leprosum (ENL).

- This is mediated through humoral hypersensitivity and there is no alteration of cell-mediated immunity.
- It usually occurs in lepromatous and borderline lepromatous leprosy during the active phase of treatment. Although it can appear without any treatment also.

Clinical Features

- Recurrent, tender, erythematous nodules (Figs 10.18 and 10.19) appearing suddenly on any part of the body with constitutional symptoms like fever, malaise and joint pains.

Sometimes iridocyclitis, orchitis, swelling in the joints or persistent albuminuria may be present.

Diagnosis

Slit Smear Examination

Smears taken from the lesions (commonly from the ear lobes, elbows or knees) are stained with Ziehl–Neelsen technique and seen under the microscope. The acid-fast bacilli appear red against a blue background.

Histopathology

Histopathology shows pathognomonic granuloma and the nerve involvement.

Lepromin Test

It is used to determine the type of leprosy a person is having. Lepromin positivity indicates good immunity to *M. leprae*.

Treatment

- Leprosy patients need moral support and reassurance, so they gain self-confidence and self-respect.
- Leprosy is far less infectious than even the common cold or sore throat.
- The treatment recommended by WHO is presented in Table 10.4.

Table 10.4 Medical treatment of leprosy recommended by WHO

Paucibacillary (TT, BT and indeterminate) patients(5 or < lesions): • Dapsone: 100 mg daily for 6 months • Rifampicin: 600 mg once in a month For multibacillary (BB, BL and LL) patients for 2 years (> 5 lesions) • Dapsone: 100 mg, daily. • Rifampicin: 600 mg, once in month. • Clofazimine: 100 mg, on alternate days. • Clofazimine: 300 mg, once in month.

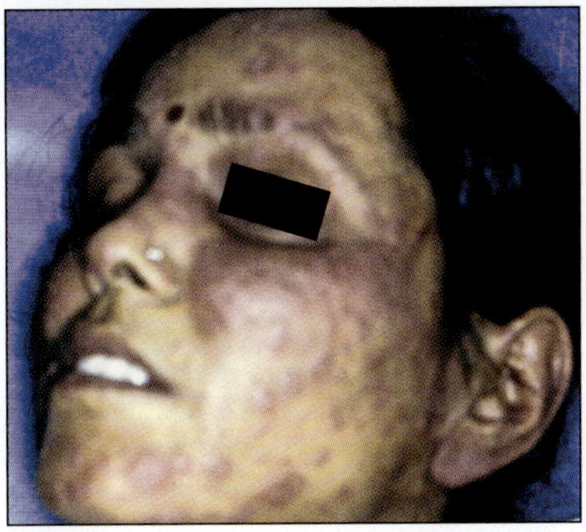

Fig. 10.19 Erythema nodosum leprosum (ENL)

- The author however feels that rifampicin should be given in a dose of 600 mg, daily to all the patients and the treatment must be continued till all the lesions have cleared completely, clinically as well as histopathologically. Rifampicin has bactericidal activity and with oral 600 mg daily, it makes the patient non infective in 4–6 weeks. With the interrupted doses, there is a risk of development of resistance to rifampicin.

Newer Drugs

- Ofloxacin.
- Minocycline.
- Sparfloxacin.
- Clarithromycin.

Indication

- Used for treating resistant cases.
- Those who cannot tolerate the commonly used drugs.

Treatment of Type I Reaction

Systemic corticosteroids, especially when there is nerve involvement, to prevent the paralysis.

Treatment of Type II Reaction:

- Thalidomide: 100–400 mg a day.
- Oral corticosteroids.
- Clofazimine: 100–300 mg daily.

Side effects

With Dapsone

- Anaemia.
- Methaemoglobinaemia.
- Hepatotoxicity and jaundice.

With Rifampicin

- Hepatotoxicity.
- Flu like syndrome.

With Clofazimine

Clofazimine is a dye. It has both antileprosy and anti-inflammatory action. On prolonged use, it has the following side effects:

- Discolouration.
- Ichthyosis like scaling (Fig. 10.20).
- Gastrointestinal upset.

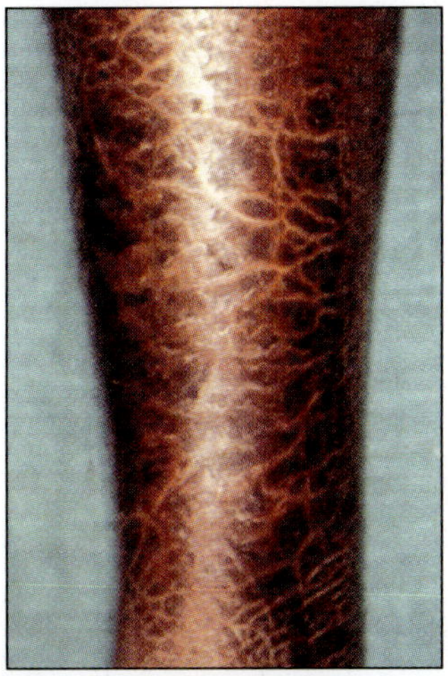

Fig. 10.20 Ichthyosis due to clofazimine

Thalidomide

Teratogenic drug.
Contraception is a must during its use.

Leprosy Vaccines

The development of leprosy vaccines is hindered by the inability to grow *M. leprae* in artificial media. Several candidate vaccines are being investigated, some of them are as follows:

- BCG
- BCG+killed M. leprae
- Killed M. leprae
- Mw
- ICRC bacillus
  Leprosy vaccines have been useful in:

Immunoprophylaxis

To reduce the chance of development of leprosy, e.g., in contacts.

Immunotherapy

Along with chemotherapy, in highly bacillated patients, so as to hasten the clearance of bacillus.

Chapter 11

Fungal Infections

INTRODUCTION

Fungal infection of the skin is very common in India due to the warm and humid climate in most of the parts of the country. The incidence of fungal infection is more during the summer and rainy seasons. Common fungal infections of the skin are presented in Table 11.1.

Table 11.1 Common fungal infections of the skin

Fungal Infection	Fungus Responsible
Dermatophytoses or ringworm	Dermatophytes
Pityriasis versicolor	Malassezia furfur
Candidiasis	Candida

DERMATOPHYTOSES OR RINGWORM

Etiology

- Most common fungal infection of the skin.
- Caused by any one of the following dermatophytes:
  - i) Microsporon.
  - ii) Trichophyton.
  - iii) Epidermophyton.

The clinical features and nomenclature of the dermataphytoses depend upon the site of involvement.

Tinea Capitis

When the fungus involves the scalp (Fig. 11.3), it is called tinea capitis.

Age

This condition is very common in children.

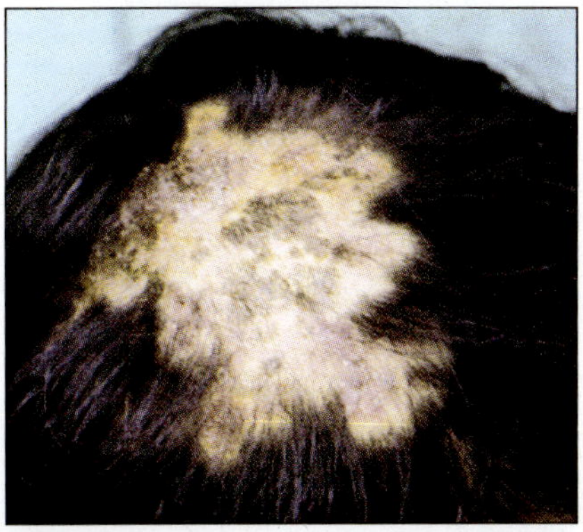

Fig. 11.1 Tinea capitis: kerion

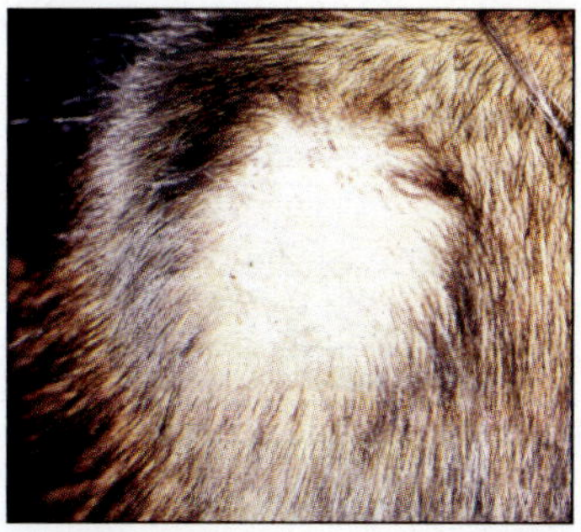

Fig. 11.2 Kerion: after treatment

Clinical Features

- Manifests as localised form of partial alopecia associated with itching, erythema and scaling.
- The hair in the patch is dry, lusterless, brittle and broken at varying lengths.
- In some patients, there is localised and painful boggy swelling on the scalp (Figs 11.1 and 11.2), called **kerion**.
- In **black dot tinea capitis**, the hairs are broken at the level of the skin surface producing the picture of black dots in an area of alopecia.
- **Favus** presents as a localised area of loss of hair with plenty of pus discharge and crusting. The presentation is endemic in Kashmir and caused by *T. schoenleinii*.

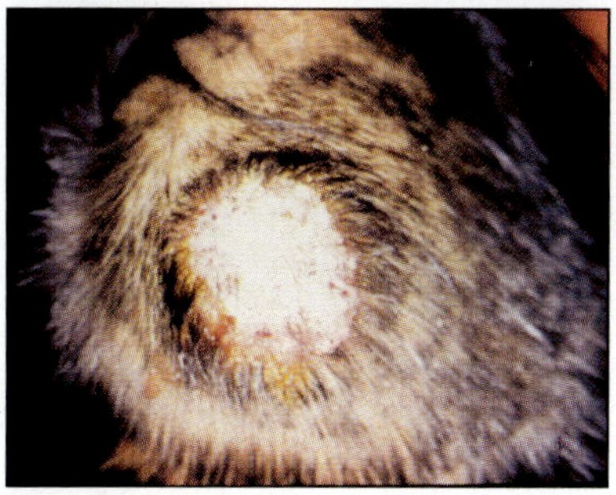

Fig. 11.3 Tinea capitis

Tinea Barbae

In this condition, the fungus involves the coarse hair of beard and moustache.

Age and Sex

Adult males.

Clinical Features

- Red inflammatory papules or pustules are seen associated with exudation and crusting.
- Hair in the lesion become loose and can be removed without much pain.
- Less severe infections consist of dry, circular, reddish and scaly lesions with lusterless hair stumps which are broken close to the surface of skin.

Tinea Corporis

It is the fungal infection of the trunk (Figs. 11.4–11.8) and extremities.

Clinical Features

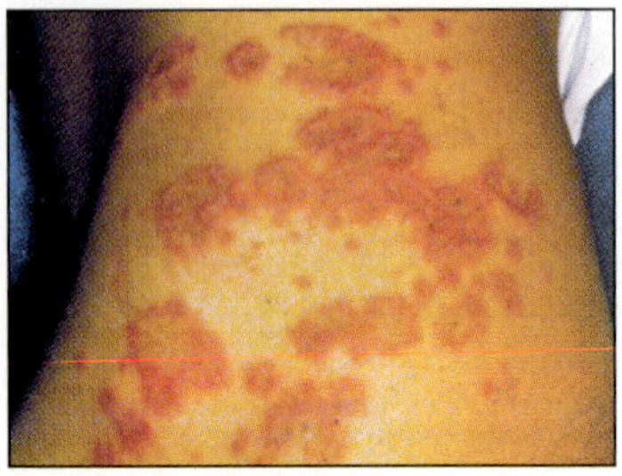

Fig. 11.4 Tinea corporis: abdomen

Severely itchy, circular or irregular lesions with well-defined active borders; the border consists of papulovesicles (Figs. 11.5 and 11.10) while the central part of the lesion shows erythema, scaling and occasionally hyperpigmentation (Fig. 11.6)

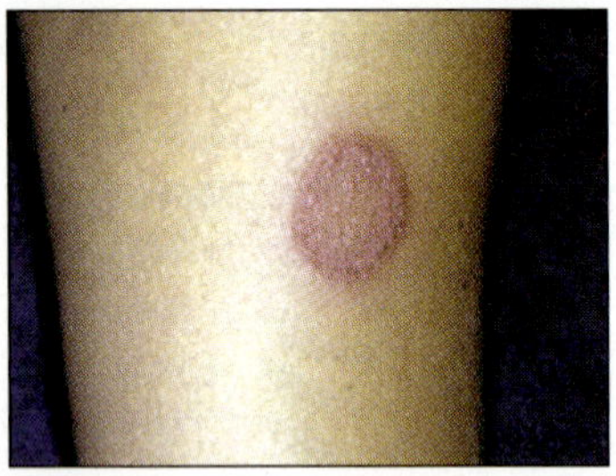

Fig. 11.5 Tinea corporis: active periphery

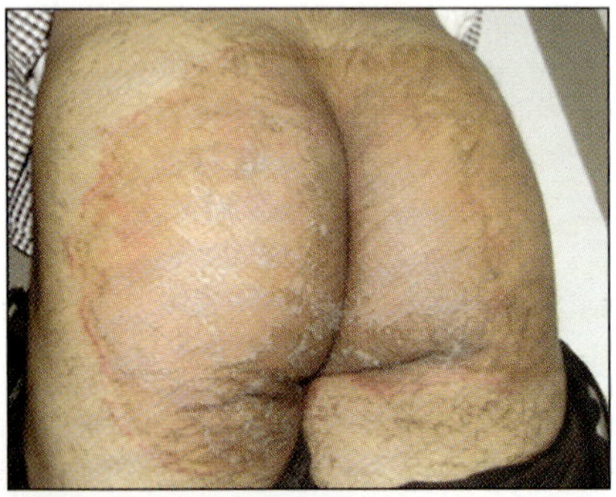

Fig. 11.6 Tinea corporis: buttocks (scales)

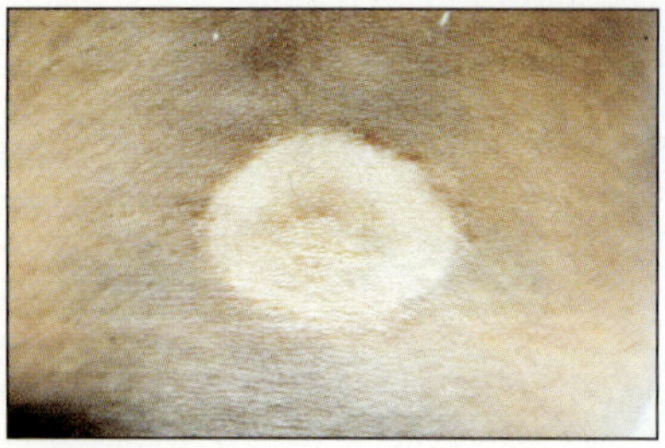

Fig. 11.7 Tinea corporis in 10 days old child

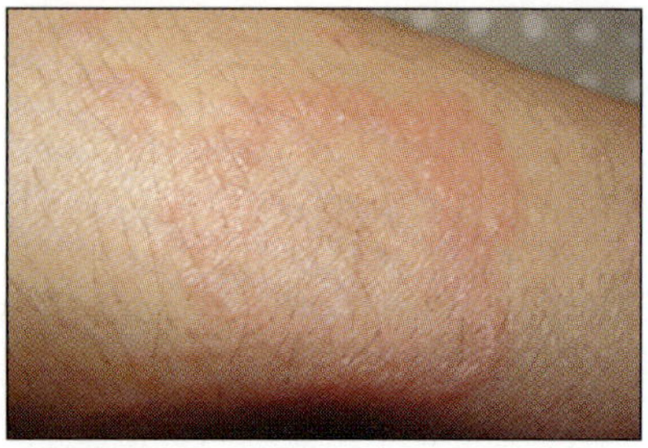

Fig. 11.8 Tinea corporis: vesicle

Tinea Cruris

Lesions similar to tinea corporis are seen in the groin. It usually occurs in adults wearing synthetic clothes such as **terylene and nylon** that tend to accumulate heat and humidity in the skin.

Clinical features

- Scaling is variable, vesiculation is rare (Figs. 11.9 and 11.10).
- Central clearance is usually present.

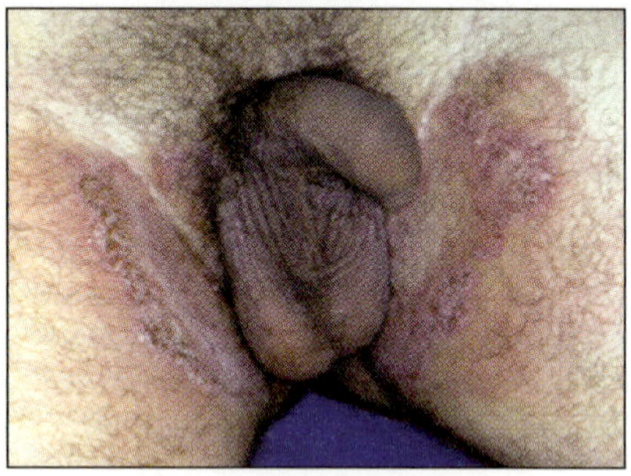

Fig. 11.9 Tinea cruris

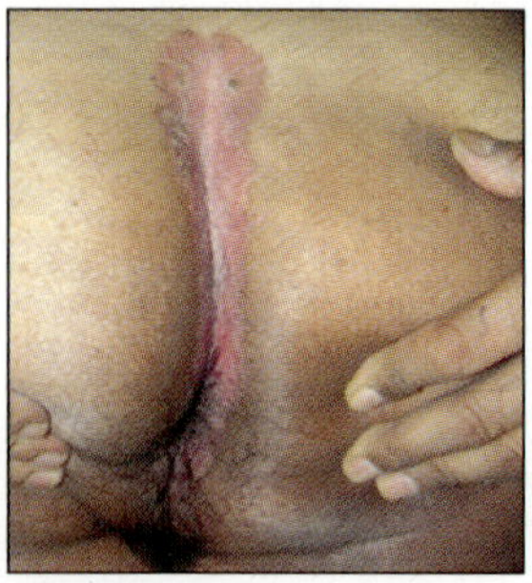

Fig. 11.10 Tinea interdigitale

Tinea Faciei

Infection of the skin of face excluding the moustache and beard areas (Figs. 11.11 and 11.12).

Age and Sex

Adult male.

Clinical Features

The lesions are similar to tinea corporis with the presence of itching and scaling.

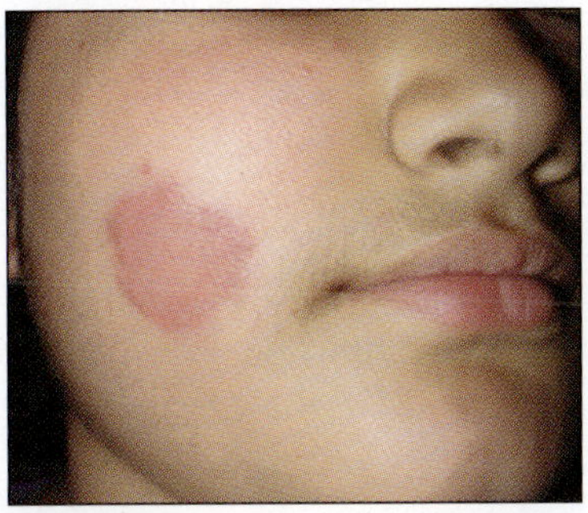

Fig. 11.11 Tinea Faciei

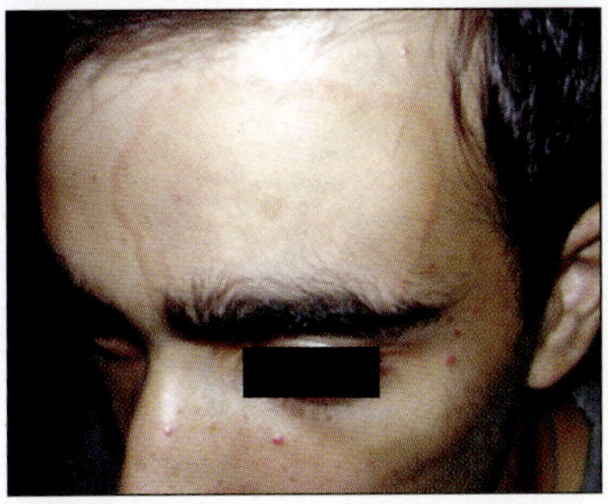

Fig. 11.12 Tinea forehead

Tinea Incognito

Topical application of the steroids alters the appearance of the lesions and they are then called tinea incognitio (Figs 11.13 and 11.14) with scaling and erythema present without itching.

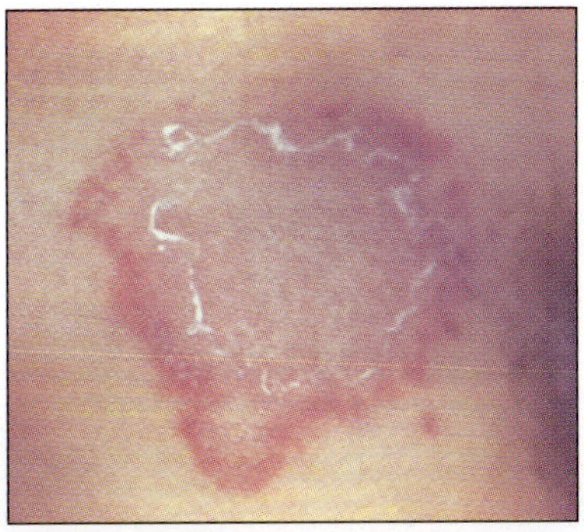

Fig. 11.13 Tinea incognitio

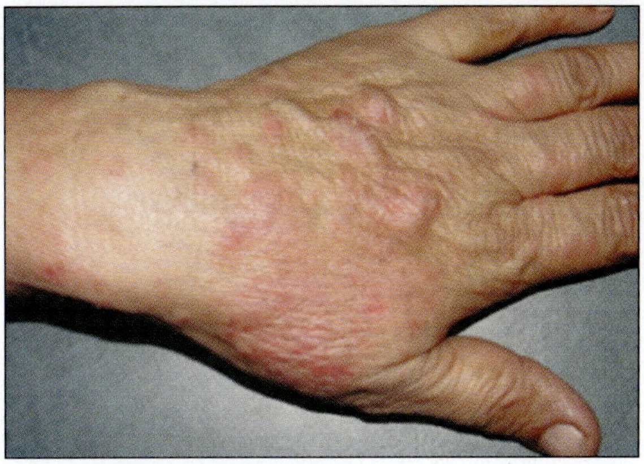

Fig. 11.14 Tinea Incognitio: hand

Tinea Manuum

- It presents on the palm(s) as a circumscribed or diffuse area of scaling, fissuring and papulo-vesicles with severe itching.
- It is usually unilateral, but occasionally it may involve both palms.

Tinea Pedis

It is a fungal infection of the soles or toes.

Clinical Features

- Commonest presentation is peeling, maceration and erythema of the clefts and occasionally the undersurface of the toes with or without itching and papulo-vesiculation (Tinea interdigitale).
- Common in persons who wear shoes and nylon socks in summer.
- Infection of the soles manifests as a circumscribed area of scales, fissures, papulo-vesicles or even pustules associated with severe itching and some hyper pigmentation.
- Occasionally, both the soles may develop recurrent eruptions of severely itchy vesicular lesions.

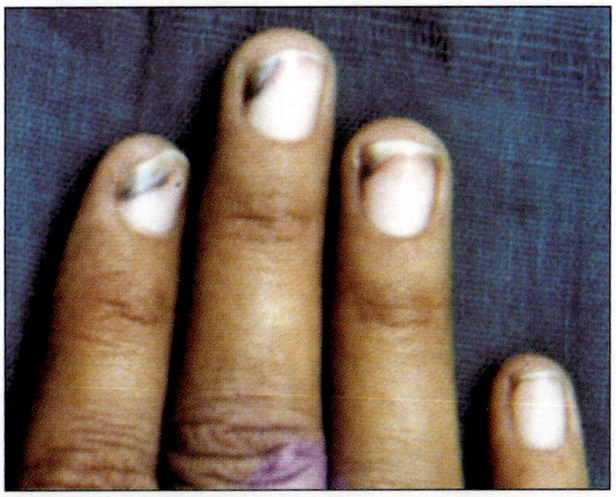

Fig. 11.15 Tinea unguium

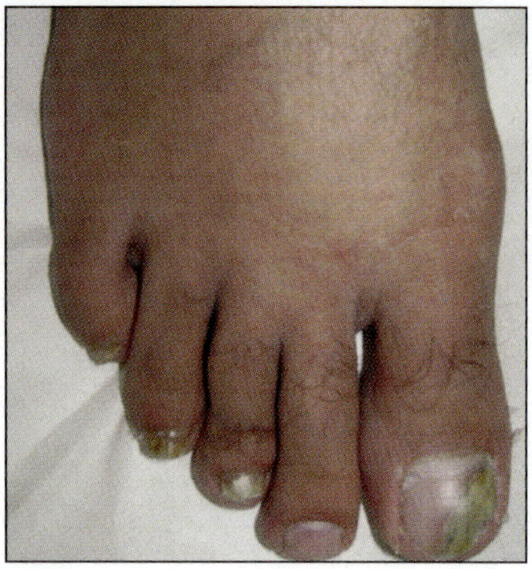

Fig. 11.16 Tinea unguium

Tinea Unguium

This is an infection of nail(s) (Fig. 11.15–11.17).

Clinical features

- Usually starts with infection of a single nail, other nails may also get infected in the due course.
- It primarily involves the nail bed.
- Starts from the distal portion and progresses proximally.
- The nail may become dark brown or black.
- Deposition of powdery material under the nail plate lifts it up.
- When the nail plate is primarily involved, it becomes brittle and disintegrates from the distal portion and looks as if it has been eaten away (Fig. 11.17).
- The remaining part of the nail plate may become thickened, dull and discoloured.

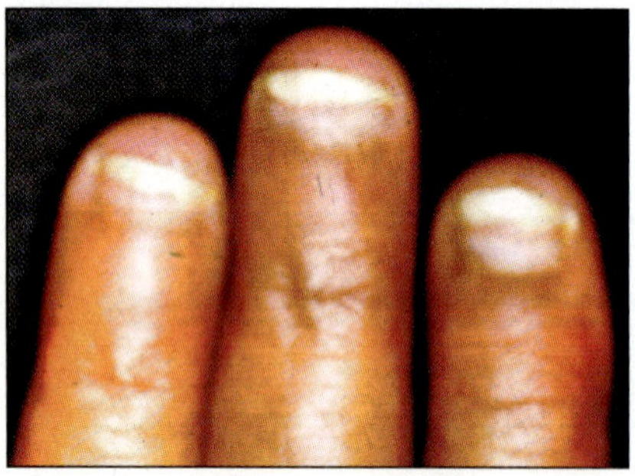

Fig. 11.17 Tinea unguium: half-eaten-away nails

Diagnosis

- Diagnosis of dermatophytoses is confirmed by seeing the fungal hyphae or the spores under 10 X magnification of microscope in the scrapings from the skin, nails or hair in a 10% KOH solution. Tinea cruris and corporis show branching hyphae while the capitis will show spores within or around the hair.
- Culture on Sabouraud's dextrose agar produces growth of fungal colonies within 2–4 weeks.
- Wood's lamp examination will show fluorescence of different colours. Tinea capitis will emit green fluorescence on exposure to Wood's lamp in contrast to the yellow fluorescence of pityriasis versicolor and coral pink of erythrasma. Wood's lamp enhances the epidermal pigmentation.

Treatment

- Clean the area with soap and water regularly.
- For tinea cruris or tinea pedis, avoid using terylene or nylone clothes at least during summer season; wear cotton clothes.

Topical Antifungal Drugs

Used for infection of glabrous skin, i.e., for tinea corporis, tinea cruris, tinea faciei and tinea interdigitale for 2–3 weeks, or till all the evidence of infection has disappeared (Table 11.2).

Table 11.2 Topical antifungal drugs

Imidazoles	• Miconazole 2%. • Clotrimazole 1%. • Econazole 1%. • Ketoconazole 2%.
Allylamines	• Ciclopirox olamine 1%. • Terbinafine 1%. • Amorolfine 5%. • Nail Lacquer (morpholines). • Butenafine 1%.

Oral antifungal drugs

Patients having tinea capitis, tinea manuum, tinea pedis, tinea unguium, widespread skin lesions or lesions not responding to topical therapy should be treated with one of the oral anti-fungal drugs (Table 11.3).

Table 11.3 Oral antifungal drugs

Griseofulvin: 250 mg, twice daily after meal. Ketoconazole: 200 mg, daily. Fluconazole: 150–200 mg, daily. Itraconazole: 100 mg, daily. Terbinafine: 250 mg, daily.
Duration of treatment 1 month for tinea capitis. 6–12 months for tinea unguium. The treatment should be given till the lesions clear completely

Griseofulvin is absorbed easily from the gastrointestinal tract, especially if taken after a fatty meal which is supposed to facilitate its absorption.

Side Effects of Antifungals

- Transient headache.

Table 11.4 Differences between pityriasis versicolor, leprosy and vitiligo

Pityriasis Versicolor	Leprosy	Vitiligo
Always macular.	Hypopigmented lesions, may be atrophic.	Well defined, depigmented or hypopigmented lesions.
Branny perifollicular scales.	Scaling seen in subsiding reaction.	No scaling seen.
Clears with treatment.	Subsides on treatment.	Perifollicular repigmentation seen on treatment.
There is no loss of sensations.	Loss of sensations seen.	Loss of sensations is not seen.
No loss of hair.	Hair may be lost.	Leucotrichia may be present.

- Photosensitivity.
- Contact dermatitis may be caused by topical preparations.

Pityriasis Versicolor

Etiology

Caused by *Malassezia furfur*. It is believed to be the hyphal phase of *Pityrosporum orbiculare*, which is normally present on the skin.

Clinical Features

- Usually slightly scaly, hypopigmented macules (Fig. 11.18–11.19) are seen. Sometimes one can see erythematous lesions (Fig. 11.20)
- Earliest lesions are usually located around the hair follicles. But they soon coalesce to form large areas.

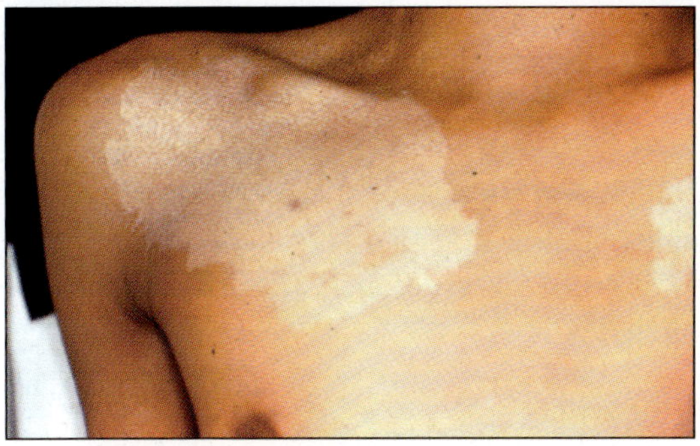

Fig. 11.18 Pityriasis versicolor

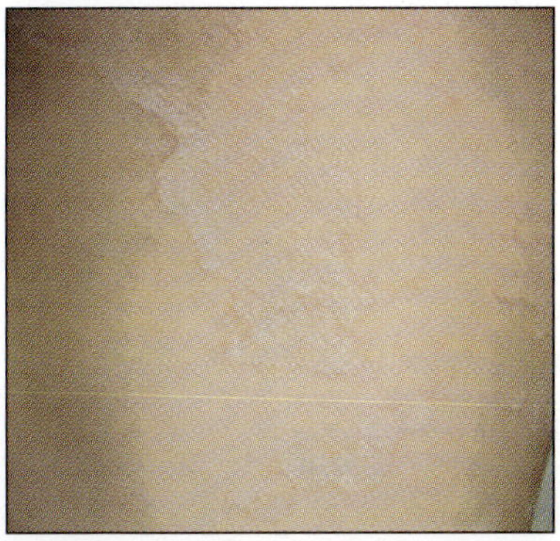

Fig. 11.19 Pityriasis versicolor

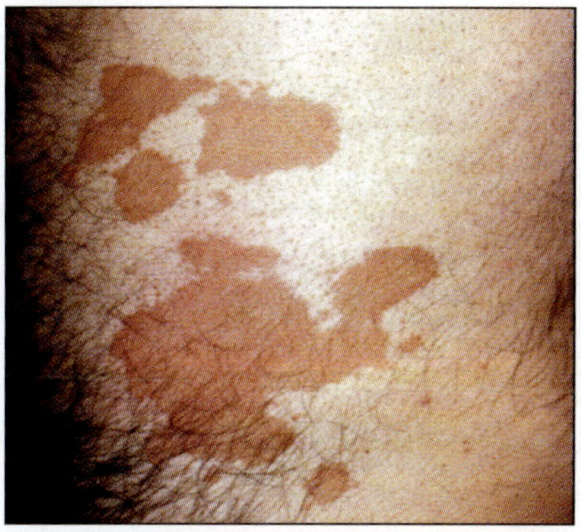

Fig. 11.20 Pityriasis versicolor: erythematous lesions

Sites

- Mainly seen on upper trunk, shoulder, upper arms and neck.
- Sometimes present on lower trunk also.
- Earliest lesions are usually located around the hair follicles, but they soon coalesce to form large areas.

Diagnosis

- *Malassezia furfur* can easily be demonstrated in the scrapings from the lesions in a 10% KOH solution (**spaghetti and meat ball appearance**).
- It has not been grown on artificial media.

The condition is to be differentiated from leprosy and vitiligo (Table 11.4).

Treatment

Treatment of pityriasis versicolor is presented in Table 11.5.

Table 11.5 Treatment of pityriasis versicolor

Local
Sodium thiosulfate: 25% at night, daily for 2–3 months.
Selenium sulphide: 2% shampoo applied daily at night, for 3–5 days.
Miconazole: 2%, clotrimazole 1% or ketoconazole 2%, twice daily for 3–4 weeks. Fungus usually disappears in 3–4 weeks. Hypopigmented area takes more time to return to normal.
Systemic
Ketoconazole: 200 mg or fluconazole 150 mg orally, for 3–5 days.

Candidiasis

Majority of the cases are caused by *Candida albicans.* Occasionally, other species of *Candida* may also be responsible. The fungus is present as a commensal in the following areas:

- Skin.
- Mouth.
- Gastrointestinal tract.

It becomes pathogenic in the presence of certain conditions (Table 11.6).

Table 11.6 Conditions which can precipitate candidiasis

Heat and humidity.
States of immune deficiency.
Diabetes mellitus.
Prolonged oral treatment with tetracylines.
Immuno-suppressive drugs.

The clinical manifestations and nomenclature of candidiasis depend on the site of involvement

Thrush

Infection of oral cavity with *Candida albicans.*

Clinical Features

It is seen as a sharply defined, curdy-white, pseudo-membranous deposit (Figs. 11.21 and 11.22), having diffused redness on the base. The condition is commonly seen in the following cases:

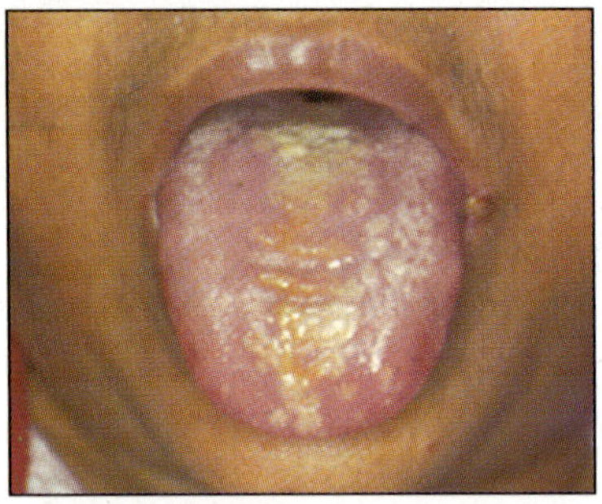

Fig. 11.21 Candidiasis: tongue

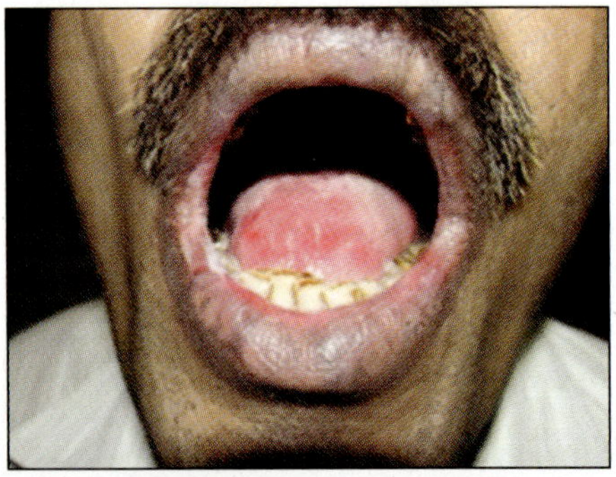

Fig. 11.22 Candidiasis: tongue

- Infants.
- Extremely debilitated individuals.
- Individuals undergoing treatment with immuno-suppressive drugs.

Intertrigo

Infections of the skin folds such as groins, under breast, interdigital space of toes or fingers.

Clinical Features

- Localised areas of erythema and maceration seen (Fig. 11.23) with itching and burning.
- Edges are ill-defined and satellite lesions are seen.

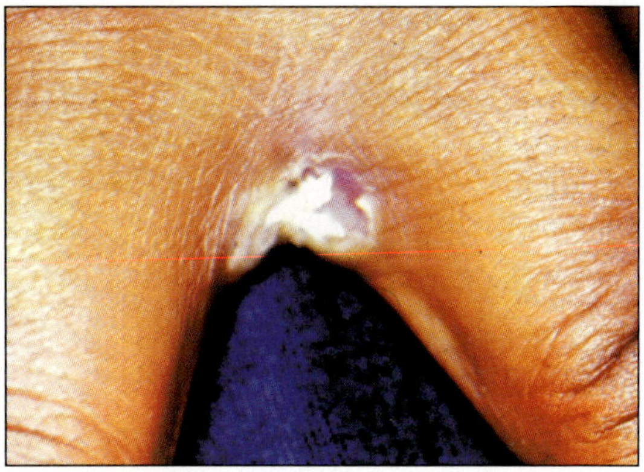

Fig. 11.23 Intertrigo

Angular Stomatitis

Infection of angle of mouth due to *Candida albicans.*

Clinical Features

- Proliferative lesions with maceration are seen at the angles of mouth (Fig. 11.24).
- It has to be differentiated from vitamin B complex deficiency.

Vulvo-vaginitis

It is the infection of vaginal cavity with *Candida albicans.*

Clinical Features

- There is itching, soreness and erythema of the vulva and the vaginal (Fig. 11.25) mucous membrane with the presence of thick creamy white discharge.
- This condition is commonly seen during the following states:
  - i) Pregnancy.
  - ii) In individuals who are on contraceptive pills.
  - iii) Individuals on systemic tetracyclines.
  - iv) Individuals on immunosuppressive drugs.

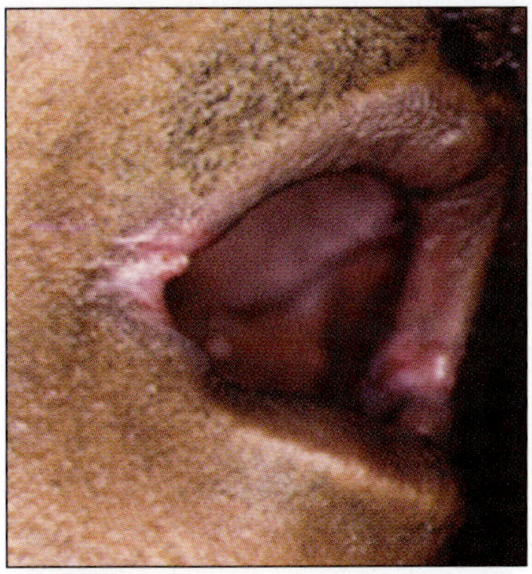

Fig. 11.24 Angular stomatitis

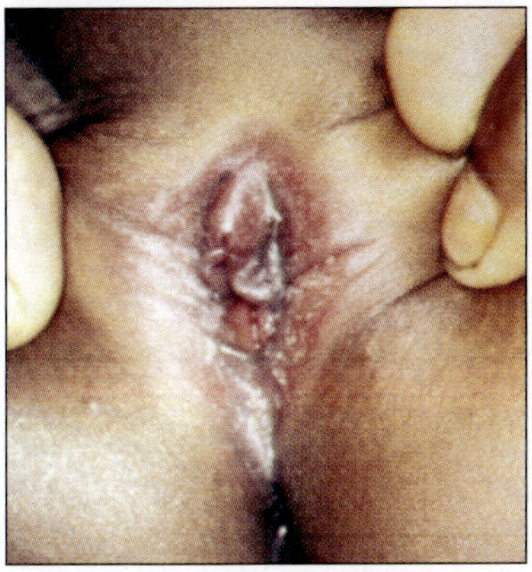

Fig. 11.25 Vulvo-vaginitis

Balanoposthitis

This is the fungal infection of the glans penis and the prepucial mucosa.

Clinical Features

- There is pain, erythema and maceration (Fig. 11.26).
- Prepucial opening may become narrow (Fig. 11.27) and develop fissures on opening.
- The infection is generally acquired during contact with an infected female.
- Diabetics are prone to develop the lesion.

Plasma Cell Balanitis of Zoon

The disease was first described by Zoon in 1952. This disease is called plasma cell balanitis in males and plasma cell vulvitis in females due to the presence of numerous plasma cells visible on skin biopsy.

Etiology

- Not known.
- It is an idiopathic benign penile lesion.
- May be a reactive response to an infection, irritation or injury.

Clinical features

- It usually presents as a persistent, well defined irritable glistening orange red plaque on the glans.
- It may be symptomless, or the patient may complain of tenderness and/or slight itching (Fig. 11.28).

Diagnosis

Skin biopsy and histopathological features confirm the diagnosis.

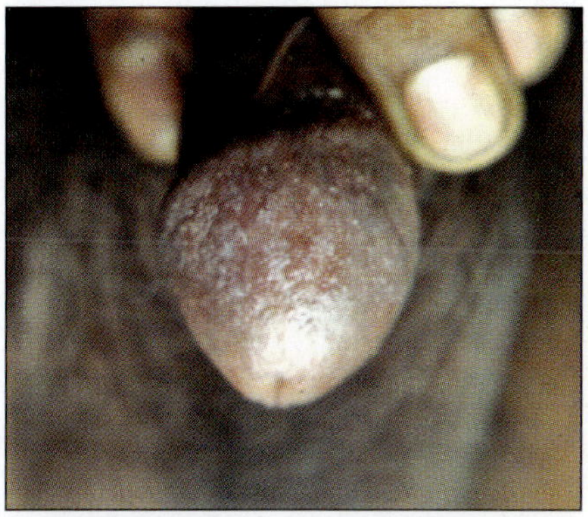

Fig. 11.26 Candidal balanitis

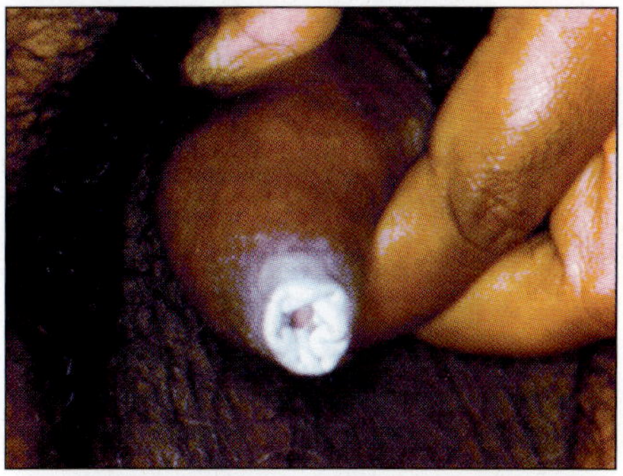

Fig. 11.27 Pinhole meatus in candidal balanoposthitis

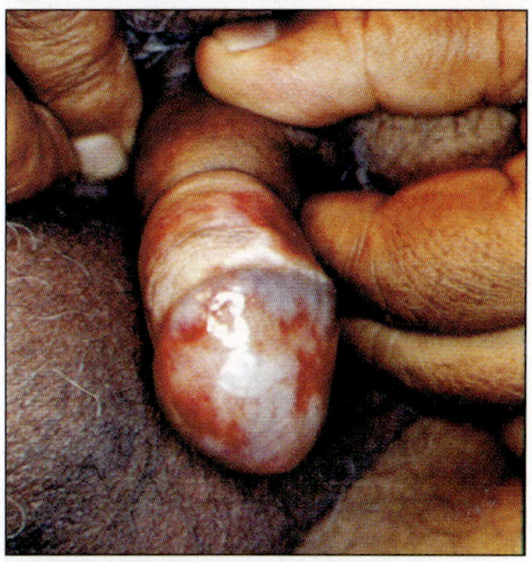

Fig. 11.28 Plasma cell balanitis of Zoon

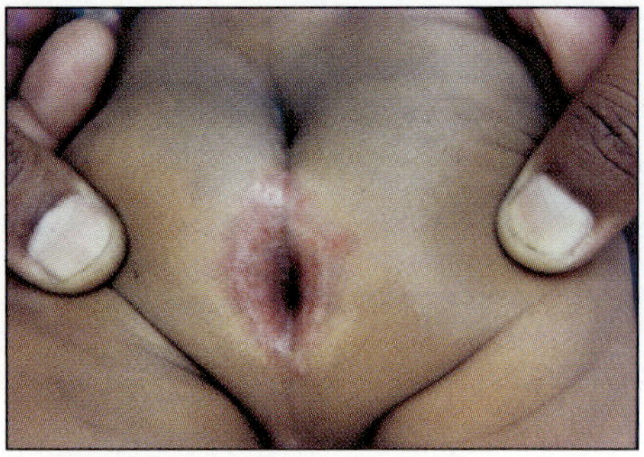

Fig. 11.29 Perianal dermatitis

Chronic paronychia

This is commonly seen in the following individuals:

- Housewives.
- Washermen.
- Bakers.
- Individuals whose profession involves excessive immersion of their hands in water and alkalies. Diabetics are prone to develop these lesions.

Clinical Features

- There is an asymptomatic erythematous swelling of the posterior nail fold (Figs. 11.30 and 11.31) of one or more fingers.

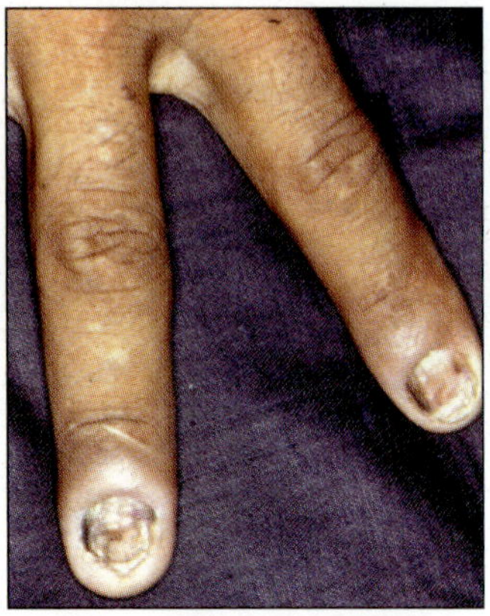

Fig. 11.30 Chronic paronychia

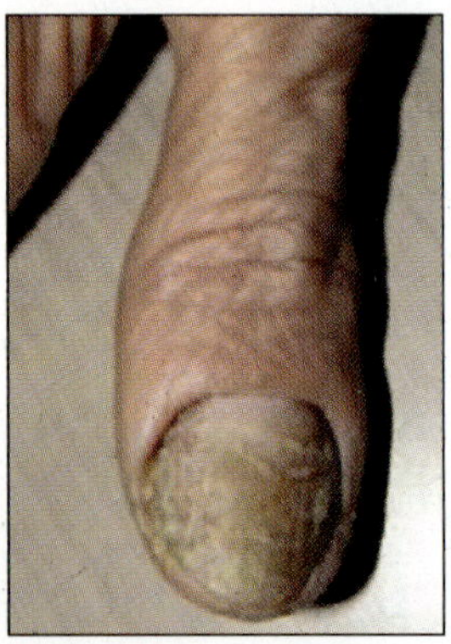

Fig. 11.31 Chronic paronychia

- Irregularities in the thickness of the nail plates occur due to the inflammation in the nail matrix.
- Sometimes a bead of pus appears from underneath the nail fold on expression.
- Occasionally, the area may be tender.

Diagnosis

By demonstrating the candidal mycelia and pseudohyphae from the scrapings or discharge in 10% KOH solution.

Treatment of candidiasis

- All the predisposing factors, local or systemic, must be controlled.
- Underlying diseases, such as diabetes mellitus, should be controlled.
- Local hygiene must be maintained.
- The affected parts should be kept dry as far as possible.
- Topical miconazole, clotrimazole, econazole, ketoconazole, gentian voilet 1% and nystatin 1% are effective against candida. Local massage with a mixture of topical antifungal, antibiotic and corticosteroids cream, twice daily, clears the plasma cell balanitis in 7–10 days.
- Oral ketoconazole 200 mg, or fluconazole 150 mg daily, is given for widespread lesions.
- Vaginal candidiasis is treated with pessaries containing nystatin, miconazole or clotrimazole, once a day for 6–7 days.
- Treatment of sexual partner is essential.
- **Chronic paronychia** responds best to local massage with a cream under the nail fold which contains a combination of nystatin or miconazole, antibacterial agent and corticosteroids. Nails should be kept dry as far as possible.

Mycetoma

Etiology

It is an infection of the subcutaneous tissue caused by fungi, which is divided into two groups:

- **Actinomycotic**—now considered to be bacteria rather than fungi.
- **Eumycotic**—the true fungi.

Clinical Features

- Painless subcutaneous nodules are present. They rupture through the overlying skin, producing multiple sinuses (Fig. 11.32) discharging granules

which may be yellow, black, white or red, depending upon the causative fungus.
- If untreated it involves and destroys the adjacent bones.

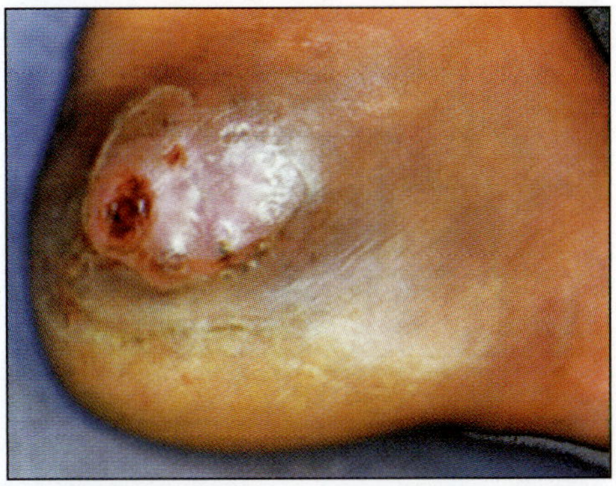

Fig. 11.32 Mycetoma: foot

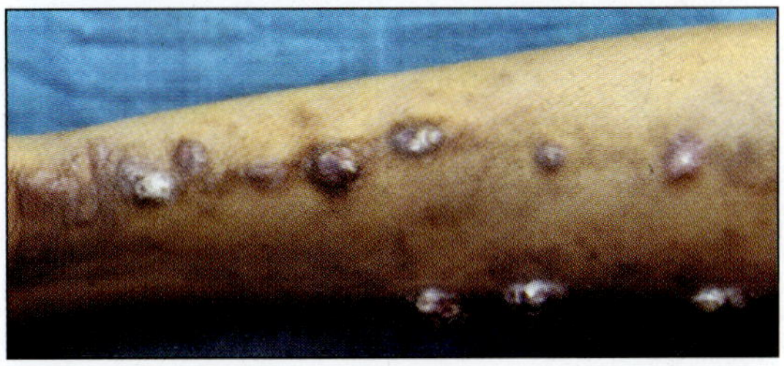

Fig. 11.33 Sporotrichosis: linear lesion

Sites

- Usually affects the foot and most of the times it follows some trauma.
- Sometimes other parts of the body may also be affected.

Diagnosis

- Microscopic examination of the granules to establish the fungal diagnosis.
- Culture of the organism.
- Histopathology of the involved skin showing a chronic inflammatory reaction.

Treatment

Actinomycotic mycetomas respond to the following:
- Sulphonamides.
- Tetracyclines.
- Antifungal agents, like ketoconazole and fluconazole.

Eumycetomas usually do not respond to medicines. Some cases improve with ketoconazole/fluconazole. Surgical debridement is attempted for symptomatic relief. In extreme cases, amputation of the area is to be done.

Sporotrichosis

This is a chronic subcutaneous fungal infection of the lymphatics caused by *Sporothrix schenckii*. Causative fungus is usually introduced into the skin by trauma.

Clinical Features

- The lesions are usually seen on exposed parts.
- It presents as nodules or pustules, in linear fashion which appear at an interval of a few days, along the lymphatics (Fig. 11.33).
- Regional lymph nodes may get involved and break-down.

Diagnosis

- Clinical presentation.
- The fungus can be cultured on common agar media.

Treatment

- Potassium iodide (saturated solution): 5 drops initially, increasing to 50 drops, thrice a day is the drug of choice
- The other drugs used are itraconazole, 100–200 mg daily; ketoconazole and amphotericin-B intravenously.

Chapter 12

Viral Infections

Viruses are electron-microscopic organisms and require a living host for their propagation. Most of the viruses automatically induce immunity in the individual. Several viral infections are self-limiting and also produce a lifelong immunity. Second attacks are rare, barring a few exceptions. Common skin diseases attributed to viral infections are presented in Table 12.1.

Table 12.1 Common viral infections

- Verrucae or warts.
- Molluscum contagiosum.
- Chickenpox.
- Herpes zoster.
- Herpes simplex.

Verrucae

Synonym

Warts.

Etiology

Warts occur when the skin is infected by warts virus or **human papilloma virus** (HPV). HPV are a type of DNA viruses.

Transmission

- It has a very low infectivity. Casual contact with an infected individual is unlikely to result in the disease.
- Infection is transmitted by direct or close contact with infected individuals.
- Virus enters into the skin through minor and microscopic injuries.

Age

Both the adults and children may get afflicted.

Clinical Features

- The lesions are asymptomatic, have irregular verrucous surface and keep on growing slowly.
- The number of warts varies from one or two to several hundred.

Table 12.2 presents different varieties of warts, based on their clinical features.

A large numbers of warts are seen in the following conditions:

- Individuals with depressed cell-mediated immunity.
- Individuals undergoing treatment with immunosuppressive drugs.
- Hodgkin's disease.
- Malignant lymphomas.
- Lymphocytic leukaemia.

Table 12.2 Varieties of warts, based on their clinical features

Common warts or verruca vulgaris.
Plane warts or verruca plana.
Filiform warts.
Plantar warts.
Genital warts or condyloma acuminata.

Common Warts or Verruca Vulgaris

This is the most commonly seen form of warts.

Clinical Features

- Seen as firm, skin-coloured papules of various sizes with verrucous surface (Fig. 12.1)
- The surface is stippled with black dots (the thrombosed capillaries).

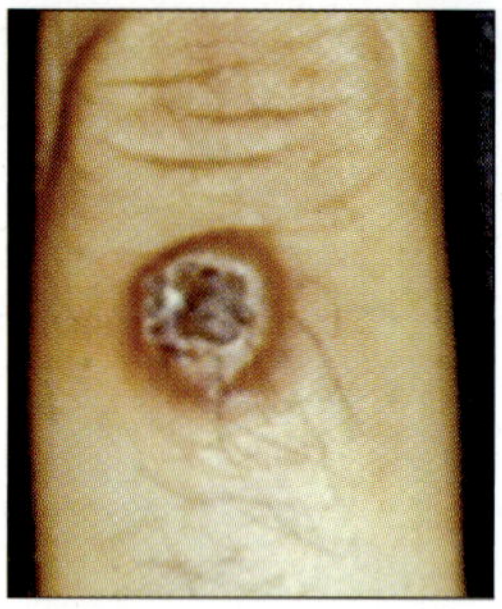

Fig. 12.1 Common wart

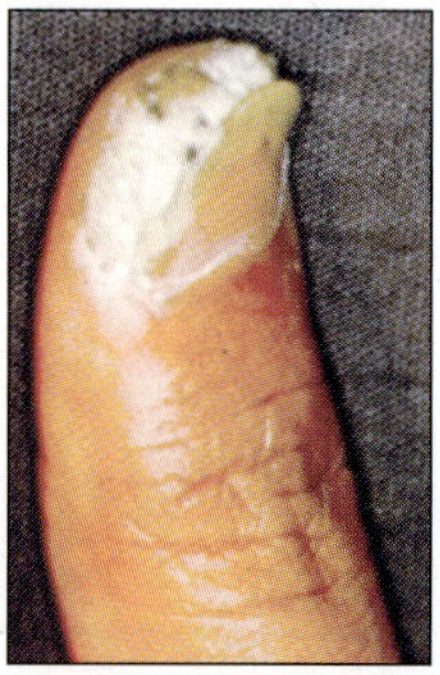

Fig. 12.2 Periungual common wart

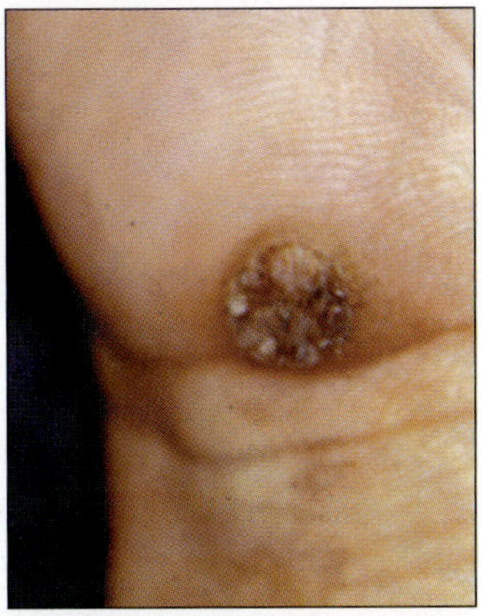

Fig. 12.3 Common wart: wrist

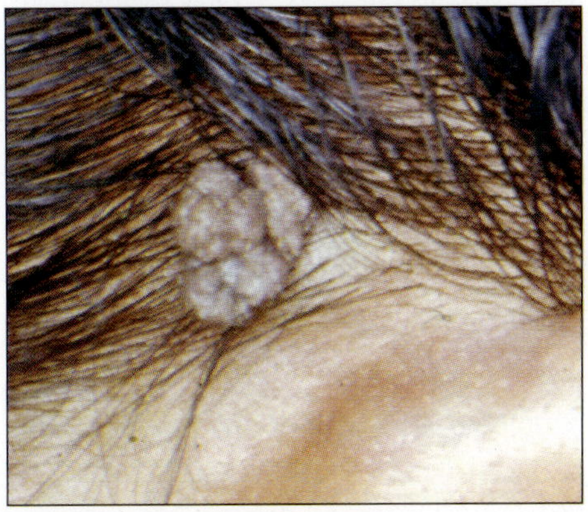

Fig. 12.4 Common wart: scalp

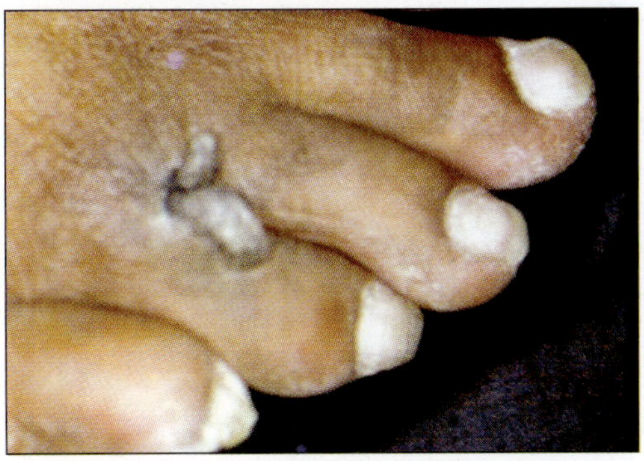

Fig. 12.5 Common wart: horny projection

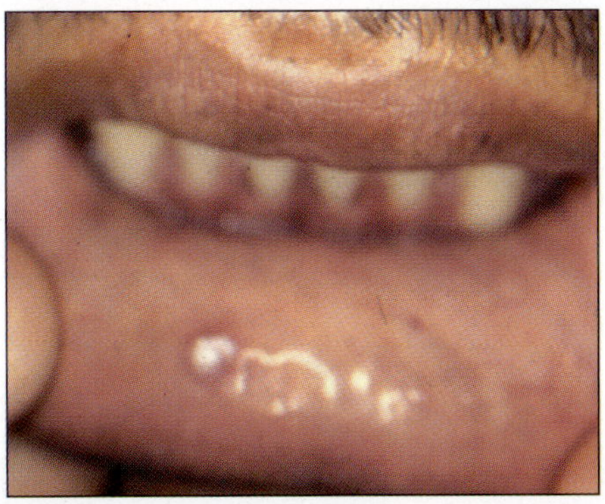

Fig. 12.6 Common wart: mucosa of lip

Sites

Most commonly present on the dorsum of the hands and fingers, though it can occur on any part of the body (Figs 12.2–12.8).

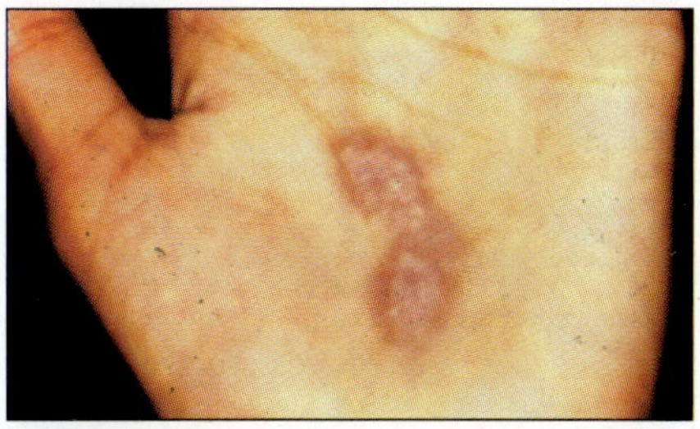

Fig. 12.7 Warts on palm

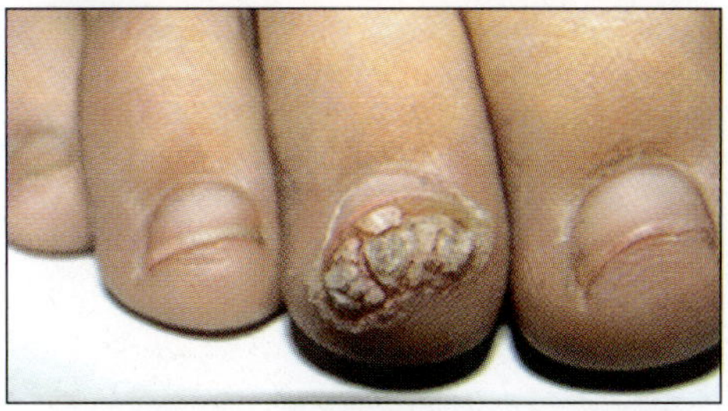

Fig. 12.8 Wart: toe

Plane Warts or Verruca Plana

Clinical Features

Seen as skin-coloured, slightly raised, flat-topped papules (Figs 12.9–12.12).

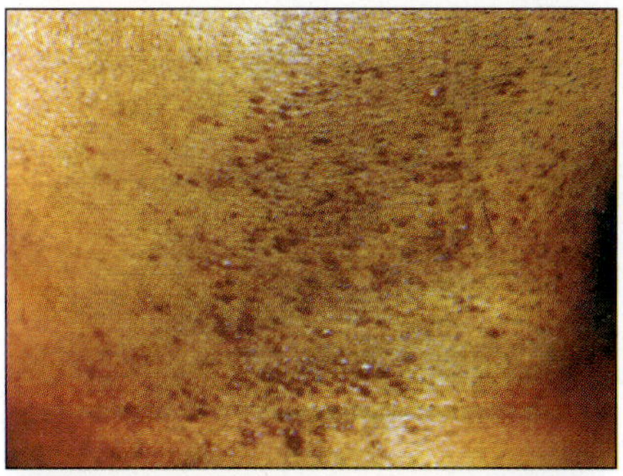

Fig. 12.9 Plane warts: neck

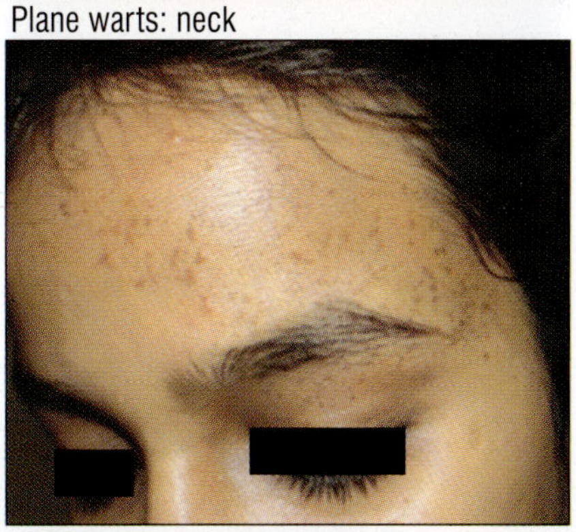

Fig. 12.10 Plane wart forhead

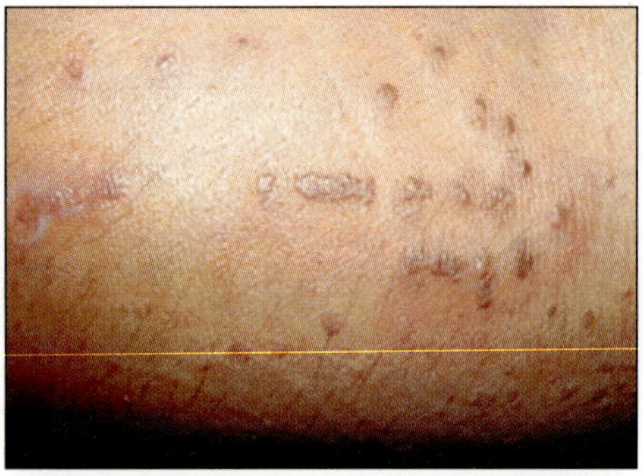

Fig. 12.11 Plane warts

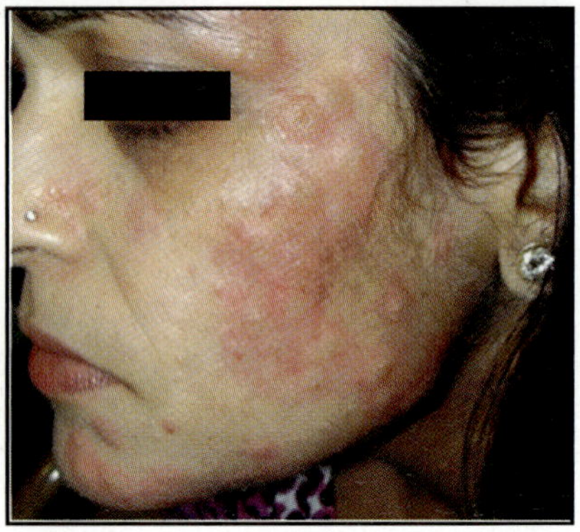

Fig. 12.12 Plane wart after cryotherapy

Sites

Usually present on the dorsum of hands and face of children.

Filiform Warts

Clinical Features

These warts are seen as finger-like projections with irregular surfaces (Figs 12.13–12.15).

Sites

Warts are seen on the neck, face and scalp.

They need to be differentiated from skin tags or achrocordon (Table 12.3).

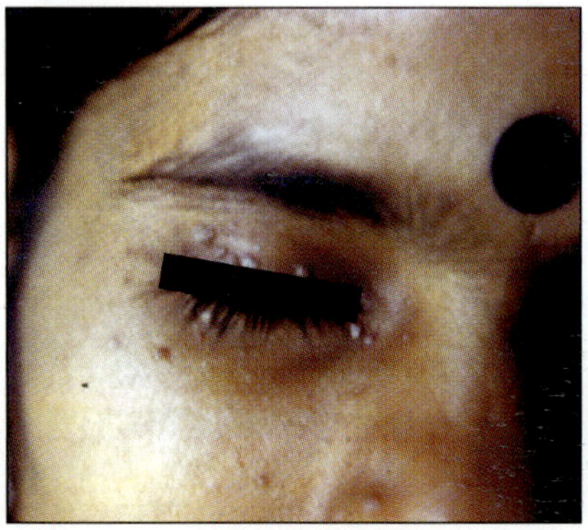

Fig. 12.13 Filliform warts: around eye-lid

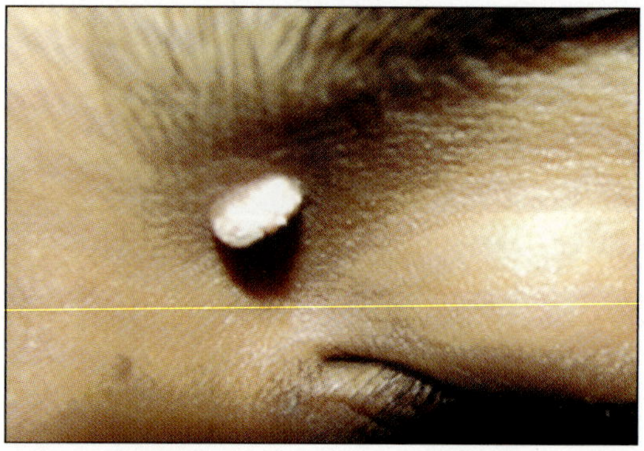

Fig. 12.14 Wart eye

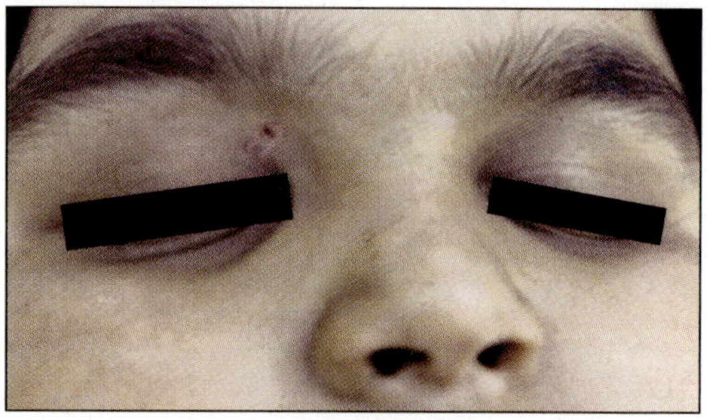

Fig. 12.15 Warts eyelid: after cauterisation

Table 12.3 Difference between filiform warts and achrocordon

Filiform warts	Achrocordon
Finger-like projection.	Projection with a narrow base. Smooth surface.
Irregular surface. Seen on neck, face and scalp.	Commonly seen on neck, axillae and groins.

Plantar Warts

Clinical Features

Warts are seen on the sole as skin-coloured, well-defined area(s) with irregular surface (Figs 12.16 and 12.17).

A wart is separated from the surrounding skin of the sole by a well-defined margin.

The lesions are occasionally painful.

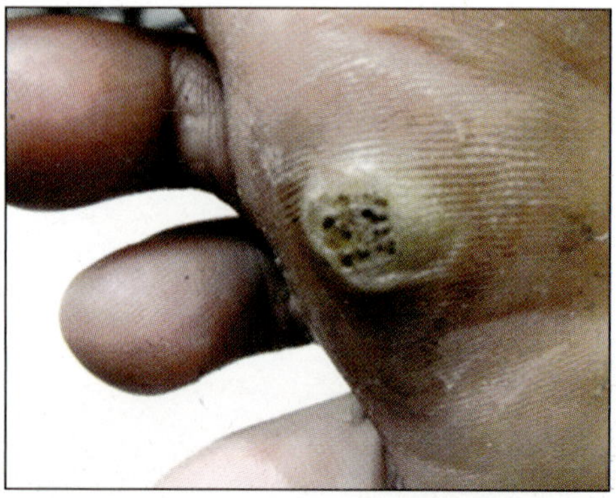

Fig. 12.16 Plantar wart: sole

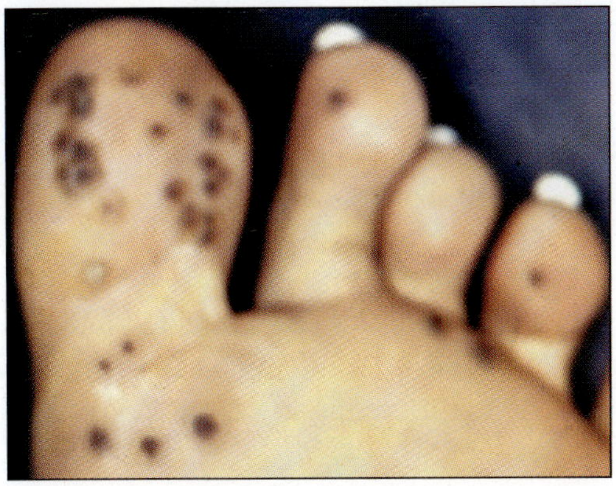

Fig. 12.17 Plantar warts: after cryo treatment

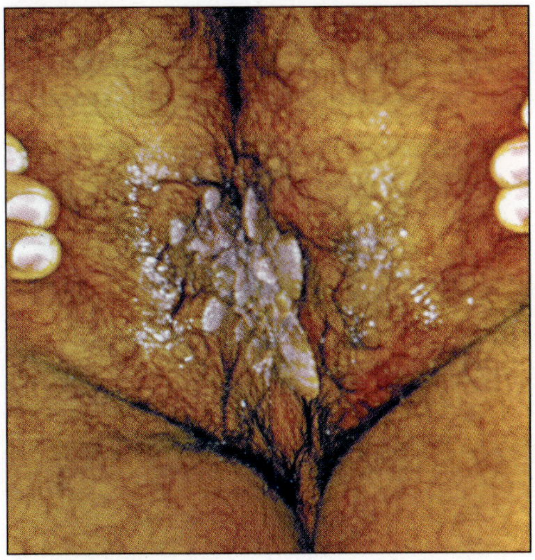

Fig. 12.18 Perianal warts

Sites

- They are present on any part of the sole.
- They need to be differentiated from a callosity or corn (Table 12.4).

Table 12.4 Differences between plantar warts and corns

Corns	Plantar Warts
Occur at the points of pressure.	Occur anywhere on the sole.
The surface is smooth and continuous with the surrounding skin of the sole.	Seen as skin-coloured, well defined area with irregular surface, separated from the surrounding skin.
Paring the lesion reveals keratinous core.	Paring reveals a loss of blood vessels.

Genital Warts or Condyloma Acuminata

Etiology

The virus causing genital warts is antigenically different from the virus causing warts on the other parts of the body.

Transmission

Usually transmitted through sexual exposure.

Clinical Features

- Fungating masses of verrucous tissue are seen on glans penis, corona, mucosal surface of prepuce, and occasionally, in the urinary meatus in males (Fig. 12.19).
- In females, the lesions are seen on the vulva and vaginal openings (Figs 12.20–12.23), whereas in patients practicing anal sex, they are seen in and around the anus (Fig. 12.18).
- Due to the moisture in the genital area, it tends to grow faster than the other varieties of warts, more so during pregnancy.

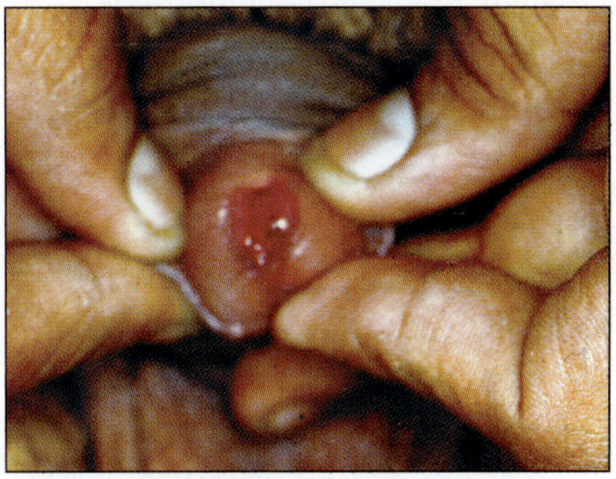

Fig. 12.19 Intra-meatal warts

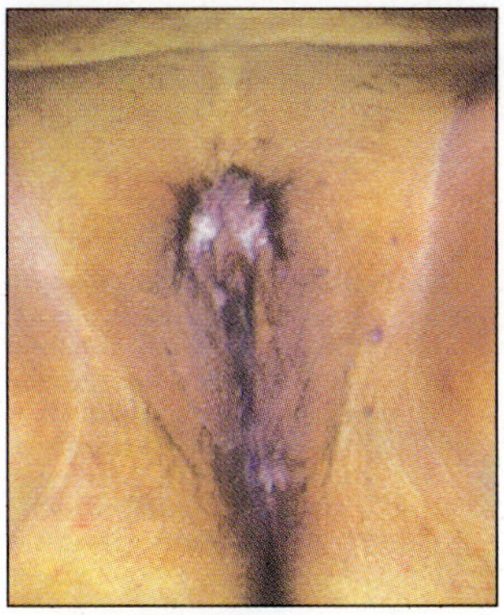

Fig. 12.20 Genital warts: female

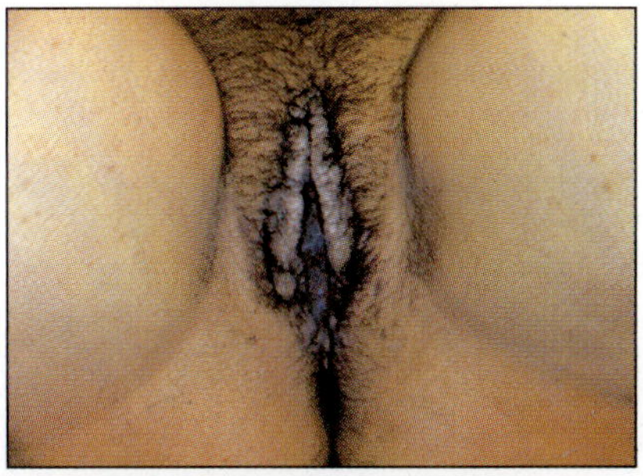

Fig. 12.21 Warts on vagina: before treatment

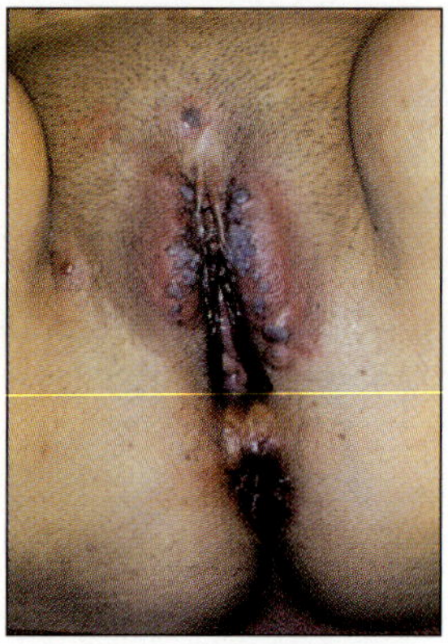

Fig. 12.22 Warts on vagina: immediately after cryotherapy

- They need to be differentiated from the condyloma lata of secondary syphilis which present as smooth moist papules at anal area along with other signs of secondary syphilis.

Treatment

Destruction of the entire infected area with:

- Chemicals such as trichloroacetic acid or phenol.
- Electric cautery.
- Cryotherapy.
- Lasers.

It is important to destroy the lesions, as much as possible, to avoid the recurrence. Treatment involves the following:

- Any recurrence of the lesions should be treated at the earliest to prevent the further spread of the infection.
- Venereal warts can also be treated with weekly application of 25% podophyllin in tincture benzoin.
- In multiple or generalised warts—levamisol, 150 mg daily on two consecutive days per week for 6–8 weeks—can be given to raise the cell mediated immunity which leads to disappearance of warts.
- Sometimes the warts disappear spontaneously, i.e., without any treatment.

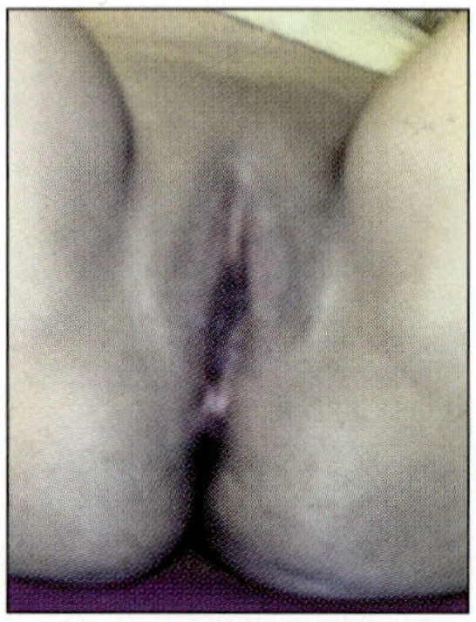

Fig. 12.23 Warts on vagina: after complete clearance

Molluscum Contagiosum

Etiology

It is caused by a large virus belonging to the pox group of viruses.

Transmission

- Occurs from contact with an infected individual.
- Auto-inoculation after infection causes the spread of the disease to different parts of the body.

Sex

- Common in children of either sex.
- When it is present on the genitals of an adult male or female, transmission is usually through sexual exposure.

Clinical Features

- Seen as asymptomatic, pearly white or pink papules with well-defined depressed centres (Fig. 12.24) known as umbilication (Figs 12.25 and 12.26).
- After trauma, or spontaneously after a few months, inflammatory changes result in suppuration and crusting leading to the destruction and disappearance of lesions.

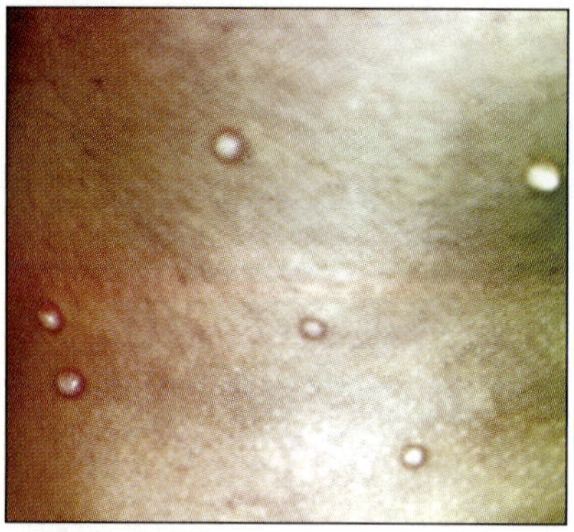

Fig. 12.24 Molluscum contasiosum

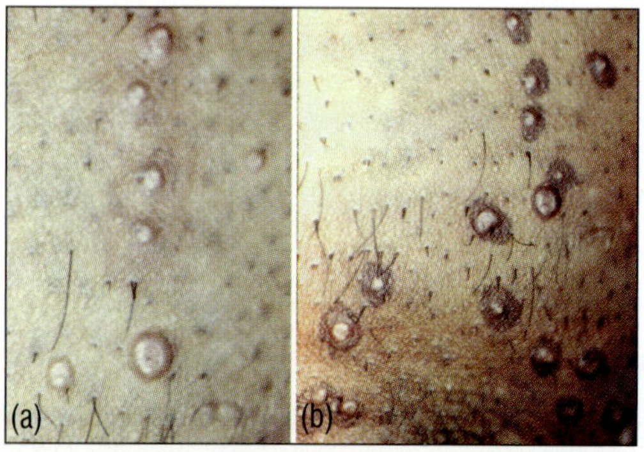

Fig. 12.25 Molluscum contagiosum: (a) before cryotherapy; (b) after cryotherapy

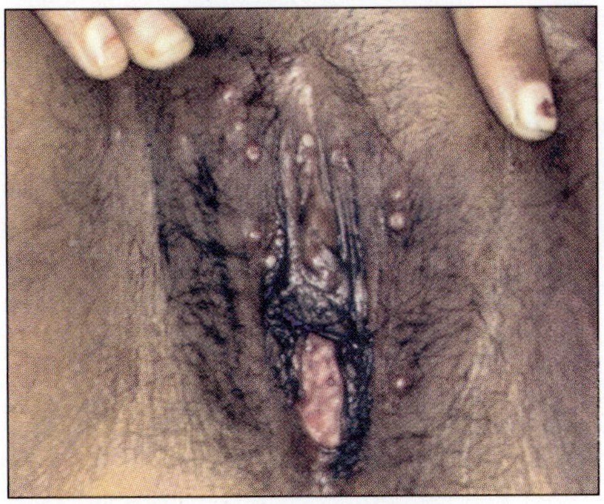

Fig. 12.26 Molluscum contagiosum: vagina

Treatment

- Lesion disappears even without any treatment in a couple of months. Persistent lesions may require treatment.
- Destruction of infected area can be carried out by the following methods:
  i) Chemicals like trichloroacetic acid or phenol.
  ii) Cryotherapy.

Measles

The disease is caused by the virus called rubeola. Skin lesions appear 7–14 days after the person is infected. It begins with high fever, cough, running nose and red, watery eyes. Within 2–3 days, white Koplik spots may appear inside the oral cavity; 3–5 day after this, a skin rash may erupt starting, as flat red spots appearing on face, hairline, neck and spreading to trunk, arms, legs and feet. It may contain watery fluid. Within a few days, the rash subsides leaving behind the crusts.

Chickenpox

Synonym

Varicella.

Etiology

Caused by *Varicella zoster* (V–Z) virus.

Transmission

- Acquired through droplet infection from the nasopharynx of the infected individual.
- Vesicle fluid contains a large number of viruses.
- Scabs are non-infectious.

Incubation period

9–23 days.

Clinical Features

- Scarlatiniform or morbiliform erythema is seen (Fig. 12.27) after 1–2 days of fever and malaise.
- Subsequently papules and tense vesicles evolve.
- They turn into pustules surrounded by red areolas.
- Within 2–4 days, dry crusts form that fall off in another 4–5 days.
- Healing occurs without or with minimal scar formation.
- Itching occurs in a few patients.
- Varicella infection confers long-lasting immunity.

Site

Centripetal distribution of lesions is seen, i.e., the lesions are more on the trunk than face, scalp and limbs

Treatment

- The patient should be kept isolated, especially from children.
- Regular bath with soap and water.
- Local application of calamine lotion as soothing agent.
- Oral antihistamines for itching.
- Systemic antibiotics for ruptured vesicles or secondary infection.
- Acyclovir—800 mg, 5 times daily for severe or in high risk patients for 5–7 days. Alternatively, famciclovir—250 mg, 3 times daily can be given for 7–10 days.

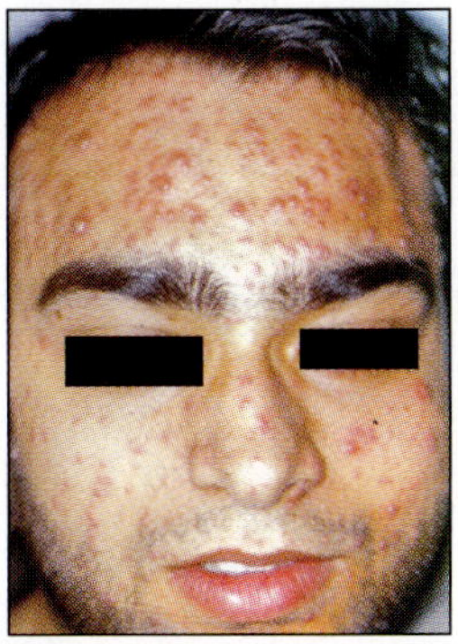

Fig. 12.27 Chickenpox: face

Herpes Zoster

Etiology

- Caused by *Varicella zoster* virus.
- After an attack of chicken pox, the virus is believed to get lodged in the posterior root ganglion(s), where it remains dormant.

- Attack occurs due to reactivation of these viruses in the posterior root ganglions.

Precipitating Factors

The precipitating factors that cause reactivation of the virus are:

- Hodgkin's disease.
- Leukemia.
- Systemic corticosteroids.
- Immunosuppressive drugs.

Clinical Features

- It starts with a severe pain that is localised to a nerve segment.
- The pain is followed by the appearance of grouped tense vesicles situated on an erythematous base (Figs. 12.28–12.30).
- Eruptions are limited to a single neural segment on one side of the body, i.e., unilateral (Fig. 12.31).

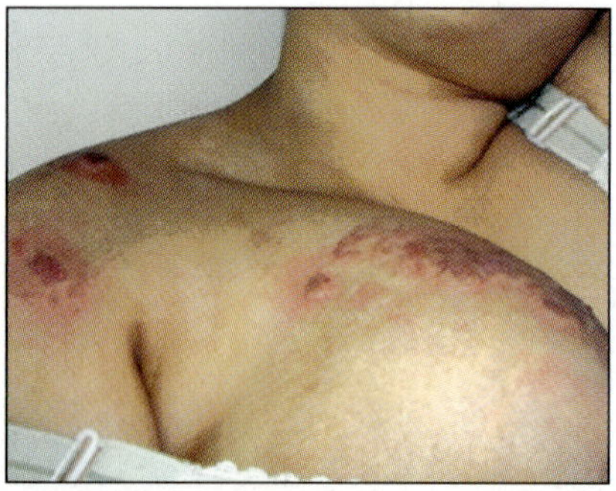

Fig. 12.28 Herpes zoster: early lesions and erythema

- Occasionally, in conditions like Hodgkin's disease and leukaemia, treatment with corticosteroids, immunosuppressive drugs or sometimes even in normal patients, the vesicles may be found in other parts of the body called **disseminated herpes zoster**.
- The vesicles become pustular and form a crust.
- Crusts fall-off and the lesions heal in 7–10 days with minimal or no scarring.

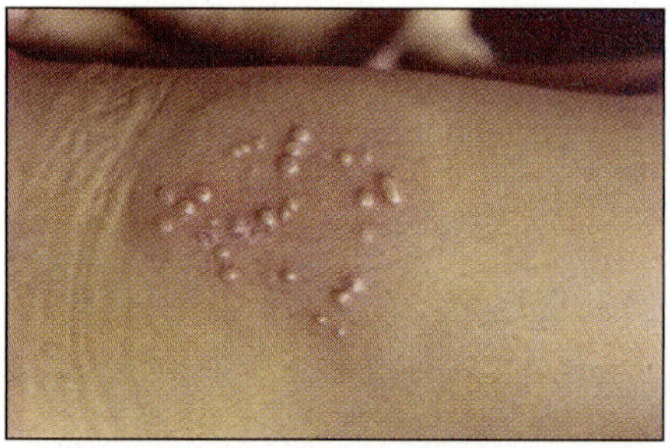

Fig. 12.29 Herpes zoster: grouped vesicles

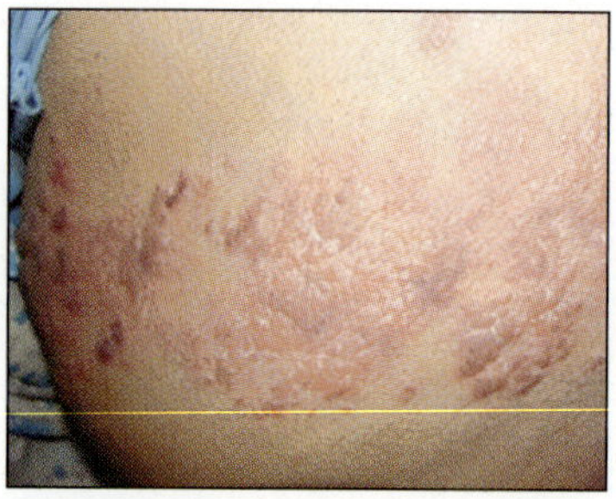

Fig. 12.30 Herpes zoster: vesicles

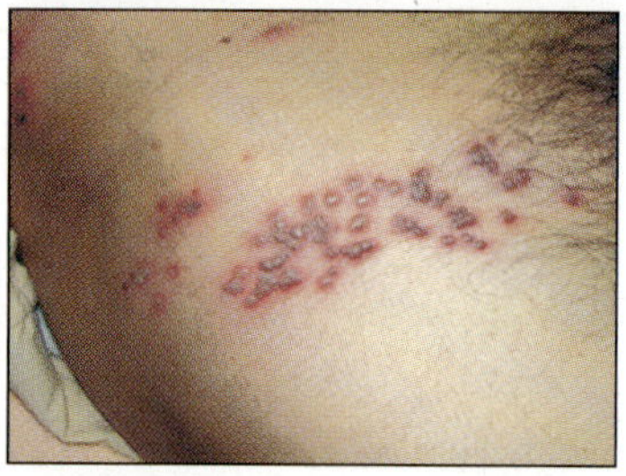

Fig. 12.31 Herpes zoster: black crust with scar

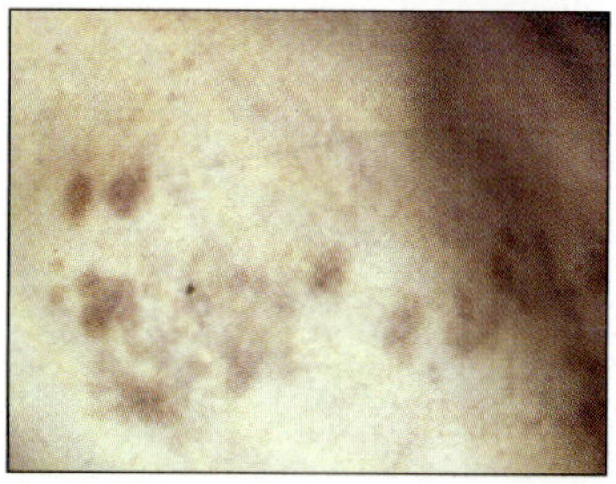

Fig. 12.32 Herpes zoster: pigmentation after healing

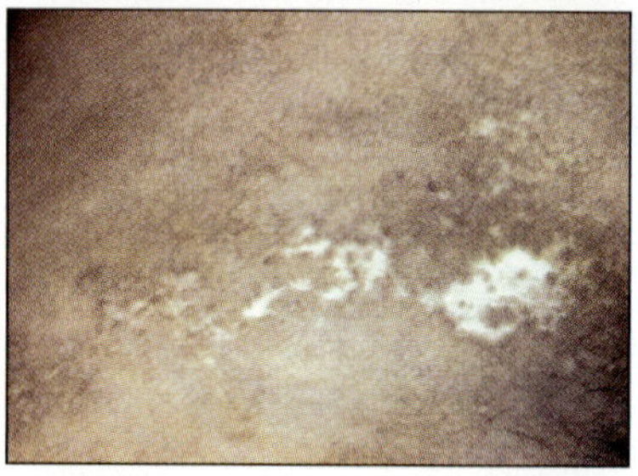

Fig. 12.33 Herpes zoster: leucoderma after healing

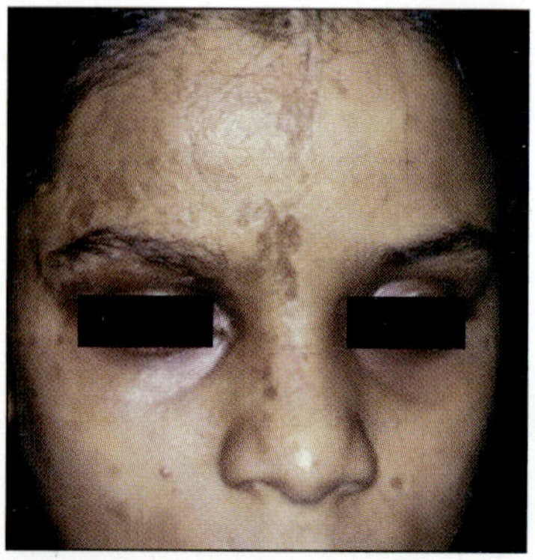

Fig. 12.34 Herpes zoster: post scar

Complications

Infection, scarring and (rarely) keloid formation occurs.

Post-herpetic neuralgia: Old people are prone to develop severe neuralgic pain at the site of eruptions, even after the lesions have healed. The pain can persist for several months.

Treatment

Vesicles dry up spontaneously in 7–10 days, leading to life-long immunity.

The treatment is aimed towards the following:

- Relieving pain.
- Reducing erythema.
- Preventing post-herpetic neuralgia.
- Proper cleaning of the area.
- Local application of calamine lotion as soothing agents.
- Systemic analgesic, anti-inflammatory agents to relieve the pain.
- Topical or systemic antibiotics, if lesions get ulcerated or secondarily infected. One of the following may be administered:
  - i) Oral acyclovir: 800 mg, five times daily, for disseminated herpes zoster for 7–10 days.
  - ii) Famciclovir: 250 mg, thrice daily, for 7–10 days.
  - iii) Valacyclovir: 1 gm, thrice daily, for 7–10 days.

Herpes Simplex

Etiology

Caused by a virus called *Herpes hominis*.

Antigenically two different types of *Herpes hominis* are found.

Type I or HSV1 which causes *Herpes labialis* and other non-genital infections.

Type II or HSV2 which causes genital herpes.

Transmission

- Through droplet infection and direct contact.
- Genital herpes is transmitted through sexual contact.
- Two types of the disease are seen:
  - i) Primary herpes simplex.
  - ii) Recurrent herpes simplex.
- After primary infection, the virus probably persists throughout life in sensory ganglion.

Primary Herpes Simplex

This disease occurs when the patient has been exposed to the virus for the first time.

Clinical Features

- Various clinical manifestations are as follows:
  - i) Acute gingivo-stomatitis.
  - ii) Balano-posthitis.
  - iii) Vulvo-vaginitis.
  - iv) Cervicitis.
  - v) Kerato-conjunctivitis.
- **The condition is generally misdiagnosed and missed.**
- Usually, an acute condition is associated with:
  - i) Malaise.
  - ii) Restlessness.
  - iii) Fever.
  - iv) Enlargement of regional lymph nodes.
- Grouped, slightly bigger vesicles at the site of infection which rapidly form ulcers covered with a white or yellow pseudomembrane (Fig. 12.41).

Recurrent Herpes Simplex

Clinical Features

- After the initial infection, the patient continues to get multiple grouped small vesicles and ulcerations (Figs 12.35–12.36).

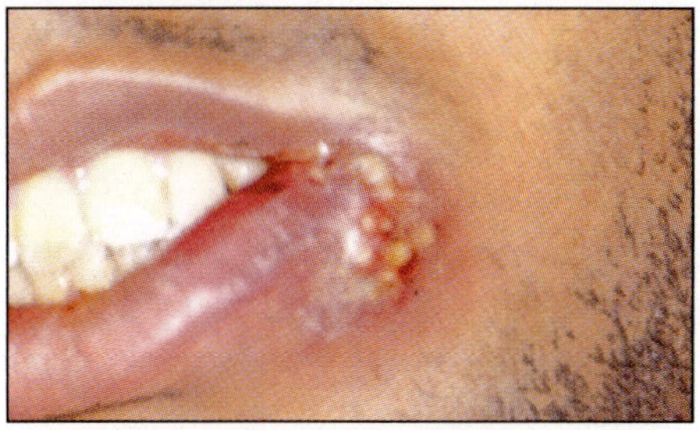

Fig. 12.35 Herpes simplex: angle of mouth

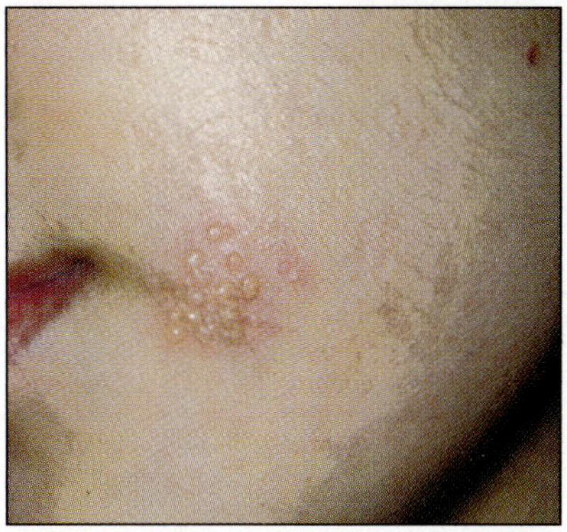

Fig. 12.36 Herpes simplex: vesicles

- The lesions may or may not be associated with a burning sensation.
- No erythema is seen at the base.
- No constitutional symptoms are present.

- The lesions are situated on, or around the mucocutaneous junctions (Figs 12.37–12.40). The affected areas are:
  - i) Mouth.
  - ii) Nose.
  - iii) Genitals.
- Hands, thighs and forehead are also affected, though their involvement is seen very rarely.
- Herpes simplex needs to be differentiated from herpes zoster infection (Table 12.5).

Table 12.5 Difference between herpes zoster and herpes simplex

Herpes zoster	Herpes simplex
Pain before eruption.	Burning and stinging prior to eruption.
Grouped vesicular lesions on an erythematous edematous base.	Grouped vesicular lesions on very mildly erythema-tous base.
Dermatomal distribution.	Does not correspond to dermatomes.
Single episode.	Recurrent lesions at same site.

Diagnosis

Tzanck smear shows multinucleated giant cells and fluorescent antibody stained smear will show apple green fluorescence

Treatment

- Ulcers heal spontaneously within a week's time.
- For genital herpes, counselling and education about sexual abstinence (till the lesions heal), use of barrier methods and presumptive treatment of partners is an important component of treatment.
- Secondary infection is treated with topical or systemic antibiotics.
- Severe or disseminated lesions are treated by acyclovir —400 mg, given orally, five times daily for 5–7 days.

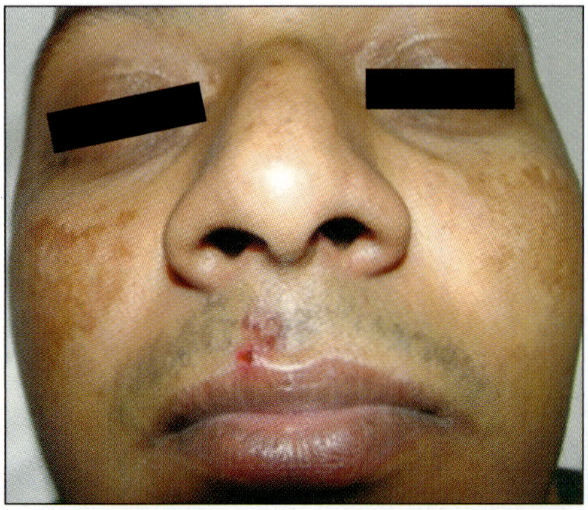

Fig. 12.37 Herpes simplex ulcer: upper lip with chloasma

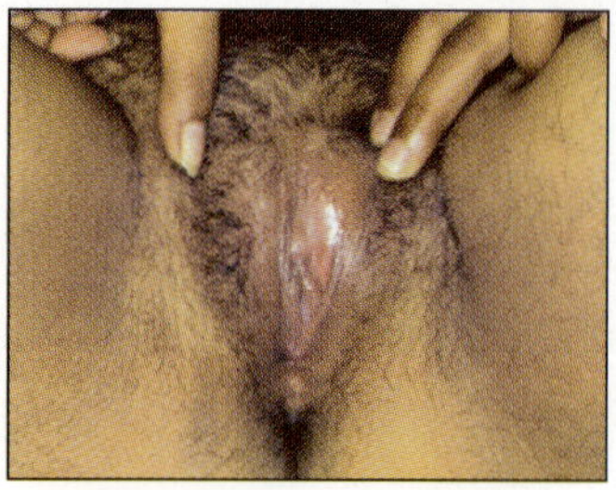

Fig. 12.38 Herpes simplex: labia

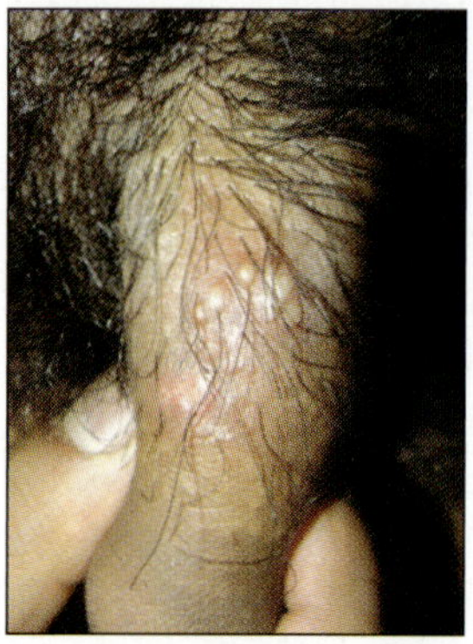

Fig. 12.39 Herpes vesicles on the shaft of penis

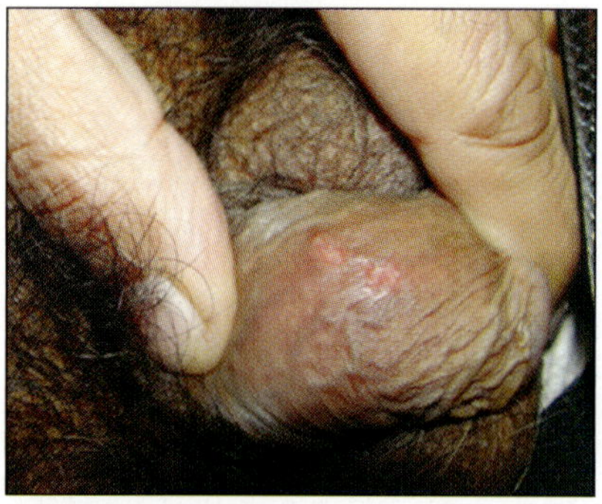

Fig. 12.40 Herpetic ulcer: penis

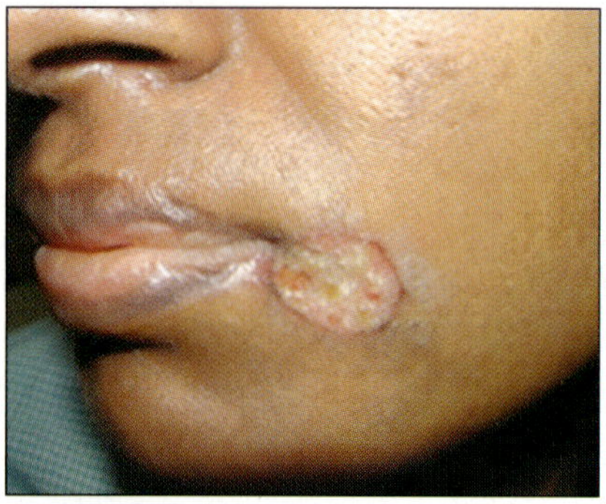

Fig. 12.41 Herpes simplex in HIV

- Recurrence can be suppressed by the long-term use of acyclovir, 200–400 mg twice daily.
- Solvent ether facilitates the healing of the lesions and reduces the recurrence due to its fat dissolving property which makes the herpes virus ineffective.

Chapter 13

Diseases due to Arthropods

Arthropods include million of species and comprise the largest group in the animal kingdom. Common arthropods of dermatological interest are presented in Table 13.1.

Table 13.1 Common arthropods of dermatological interest

• Various flying insects • Mites • Spiders	• Lice • Ticks • Scorpions

Arthropods produce skin diseases through various mechanisms like mechanical trauma, direct injection of injurious substances, hypersensitisation, secondary infection etc. (Table 13.2). Common diseases produced by arthropods are presented in Table 13.3.

Table 13.2 Various methods through which the insects produce skin diseases

• Mechanical trauma. • Direct injection of injurious substances. • Hypersensitisation. • Secondary infections.

Table 13.3 Dermatoses produced by arthropods

Insect bites Lichen urticatus Scabies Pediculosis • Pediculosis capitis • Pediculosis corporis • Pediculosis pubis

INSECT BITES

Common insects causing skin reactions are as follows:

- Mosquitoes.
- Fleas.
- Ticks.
- Bugs.
- Ants.
- Wasps.
- Spiders.

Effect of Insect Bites

The effect of insect bite depends upon the following:

- Active substances in the sting.
- Hypersensitivity of the individual to the specific insect.
- Antigens.

Chemicals in Insect Bites

The stings of bees and wasps contain the following chemicals:

- Large amounts of histamine.
- 5-hydroxytryptamine (5-HT).
- Kinins.

These mediators cause acute pain and extensive erythematous swelling at the site of the bites.

Reaction to Insect Bites

Bites of mosquitos, fleas, ticks, bugs and ants result in the following:

- Transient pain.
- Itching.
- Minute papules.

Characteristics of Lesions due to Insect Bites

Due to Mosquitoes

- Frequently seen during the summer and rainy seasons.
- Present on the exposed parts of the body such as the face, hands, forearms and legs.

Due to Fleas and Ticks:

The lesions may occur throughout the year and are usually limited to legs and thighs.

Due to Bugs which Infest the Beds and other Furniture:

Bugs that infest the beds and other furniture mostly cause lesions on the trunk.

Allergy/Hypersensitivity to Insect Bites

The substances introduced during the bites result in papular or papulo-vesicular lesions that might get infected by pyogenic organisms (Fig. 13.1). Multiple bites or allergy to sting can cause the following reactions:

- Fever.
- Headache.

- Fall in blood pressure.
- Shock.
- Multiple urticarial lesions.

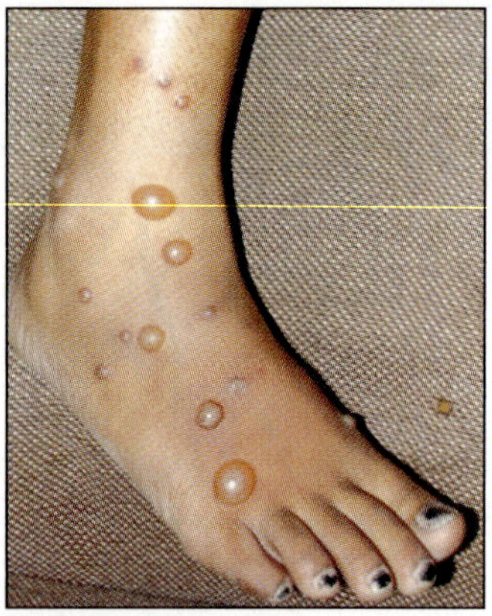

Fig. 13.1 Insect bite hypersensitivity

Lichen Urticatus

Synonym: Papular urticaria.

This occurs in children due to hypersensitivity to the antigens introduced during insect bites.

Age

2–7 years.

Clinical Features

- Recurrent, itchy papules and urticarial wheals are present.

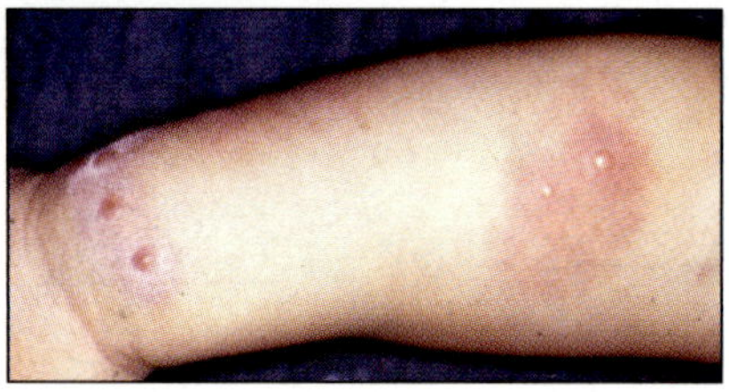

Fig. 13.2 Lichen urticatus: arm

- At some stage, it may present as papules on the surface of a wheal at the site of the bite (Figs 13.2 and 13.3).

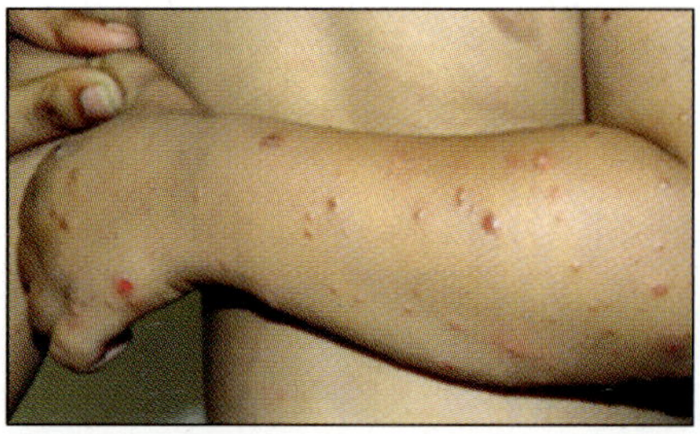

Fig. 13.3 Lichen urticatus

- Seasonal variations are seen. Lesions are more commonly seen in the summer and rainy seasons.
- As the child grows, he stops developing these lesions due to the development of desensitisation through repeated bites.

Treatment

- Guard the patient from insect bites by covering his body with full-sleeve, high-neck clothes.
- Application of insect repellant where the body cannot be covered by clothes.
- Systemic antihistamines to control the itching.

Mild Lesions

Mild lesions may be treated with topical corticosteroids and antibiotic cream.

Severe and widespread lesions

Oral corticosteroids are given.

Secondary infection

Topical/systemic antibacterial agents are prescribed.

Paederus Dermatitis

- It is a type of irritant dermatitis caused by the chemicals produced by the insect called **blister beetle**.
- Seen usually on the exposed parts.
- It manifests as an erythematous necrotic area with blistering of the skin (Figs 13.4 and 13.5).

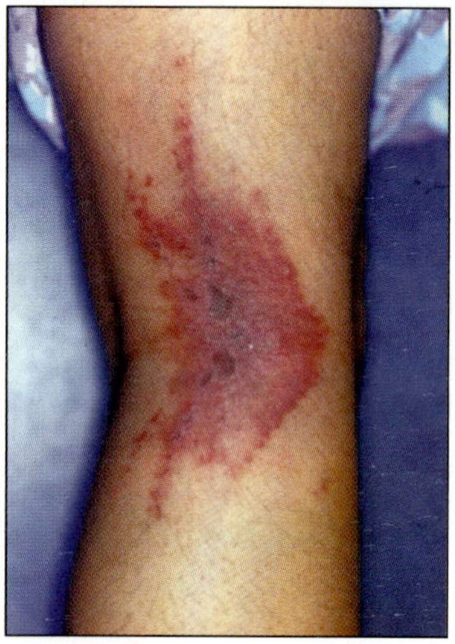

Fig. 13.4 Paederus dermatitis: cubital fossa

Treatment

- Washing the area with soap reduces blistering.
- Topical application of corticosteroids and antibiotic cream.

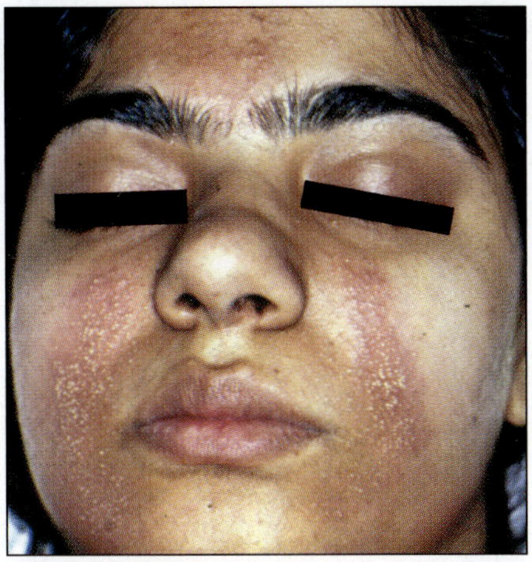

Fig. 13.5 Paederus dermatitis: face

Scabies

It is a skin infestation caused by a mite called *Sarcoptes scabiei*. There are 10–15 varieties of *Sarcoptes (Acarus) scabiei*.

Etiology

- Most of the cases are caused by the hominis variety of mite.
- Animal Scabies: Sometimes the mite that is responsible for causing scabies in the dog, cat, cattle, sheep, horse or other animals can also infest the human beings.

Transmission

- Through close personal contact, e.g., sitting and sleeping together.
- Mites spread and cause epidemics during wars, natural calamities and social or religious congregations.

Pathogenesis

- On being transferred to a new host the pregnant female excavates a sloping **burrow** in the stratum corneum and lays eggs into the tunnel.
- These eggs hatch into larvae in 2–4 days. The larvae undergo three moults to mature into adult males and females.
- After copulation which occurs in the pocket, the male mite dies. The female excavates a burrow in the stratum corneum to repeat the cycle.
- Some of the pregnant females get transferred to other individuals during these cycles and result in the spread of the scabies.
- Total number of *Sarcoptes scabiei (acarus)* are 10 to 15.

Incubation Period

2–3 weeks.

Clinical Features

- Disease can be asymptomatic for the first few weeks.
- It occurs due to development of hypersensitivity to mite(s) or its products.
- Itchy, scattered papules and papulo-vesicles develop in the interdigital clefts (Fig. 13.6) of the hands and the flexors of wrists (Fig. 13.7).
- The lesions are also seen in the following areas:
  - i) Elbows.
  - ii) Anterior axillary folds (Fig. 13.16).
  - iii) Abdomen.
  - iv) Natal cleft.
  - v) Shaft and glans of penis (Fig. 13.8–13.9).
  - vi) Scrotum in the males (Figs 13.10 and 13.11).
  - vii) Around nipples in the females.
- Face is usually spared. Face may be involved in infants (Figs 13.12, 13.13) along with palms, soles (Fig. 13.17) and legs.
- In cleaner individuals (the uncomplicated cases), the lesions occur only on trunk.
- Eczematisation, exudation and crusting is very common in infants (Fig. 13.14).
- Indurated nodules on the shaft of penis (Fig. 13.15) and scrotum which are often intensely irritable and persist for weeks or months, are seen in some cases.

Burrows

- Burrows may be seen in some cases as grey or skin-coloured ridges, 5–15 mm long and often curved or S-shaped.

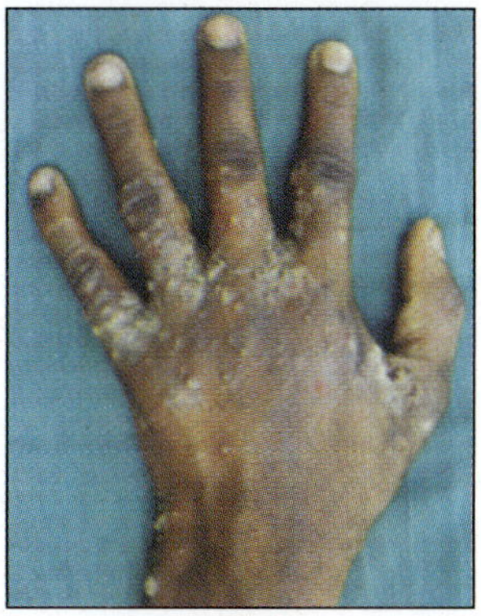

Fig. 13.6 Scabies: interdigital cleft

- Burrows are characteristic lesions of scabies.
- They represent tunnels made by mites in the stratum corneum.

- These are very few in number and occur most frequently on the sites presented in Table13.7.
- Secondary infection is very common and may present as pustules with or without crusting.

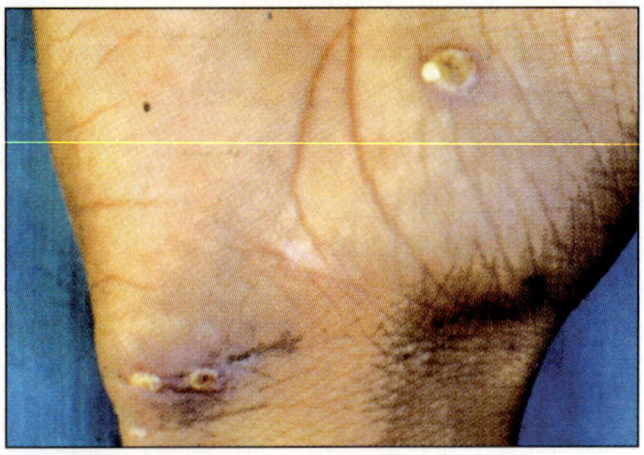

Fig. 13.7 Scabies: flexor of wrist

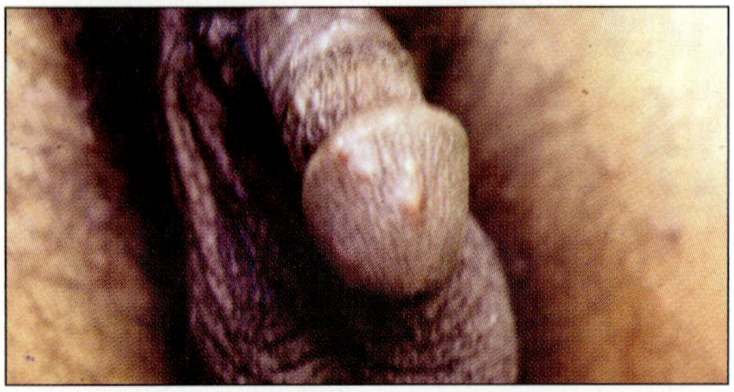

Fig. 13.8 Scabies: glans penis

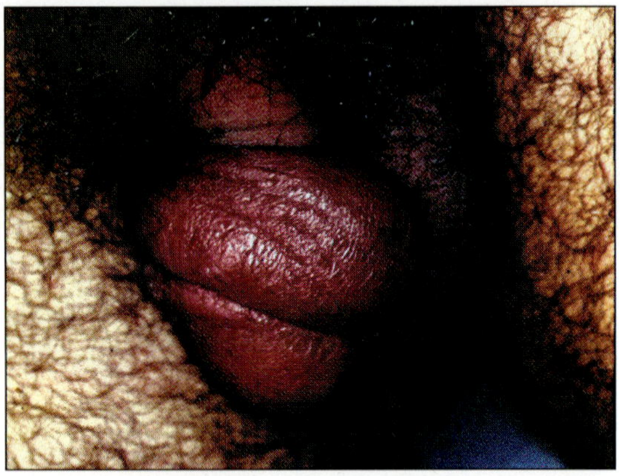

Fig. 13.9 Paraphimosis

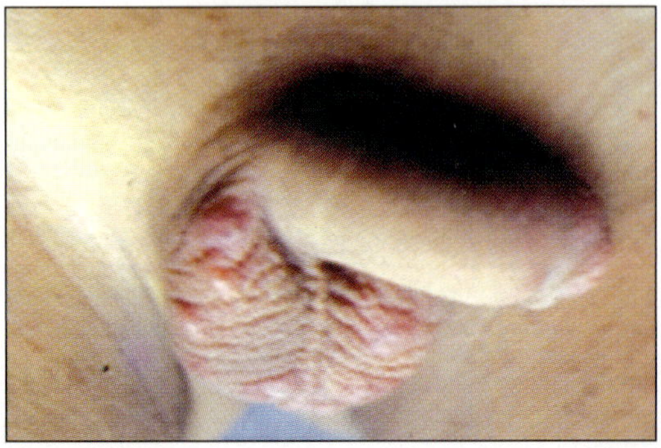

Fig. 13.10 Scabies: scrotum

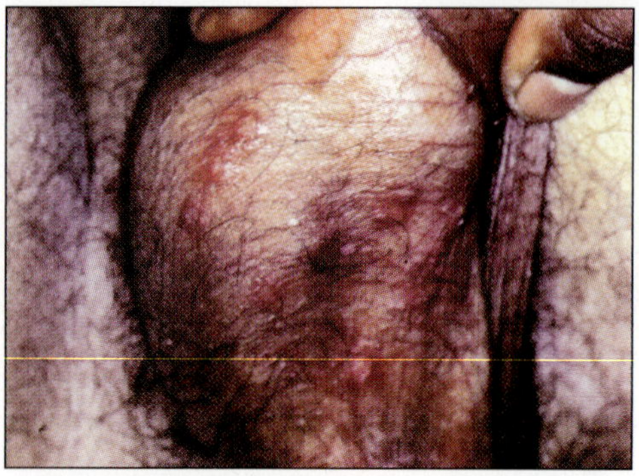

Fig. 13.11 Scabies: nodules scrotum

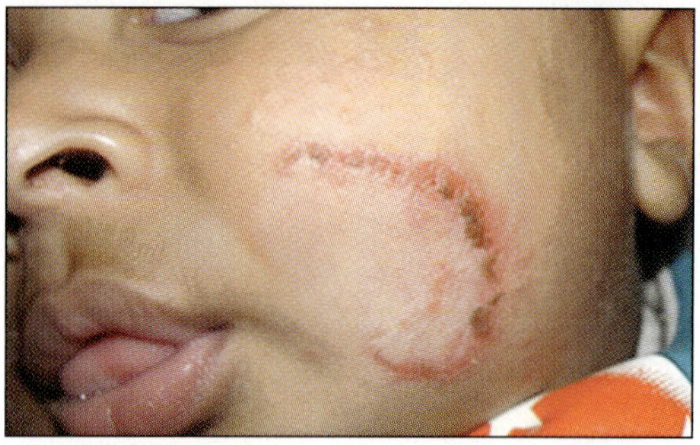

Fig. 13.12 Scabies: face

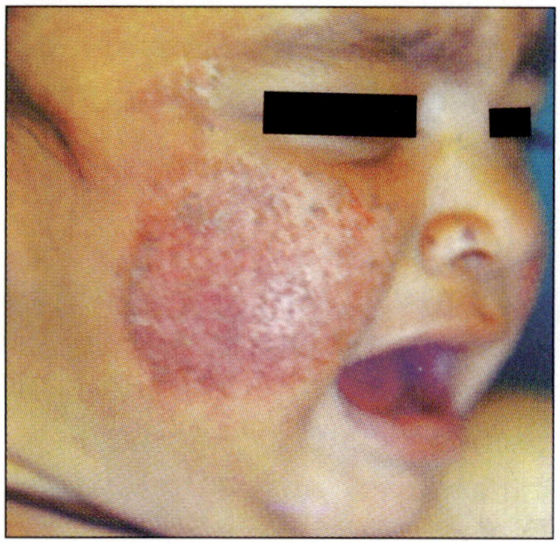

Fig. 13.13 Scabies: face of infant

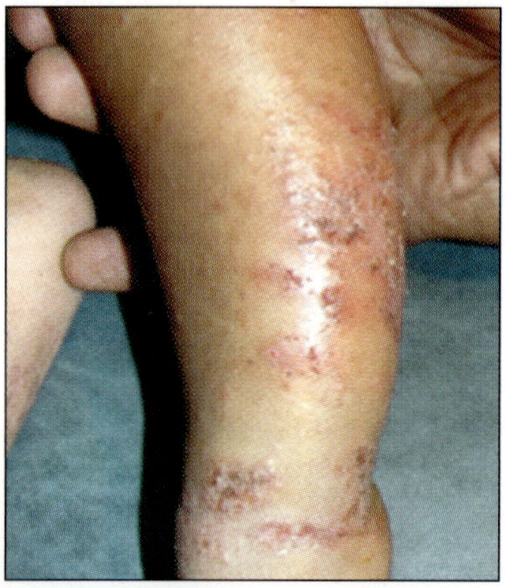

Fig. 13.14 Scabies: leg (child)

Table 13.6 Difference between scabies, lichen urticatus and infantile eczema

Scabies	Lichen urticatus	Infantile eczema
Papulo-vesiculation seen on palms and soles.	Excoriated papules on exposed parts like the extremities and face.	Palms and soles are spared.
Webs of hands, ulnar border of fore-arms, lower abdomen, genitalia may be involved.	Urticarial wheal may occur.	History of asthma.
Close contacts have typical lesions of scabies; history of atopy is not relevant.	Occurs only in children.	Family members may give history of atopy.
Not seasonal.	Usually seasonal.	May be seasonal in some cases.

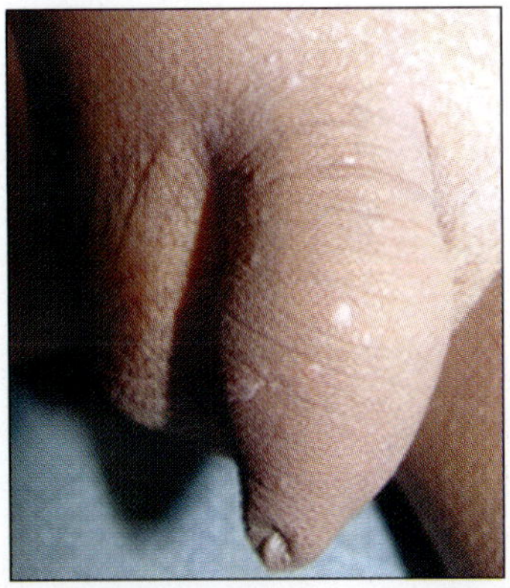

Fig. 13.15 Scabies: penis (child)

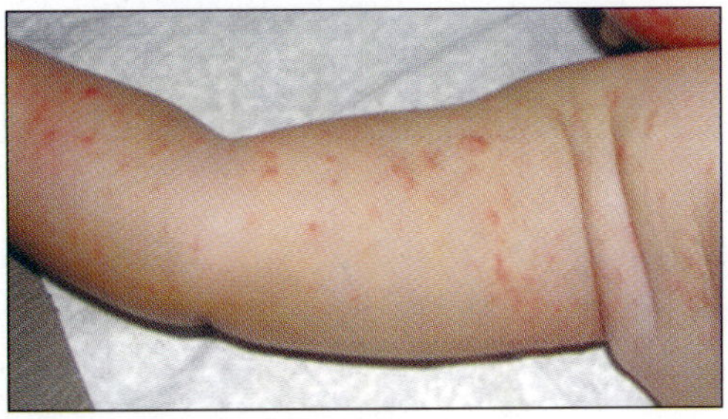

Fig. 13.16 Scabies: child (axillae)

Table 13.7 Site of presence of scabies mite

• Anterior aspect of wrist. • Ulnar border of hand. • Between the fingers. • Anterior axillary fold.	• Nipples in female. • Shaft of the penis in male. • Palms and soles in children and infants.

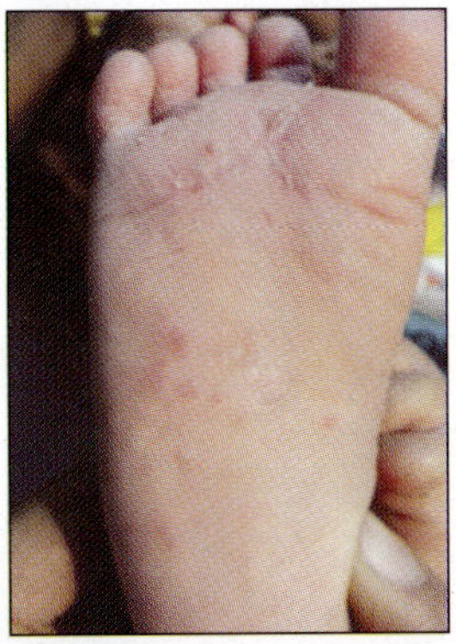

Fig. 13.17 Scabies: sole

Diagnosis

Diagnosis is often made clinically and confirmed by the identification of mites in the skin-scrappings and the presence of characteristic burrow. Scabies needs to be differentiatesd from lichen urticatus and infantile eczema (Table 13.6).

Treatment

- The patient should be treated along with other members of the family including the servants, elderly and infants, irrespective of whether they have any symptoms or not.
- Permethrine 5%, one application eradicates the disease.
- Benzyl benzoate 25%.
- Gamma benzene hexachloride 1%, is applied all over the body except face; 3 applications at 12 hourly interval are adequate.
- Sulphur precipitate 10%, in calamine lotion.
- Crotamiton 10%, cream or lotion, is applied all over body including face twice daily for 1–2 weeks.
- Ivermectin 200 mcg/kg body weight, orally in single dose is adequate.
- For secondary infection, oral antibiotics are given.
- For itching, symptomatic treatment with antihistamines is adequate.
- Eczematisation needs local and/or systemic corticosteroids.
- For itchy papules on scrotum and shaft of penis, massage with crotamiton and corticosteroids is done twice daily for 3–4 weeks.

Side Effects

- Benzyl benzoate may produce irritation.
- Gamma benzene hexachloride is contraindicated in pregnancy and infancy, while crotamiton and sulphur precipitate in calamine are safe.
- Resistance may develop to the scabicidal agents.

Crusted/Norwegian Scabies

It is a rare, but severe, form of scabies. It is extremely contagious due to a large number of mites found in and around the infected skin.

Scabies Incognitio

It is a variant of the disease in dogs, where the mites are very few in number and difficult to recover from the scrapings.

Pediculosis

Skin infestation caused by lice.

Pediculosis Capitis

Etiology

Caused by the head louse, *P. humanus capitis*, confined to the scalp hair.

Transmission

P. humanus capitis is transmitted by close contact between the members of the same family or through shared hats, caps and combs.

Pathogenesis

- During the life span of about 1 month, the female louse lays 7–10 eggs each day. The eggs, called nits, hatch in about 8 days into nymphs and require a further period of 8 days to mature into adult males and females.
- The louse is brown in colour and lives on the scalp. The nits are oval in shape and stick to the hair (Fig. 13.18).
- Their legs are adapted for grasping hair.
- The lice suck blood and inject their saliva at the site of bite.

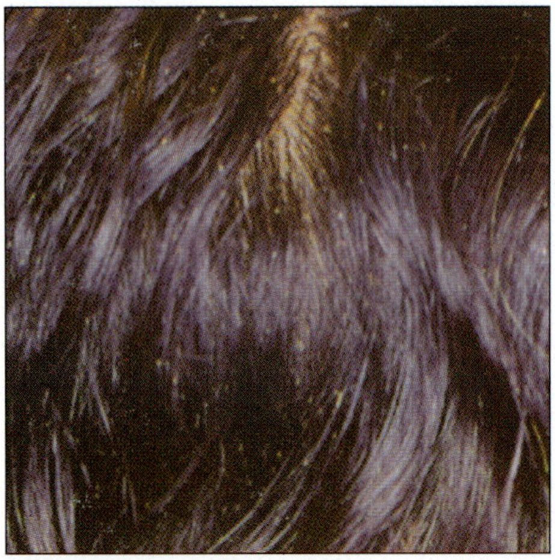

Fig. 13.18 Pediculosis capitis: nits

Clinical Features

- Itching is the most common complaint.
- It is severe around the back and sides of the scalp.
- Multiple excoriations infected with pyogenic organisms, may lead to enlargement of cervical lymph nodes and fever.

Diagnosis

Diagnosis is made on demonstration of the adult lice and/or nits. Nits stick firmly to the hair and lice slide freely along the hair shaft.

Treatment

Application of the following on the scalp:

- Gamma benzene hexachloride: 1%.
- Malathion: 0.25%, on the scalp hair, left over the night and shampooed next morning. To be repeated at weekly intervals for 2–3 weeks.
- Permethrine: 1%, only one application kills both lice and nits.
- Topical/systemic antibiotics for secondary infection.
- Antihistamines to be given for itching.

Pediculosis Corporis

Etiology

Caused by the body louse, *P. humanus corporis*. It is indistinguishable from the head louse.

It is white and lives in the seams of clothes.

Infestation is common in an individual with poor hygiene.

Transmission

Transmitted from one individual to another through close contact, e.g., exchange of infested clothes.

Clinical Features

- The lice bites the skin for feeding which results in severe itching.
- Multiple diffusely scattered excoriations and papules are present.
- Secondary pyogenic infection is seen in chronic cases.
- Lesion may be pigmented and lichenified.

Diagnosis

Demonstration of lice and their eggs in the seams of the clothes.

Treatment

All the clothes should be disinfected with:

- DDT powder 5%.
- Gamma benzene hexachloride 1%.
- Malathion 0.25%.
- Simply boiling or ironing or dry cleaning the clothes, specially the undergarments, destroys the lice.

For excoriated marks on the trunk
Corticosteroids and antibiotic cream is applied topically.

Pediculosis Pubis

Etiology
Caused by pubic or crab louse or *Phthirus pubis*.

Transmission
- Through sexual contact.
- Clothes.
- Towels.

Clinical Features
- Intense itching is usually the only presentation.
- Excoriated papules or papulo-pustules develop.

Sites
- Mainly seen on the pubic region (Fig. 13.19).

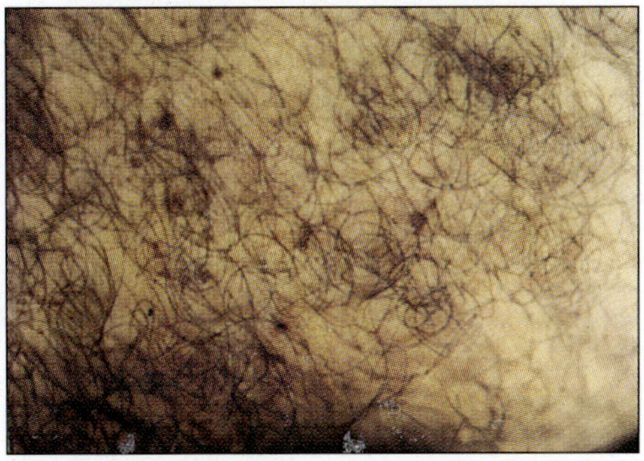

Fig. 13.19 Pediculosis pubis

- May be found in the axillae, eyebrows or eyelashes.

Diagnosis
Demonstration of adult louse sticking to the hair follicles.

Treatment
A single application of:
- Gamma-benzene hexachloride: 1%.
- Malathion: 0.25%.
- Permethrin: 1%.
- For eyelashes, petrolatum: 4–5 times daily for 7 to 10 days.

LEISHMANIASIS

Etiology

This is caused by infection with intracellular protozoa belonging to the genus Leishmania.

Transmission

Human-to-human transmission occurs through the bite by infected sand fly.

Pathogenesis

From sand fly, the infection is transmitted to humans causing the following skin manifestations:
- Cutaneous leishmaniasis.
- Mucocutaneous leishmaniasis.
- Post kala-azar dermal leishmaniasis.

Cutaneous Leishmaniasis

Synonym

Oriental sore.

Incubation Period

The incubation period is from a few weeks to months.

Clinical Features

Asymptomatic erythematous nodules are seen. They ulcerate and heal with a depressed scar (Figs 13.20–13.22).

Lesions in the chronic form do not ulcerate and last longer than 2 years.

Site

Face and hands.

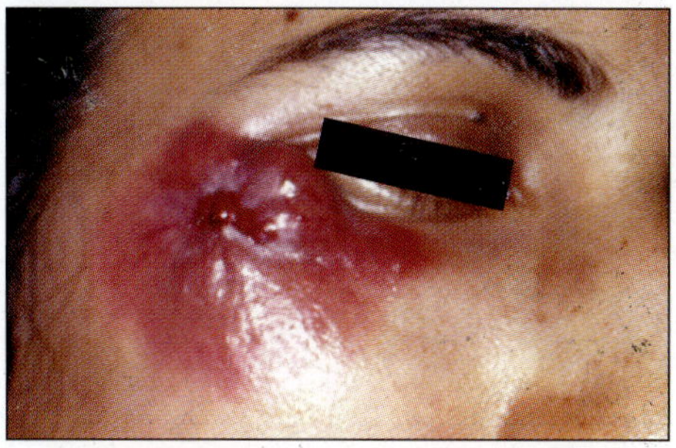

Fig. 13.20 Cutaneous leishmaniasis: face

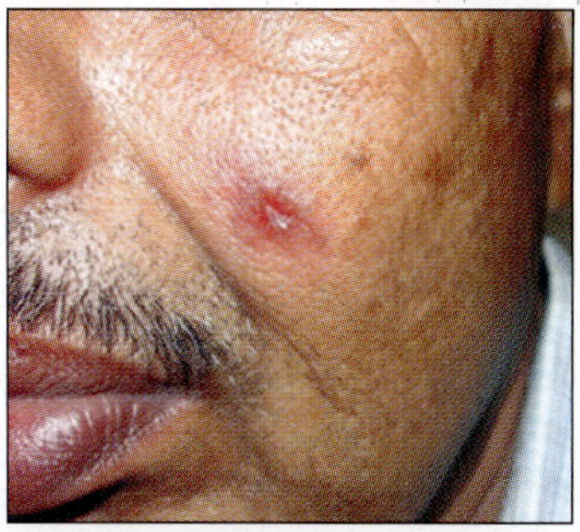

Fig. 13.21 Cutaneous leishmaniasis: face

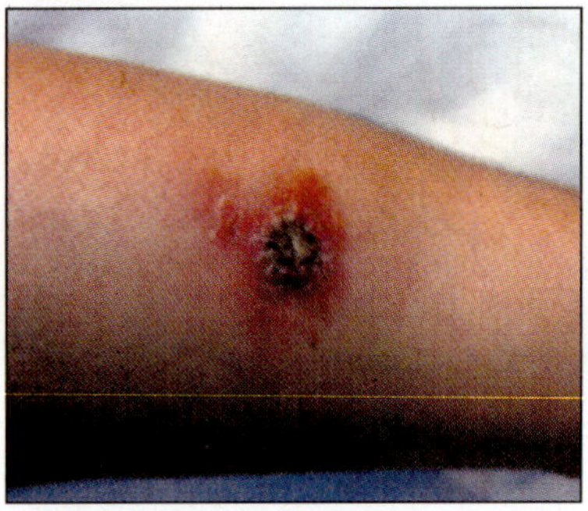

Fig. 13.22 Cutaneous leishmaniasis: arm

Mucocutaneous Leishmaniasis

Usually seen in Brazil.

Skin lesions are edematous, erythematous plaques which involve nasal mucosa after several years.

Skin lesions heal with scarring, whereas the mucosal lesions do not show a tendency for healing.

Post Kala-Azar Dermal Leishmaniasis (P.K.D.L)

Very commonly seen in the state of Bihar.

Cutaneous lesions occur between 1–5 years after the untreated or partially treated kala-azar. It manifests as the following features:

- Erythematous, juicy nodules, especially on the face (Fig. 13.23).
- Hypopigmented macules on the trunk (Fig. 13.24).

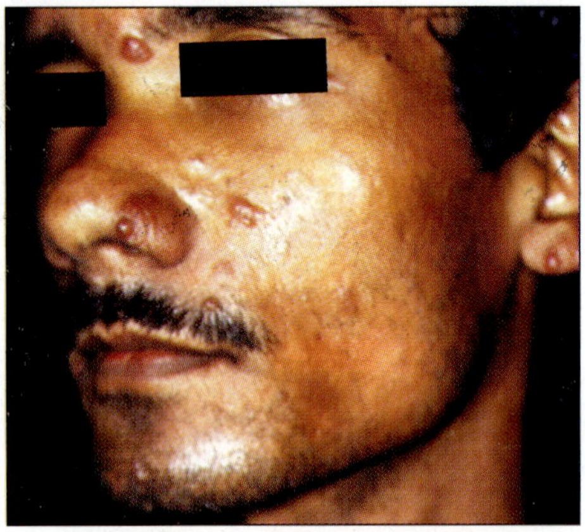

Fig. 13.23 Juicy nodules in post kala-azar dermal leishmaniasis

Treatment of Leishmaniasis

- Intramuscular/intravenous sodium stibogluconate: 20 mg/kg body weight for 20–28 days.
- Ketoconazole: 200 mg, daily.
- Itraconazole: 100 mg, daily.
- Rifampicin: 600 mg, daily till disappearance of all lesions.

CUTANEOUS LARVA MIGRANS

Synonym

Creeping eruption, ground itch or sandworms.

Etiology

More common in countries with warm climates.

Infection occurs from the infected hookworm eggs which lead to the formation of larvae.

Larvae of various other parasites may also cause the lesion.

Clinical Features

The larvae migrate under the skin surface and cause itchy, red or white lines or tracks in the skin (Fig. 13.25).

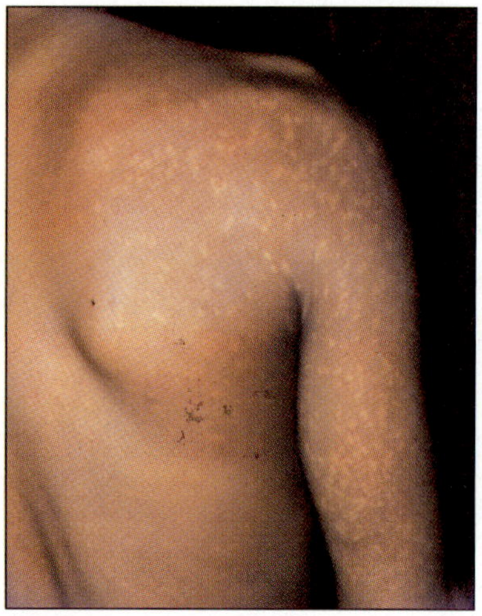

Fig. 13.24 PKDL: hypopigmented macules

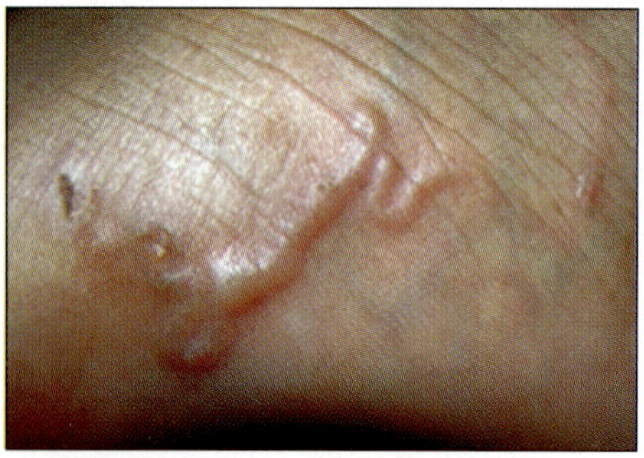

Fig. 13.25 Creeping eruption (Larva migrans)

Complication

- Bacterial infections caused by scratching.
- Rarely, spread of infection via blood to lung and small intestine.

Treatment

- Oral antiparasitic drugs like Albendazole, ivermectin or thiobendazole.
- Thiobendazole in vaseline, topically.
- Freezing by cryotherapy.

Prevention

- Wearing shoes in the endemic areas.
- Avoiding exposure to contaminated soil, sand and infected dogs.

CHAPTER 14

Diseases of the Hair

In humans, the function of hair is mainly cosmetic. Excessive loss of hair as well as excess hair, force the patients to seek medical advice. Hair growth is cyclic and approximately 1 cm per month. Approximately, 1 million hair follicles are present on the human body. Out of that, about 1 lakh hair are found on the scalp. Shaving has no effect on the growth of hair.

EMBRYOLOGY

- Rudiments of hair follicles first appear in the region of eyebrows, upper lip and chin around the ninth week of embryonic life, and in the other regions, around the fourth month.
- New hair follicles do not develop in the adult skin.

At Birth

The newborn has coarse terminal hair (long, coarse, medullated hair) on the following regions:

- Scalp.
- Eyebrows.
- Eyelashes.

Tiny vellus hair (fine, short, non-medullated) are present on the rest of the body.

At Puberty

Coarse hair develops in the axillae and pubic region in both sexes; and on the upper lip and beard region in males.

- In males, the hair all over the body tend to be coarser, especially in the upper part of chest and legs.
- With increasing age, hair follicles decrease in number and produce more vellus hair.

GROWTH CYCLE

The growth of the hair is cyclic and has the following phases:

Anagen or Growth Phase

- Hair grows at the rate of approximately 1 cm per month.
- Length of the hair at any site depends upon the duration of the anagen phase, which varies from region to region and individual to individual.
- In a young male, the duration of anagen phase shows the following ranges:
  - i) Few to several years for scalp hair.
  - ii) 4–14 weeks for moustaches.
  - iii) 6–12 weeks for hair on the arms.
  - iv) 19–26 weeks for leg hair.

Catagen Phase

At the end of anagen phase, the hair stops growing and enters into a short transitional phase which lasts approximately 3 weeks. At any time, 1% or less hair are in the catagen phase.

Telogen Phase

- Catagen phase leads to the resting phase, called telogen phase. It lasts for about 3 months.
- At the end of telogen phase, old hair fall and are replaced by new hair which follow the same cycle.
- At any time, about 13% of hair follicles are in telogen phase, though this may vary from 4–24%.

Mosaic

In humans, all the hair follicles in any region are not in the same phase of growth cycle. Many hair follicles are in anagen phase, a few are in catagen and the rest are in telogen phase. This pattern is called a mosaic pattern.

The hair which complete the telogen phase on a particular day, falls. Thus an individual loses some hair normally every day.

ALOPECIA

Alopecia is an abnormal loss of hair. Different types of alopecia are presented in Table 14.1.

Telogen Effluvium or Diffuse Alopecia

Etiology

This is the most common variety of alopecia that occurs due to premature precipitation of anagen follicles into

Table 14.1 Types of alopecia

- Telogen effluvium or diffuse alopecia.
- Androgenic alopecia or male pattern baldness.
- Alopecia areata.
- Traction alopecia.
- Trichotillomania or hair-pulling tics.
- Secondary alopecia.
- Folliculitis decalvans.
- Pseudopelade.

telogen. Common causes for telogen effluvium are presented in Table 14.2.

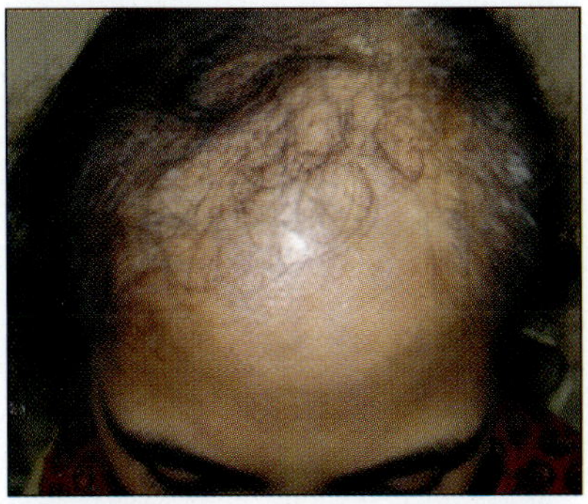

Fig. 14.1 Diffuse alopecia

Table 14.2 Causes for telogen effluvium

- Pregnancy.
- Prolonged fever, particularly due to typhoid.
- Surgical shock.
- Haemorrhage and blood donation.
- Anaemia.
- Sudden severe reduction in food intake as in crash dieting.

Severe general illnesses

- Systemic lupus erythematosus.
- Exfoliative dermatitis.
- Prolonged emotional stress.

Drugs

- Antimitotic agents.
- Anti-coagulants.

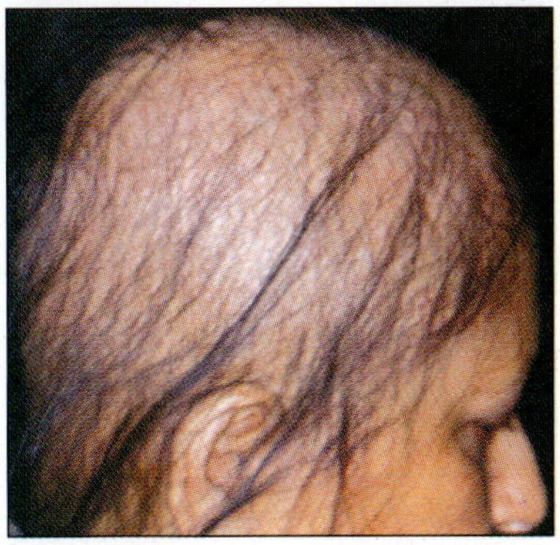

Fig. 14.2 Diffuse alopecia

- Nearly three months after such episodes of stress, these hair start falling and continue till all such hair have been lost (Figs 14.1 and 14.2).
- Severity of alopecia depends on the duration and severity of the stress and individual variation.

Treatment

- Explanation and assurance is very essential.
- Investigate and find out the exact cause.
- Treat according to the cause.
- Clean the hair regularly with shampoo.
- In due course, hair regrow to their original state.

Androgenic Alopecia or Male Pattern Baldness

Etiology

- This occurs due to androgenic stimulation of predisposed hair follicles with reduction in the anagen phase and increase in the number of telogen follicles. The size of follicles progressively reduces and terminal hair is replaced by vellus hair during subsequent cycles. Many of the vellus follicles also disappear (Fig. 14.3).
- Transmitted as an autosomal dominant character.

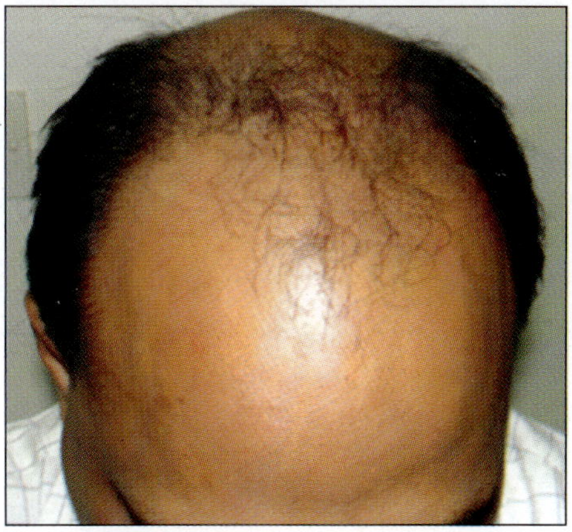

Fig. 14.3 Androgenic alopecia

Age of Onset

Varies in different individuals, but it does not start before puberty.

Clinical Manifestations

- In females, the manifestations depend upon the levels of androgenic hormones. However, no difference in the levels has been found between the men with androgenic alopecia and those with full hair.
- Initially, there is backward recession of the frontal hairline with widening of the forehead (Fig. 14.4). It may follow loss of hair from vertex. With increasing age, hair loss becomes more prominent. In some

cases, most of the hair on the scalp is lost except a rim of hair on the sides and back.

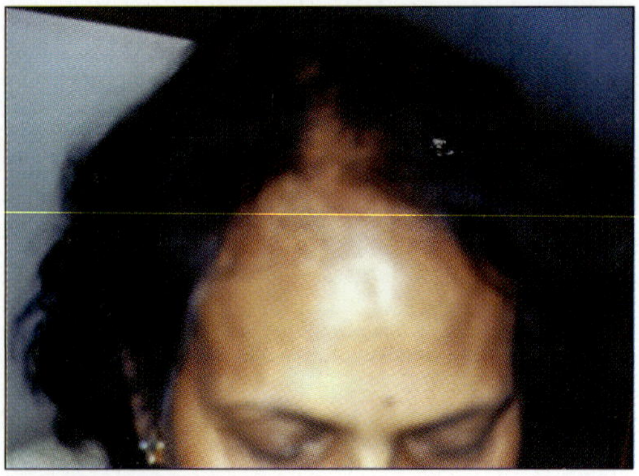

Fig. 14.4 Male pattern baldness in female

Treatment

- No effective treatment is available at present.
- Drugs found to have some use are as follows:
  i) 2–5% topical minoxidil: 1 ml twice daily for 3–6 months or more. It is an antihypertensive vasodilator medicine that is used to treat hair loss. It is equally effective in male and female androgenic alopecia.
  ii) Finasteride: 1 mg/day for at least 2 years.

Follicular unit transplant

It is a technique of hair transplantation, where the grafting is done with naturally occurring groups of 1 to 4 hairs—the follicular unit graft. Single hair graft is placed over the frontal hair line followed by grafting behind the hair line. The results with this technique are natural but may lack density.

Side Effects: Bleeding from the site along with moderate swelling for 4–5 days. Temporary numbness can accompany.

Alopecia Areata

One of the commonest problems seen in children and young adults.

Clinical manifestations

- There is a sudden appearance of single or multiple areas of complete loss of hair on the scalp (Figs 14.5–14.9).
- It is asymptomatic with smooth normal skin.
- Lesions may be localised only to one area of the scalp, or may involve the whole scalp (Fig. 14.10), eyebrows, eyelashes, beard or any other parts of the body.
- Lesions may continue to increase in size or a few new patches may appear.

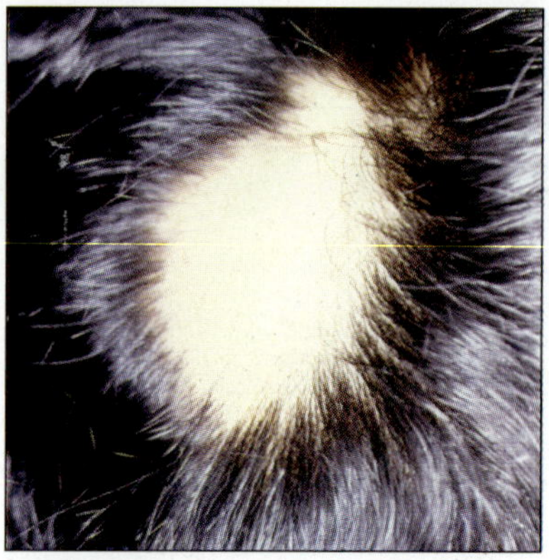

Fig. 14.5 Alopecia areata

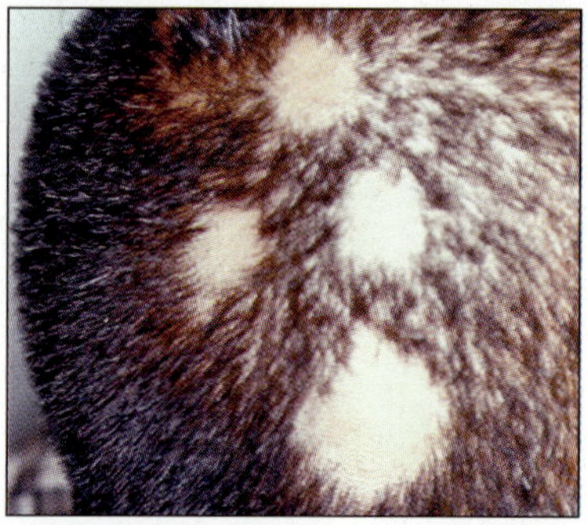

Fig. 14.6 Alopecia areata: multiple lesions

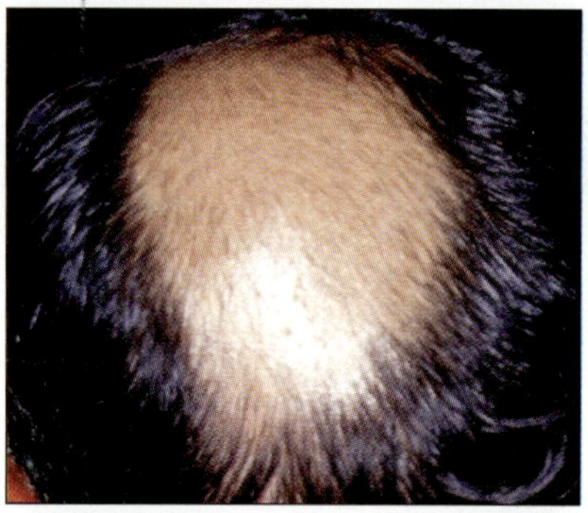

Fig. 14.7 Alopecia areata: spontaneous regrowth of a few hair

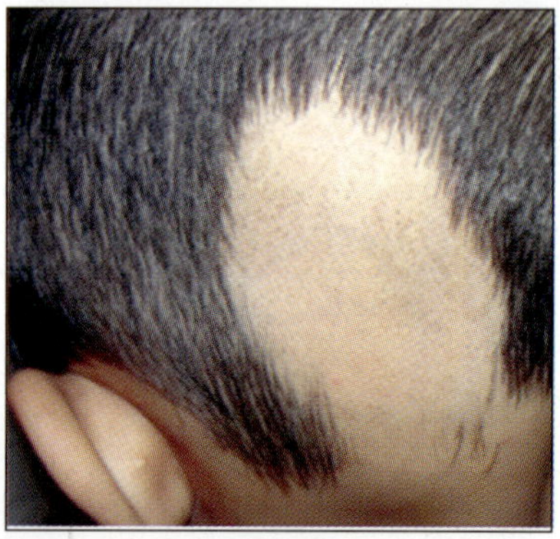

Fig. 14.8 Alopecia areata: spontaneous hair growth

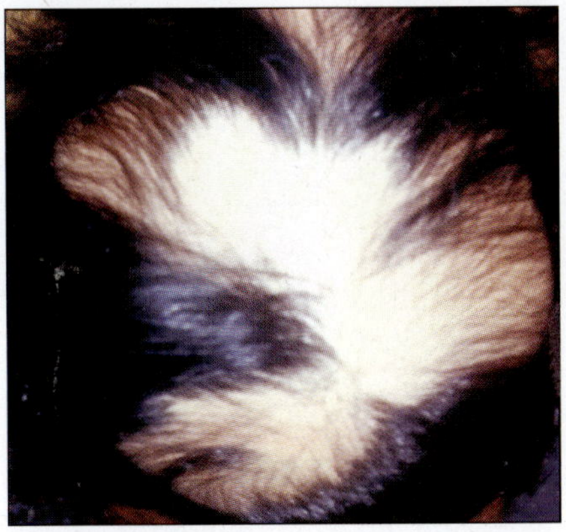

Fig. 14.9 Alopecia areata: 5 year old child

Alopecia Totalis

When there is complete loss of hair from the scalp without any loss of hair from the other parts of body (Figs 14.11–14.14).

Alopecia Universalis

In this condition, the loss of hair is complete from all over the body.

Nail Involvement

Pitting and thinning of nail plate is also present.

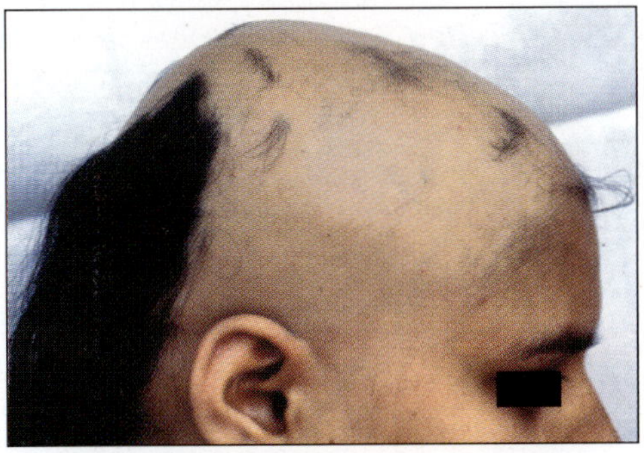

Fig. 14.10 Alopecia areata: wide spread

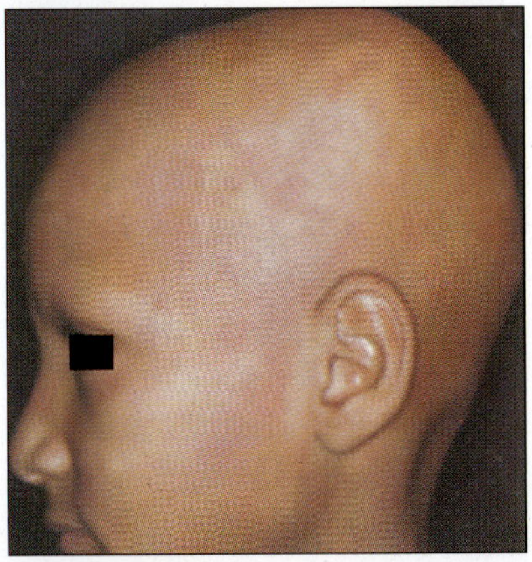

Fig. 14.11 Alopecia totalis

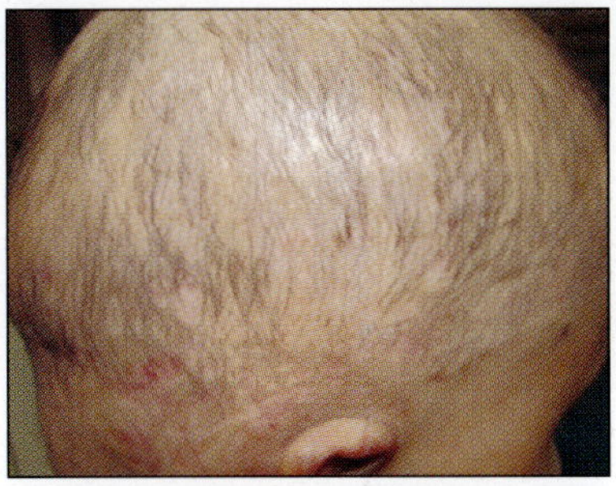

Fig. 14.12 Alopecia totalis: 3months after treatment

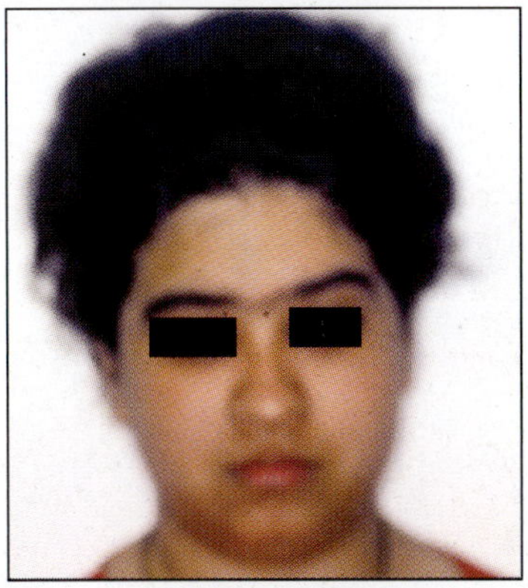

Fig. 14.13 Alopecia totalis: growth of hair 6 months after treatment

Treatment

- Majority of cases do not require any treatment and the hair regrow spontaneously usually in 3 months (Fig. 14.8).
- Indication for systemic corticosteroids: In cases where the lesions continue to increase in size or in number, or hair have not regrown in any patch even after 3 months, prednisolone (a systemic corticosteroid), 10–20 mg is given daily for 3 months. It is then slowly reduced over the next 3 months.
- Role of other treatment modalities like locally applied counter-irritants, corticosteroids, minoxidil and photochemotherapy is questionable.
- Intralesional corticosteroid should be discouraged, due to its atrophic effect.

TRACTION ALOPECIA

This occurs due to prolonged traction on the hair because of hair dressing styles in a particular religion or regions.

Clinical Presentation

- Initially, perifollicular erythema, scaling and broken hair is seen.

- Initial changes are followed by follicular scarring and permanent alopecia in the long run.

Sites

Depend on the hair styles (Figs 14.15 and 14.16).

Treatment

- Correction of hair styles.
- Initial changes revert back after correction.
- If scarring has occurred, hair does not regrow.

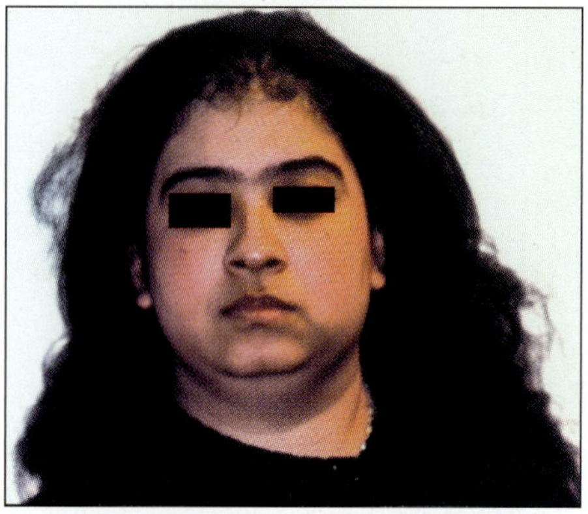

Fig. 14.14 Alopecia totalis: 2 years after treatment

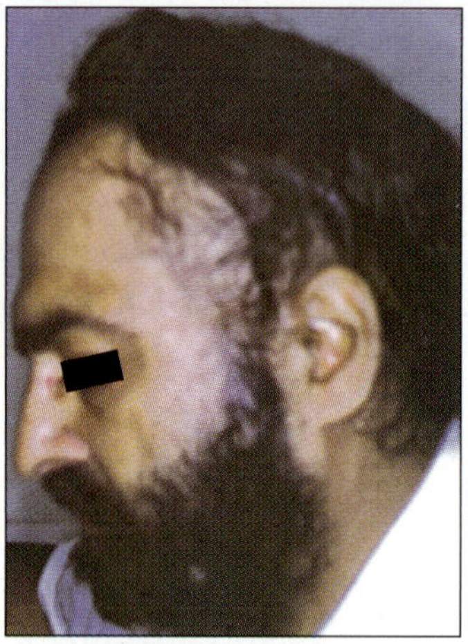

Fig. 14.15 Traction alopecia

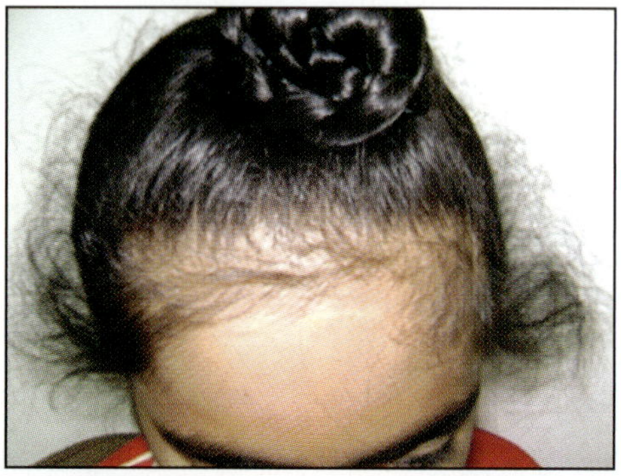

Fig. 14.16 Traction alopecia

TRICHOTILLOMANIA

Synonym

Hair-pulling tics.

Etiology

This occurs in children and adults with mild to severe emotional disturbances.

Clinical Features

Hair on the patch vary in length (Fig. 14.17) due to breakage occurring at different lengths.

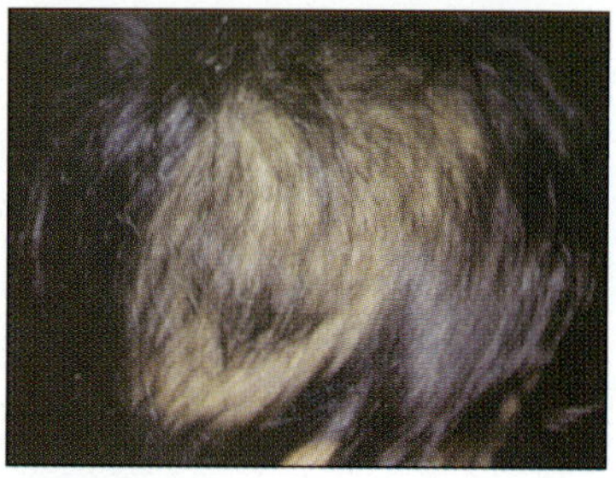

Fig. 14.17 Trichotillomania

Sites

- Scalp.
- Eyebrows.
- Eyelashes.

Treatment

- Psychological approach through repeated assurances and explanation.
- For those who do not respond, psychiatric advice is essential.

Secondary Alopecia

The loss of hair occurs secondary to some local trauma or systemic disease like:

- Mechanical trauma.
- Tinea capitis.

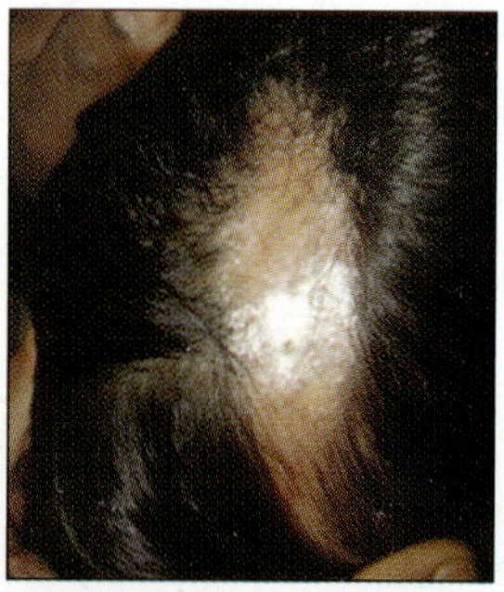

Fig. 14.18 Alopecia-cicatricial

- Lupus vulgaris.
- Carbuncle.
- Syphilis.
- Lichen planus.
- Lupus erythematosus.
- Scleroderma.

The cause of alopecia is usually clear from the signs and symptoms of the original disease

Treatment

- Do not require any special treatment.
- Outcome depends upon the progress of the original disease.
- In case of syphilis, tinea capitis and lupus erythematosus where follicles are not destroyed, hair regrows when the original disease is treated.
- In conditions like morphoea, lichen planus, lupus vulgaris and mechanical trauma, where the hair follicles are destroyed, chances of regrowth of hair are very poor.

Folliculitis Decalvans

Etiology

Inflammation of hair follicles which leads to their destruction and subsequently cicatricial alopecia (Table 14.3).

Table 14.3 Differences between cicatricial and noncicatricial alopecia

Cicatricial alopecia	Noncicatricial alopecia
Due to scarring.	Scarring absent.
Hair follicles destroyed.	Hair follicles not destroyed.
Irreversible.	Reversible.
Skin shiny and follicular openings absent.	Follicular openings visible.
Signs of inflammation like scaling, hyperpigmentation are visible.	Absent.

Clinical Features

- Small, rounded or oval patches of cicatricial alopecia (Fig. 14.18) are seen surrounded by perifollicular pustules.
- Sometimes red macules are seen. They fade away leaving behind scars.

Treatment

During Active Phase

- Systemic antibiotics in full dose.
- Corticosteroids equivalent to 15–20 mg of prednisolone, daily.
- Antibiotic are stopped after the infection disappears.

Late Phase

Corticosteroids are continued for another 2–3 months.

Pseudopelade

This term is used for a variety of cicatricial alopecia where the hair follicles are destroyed by scarring, but without any preceding folliculitis.

Etiology

- Not known.
- It can best be regarded as a pattern of follicular response to a wide variety of known and unknown insults.

Clinical Features

Asymptomatic, irregular areas of scarring alopecia seen without inflammation (foot-print-in-snow pattern) (Fig. 14.19).

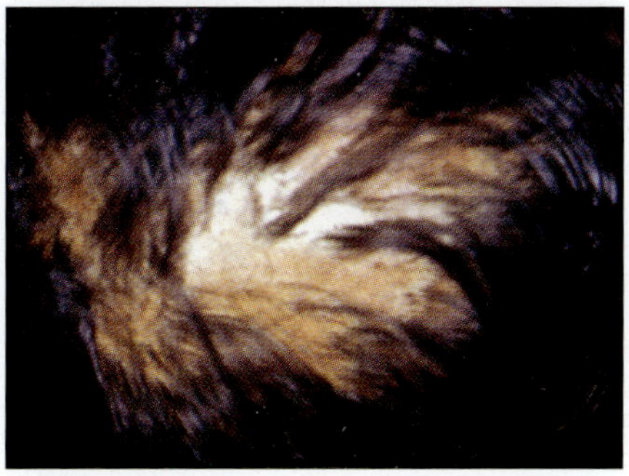

Fig. 14.19 Pseudopelade

Treatment

- The scar is irreversible.
- Hair do not regrow from the lesion.
- Progress of the disease can be halted by systemic corticosteroids, 15–20 mg, prednisolone, daily for 3–6 months.
- Hair grafting is done, once the disease is controlled.

HYPERTRICHOSIS

Excessive growth of coarse terminal hair on any part of the body is called hypertrichosis.

Sites

- Forehead.

- Neck.
- Lower back.
- Any other area of the body where coarse hair are normally not found.

Conditions associated with hypertrichosis are presented in Table 14.4.

Table 14.4 Conditions associated with hypertrichosis

1. Congenital hypertrichosis lanuginose.
2. Internal malignancies in:
   Bronchus.
   Gall-bladder.
   Rectum.
3. Underlying naevus, such as:
   Melanocytic.
   Becker's naevus.
4. Metabolic disorders.
5. Hepatic porphyria.
6. Prolonged use of drugs, such as the following:
   Corticosteroids.
   Psorlens.
   Phenytoin.
7. No apparent cause.

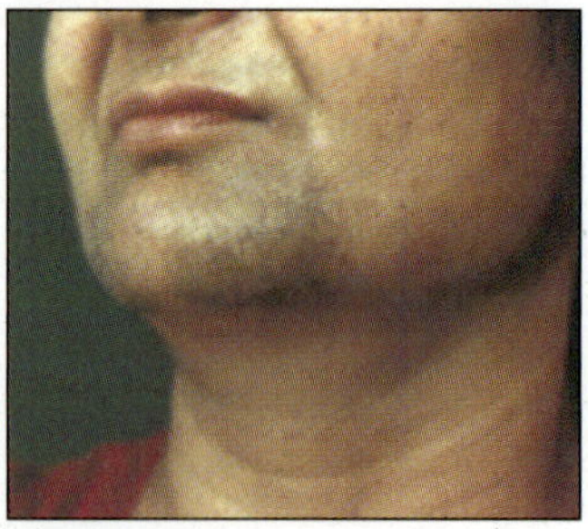

Fig. 14.20 Hirsutism

Hirsutism

In hirsuitism, coarse terminal hair are seen in females in an adult male sexual pattern (Fig. 14.20).

Etiology

In majority, the cause is not known. Hirsutism can be mild or severe.

Clinical Features

Mild Hirsuitism

The hirsutism is mild, when it is limited to a few areas without any detectable underlying endocrinological abnormality.

Severe Hirsuitism

The condition is severe, when it occurs due to an underlying endocrinological abnormality such as in certain tumours of the following organs:

- Ovary.
- Adrenals.
- Pituitary.
- Cushing's syndrome.
- Polycystic ovary syndrome.

Severe hirsuitism may be associated with the following symptoms:

- Abnormal menstruation.
- Enlargement of clitoris.
- Under developed breasts.
- Obesity.
- Enlarged polycystic ovary.

Sites

- Beard area, upper lip and upper part of chest, extremities and around the nipples.
- The pubic hair may show male pattern distribution.

Treatment

- The condition needs treatment only when it is cosmetically unacceptable.
- Underlying cause should be investigated and treated.
- In some, excess hair fall occurs spontaneously after elimination of the underlying cause.
- In majority of cases, coarse hair persist. In such cases, and cases without any known cause, hair is removed by the following measures:
  i) Electrolysis.
  ii) Threading.
  iii) Waxing.
  iv) Lasers.

PREMATURE GREYING OF HAIR OR CANITIES

Development of grey hair (Fig. 14.21) during teens or even in childhood.

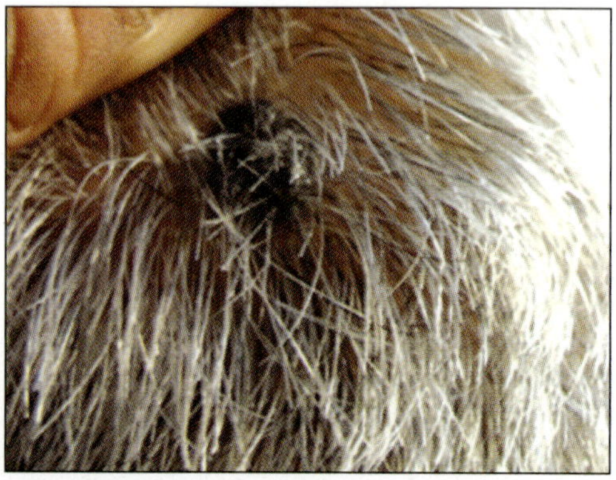

Fig. 14.21 Canities

Treatment

Oral calcium pantothenate: 100 mg, twice daily for 6–12 months, have shown to convert some hair into black in some patients.

MATTING OF THE HAIR

Synonyms

- Plica neuropathica.
- Bird's nest.

Etiology

- May occur after the use of cetrimide shampoo, which is a cationic detergent.
- Repeated manipulation of hair by psychologically disturbed women.

Clinical features

- Compact hair that is irregularly twisted and entangled (Fig. 14.22).
- Densely tangled bird nest following the use of cetrimide shampoo.
- Matting is similar to felting of fibres in wool and textile industries.

Treatment

Shaving of hair.

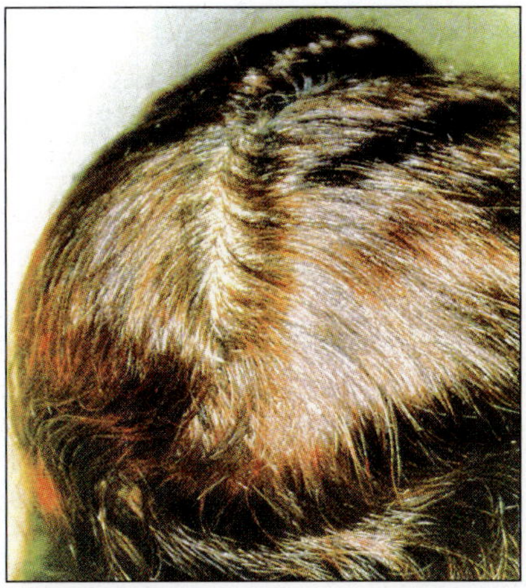

Fig. 14.22 Matting of hair

CHAPTER 15

Diseases of the Sebaceous Glands

SEBACEOUS GLANDS

Sebaceous glands are found all over the body except palms and soles. These glands are larger and numerous on chest, scalp, forehead, cheek, chin , inter scapular region, external auditory meatus and anogenital regions. On the margin of the upper lip and shaft of penis, they may present as pale-yellow bodies called Fordyce's spots.

They are holocrine glands and occur in close association with hair follicles (pilosebaceous units). Sebaceous glands produce an oily secretion called sebum.

Sebum is a complex mixture of lipids. The lipid consists of glycerides, free fatty acids, wax esters, squalene, cholesterol esters and cholesterol. Production of lipid varies with site and age.

Development

It is closely related with the development of hair follicles and epidermis.

At 10–12th week of embryonic life

Rudiments of the glands appear on the posterior surfaces of the hair pegs.

By 13–15th week

Sebaceous glands are distinguishable

By 17th week

Central cells show droplets of lipid.

Function

Sebaceous glands control the loss of water from epidermis. Thus, they protect the skin from fungal and bacterial infections.

Common diseases involving the sebaceous glands are shown in Table 15.1.

Fordyce's Spots

Named after an American dermatologist, John Addison Fordyce, it is the visible ectopic sebaceous gland.

Synonym

Fordyce granules, Fordyce disease.

Clinical Features

- Present as small, painless, raised pale papules of 1–3 mm size on vermilion border of lips, oral mucosa, shaft of penis and labia.
- Lesions on lips are normally found in 80% of people (Fig. 15.1).

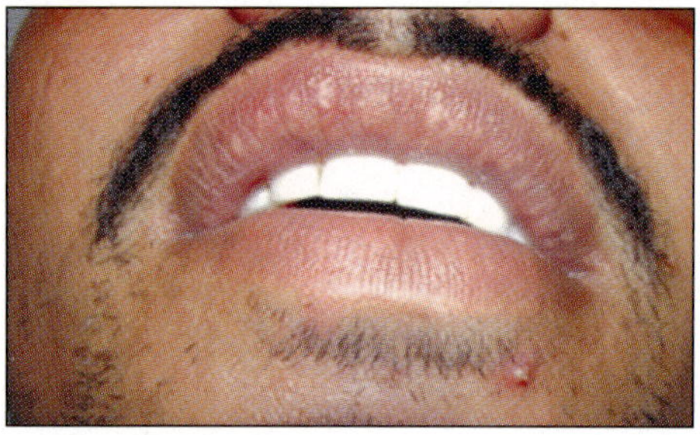

Fig. 15.1 Fordyces spot lip

Treatment

Fordyce spots are completely benign and require no treatment.

Table 15.1 Common diseases involving the sebaceous glands

Seborrhoea. Acne • Acne vulgaris. • Acneform eruptions. • Oil acne.

Seborrhoea

Definition

Excessive production of sebum is called seborrhoea.

Etiology

Exact cause is not known, but it is seen in some neurological disorders such as:

- Active stage of Parkinsonism.
- Some epileptics, especially after 40 years.
- Some cases of manic depressive psychosis.

Seborrhoea is also observed in:

- Some elderly males without any gross neurological disorder.

- Cushing's syndrome.
- Some virilising syndromes in females.

Clinical Features

- Usually noticed as oiliness of face, scalp, middle of the chest and upper back with greasy hair.
- Skin may glisten. This becomes more prominent while sweating.
- Skin is coarse and thickened with prominent follicular openings.

Course

Spontaneous recovery takes place in a few years. Recovery varies from individual to individual.

Complications

- Acne.
- Seborrhoeic dermatitis.
- Pyogenic infections.

Treatment

The associated disease should be treated.

- Isotretinoin, and to a lesser extent, antiandrogen reduce the sebum production.
- L-dopa reduces the seborrhoea in Parkinsonism.

Seborrhoeic Dermatitis

Etiology

- The exact etiology is not known. Improper cleaning and application of hair oils and greasy cosmetics can cause aggravation.
- Bacterial infections sometimes play a role.

Clinical Features

- An inflammation of sebaceous glands, it manifests as severely itchy papulo-squamous lesions.
- Persistent lesions can become lichenified.

Sites

Lesions occur predominantly on the seborrhoeic areas, especially scalp, face, eyelids, retro-auricular areas, central-upper part of chest, back, axillae and sometimes groins.

Treatment

- Repeated cleaning of the skin and hair with soaps and shampoos, respectively.
- Repeated course of systemic antibiotics with topical and systemic corticosteroids for severe lesions.
- Treatment for prolonged period is needed to prevent a relapse.

Acne

Acne Vulgaris

An inflammatory disorder of pilo-sebaceous follicles.

Etiology

Acne is believed to be caused by:

- Excessive secretion of the sebaceous glands.
- Blockage of pilosebaceus duct.
- Bacterial infection (*Propionibacterium acnes*) that can induce an inflammatory response.

Age and Sex

- Adolescents of both sexes get affected (usually appears at puberty).
- In a few patients, the acne may appear during late adolescence or adult life.
- Premenstrual aggravation of the lesions occur in many female patients.

Course

Stops appearing spontaneously by the age of 25 years. In a few patients, it continues to appear till the age of 40 years or so.

Clinical Features

Types of lesions vary from patient to patient.

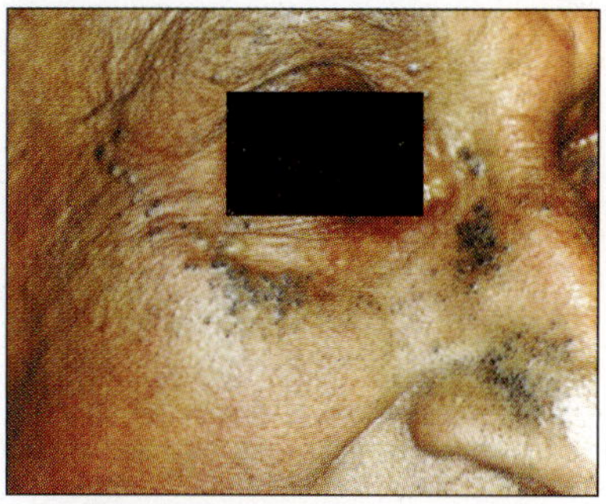

Fig. 15.2 Comedones: black head

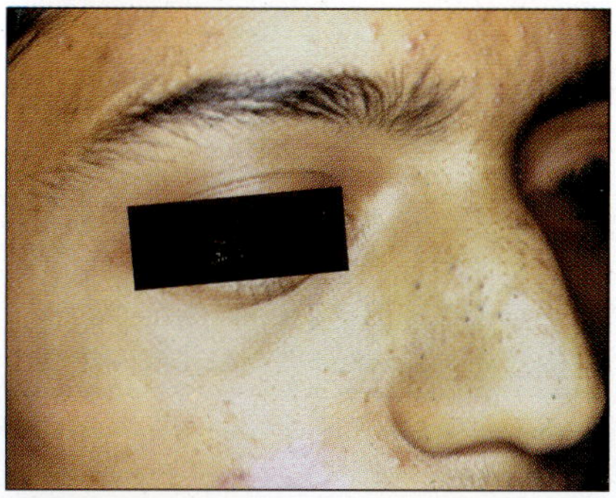

Fig. 15.3 Comedones: white head

- Characteristic lesions are the comedones which have dark horny follicular plugs.
- These may be open (called 'black head', Fig. 15.2), or closed (called 'white head', Fig. 15.3).
- Other lesions consist of papules (Fig. 15.4), with or without inflammatory changes (Fig. 15.16).

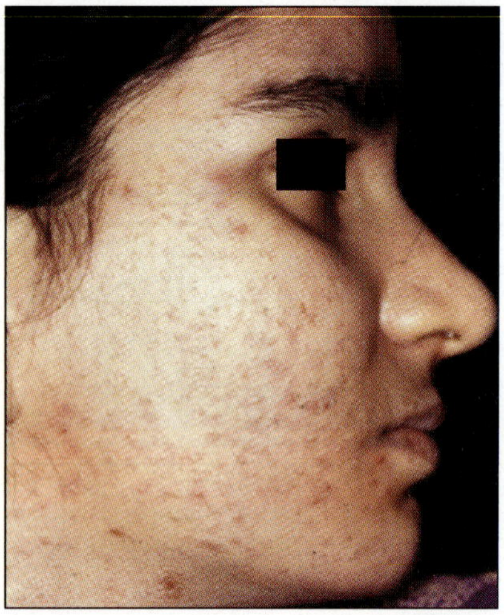

Fig. 15.4 Acne vulgaris: papules

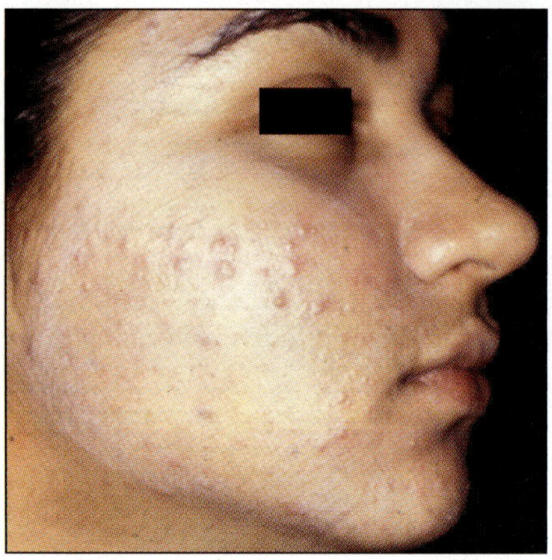

Fig. 15.5 Acne vulgaris: papulo-pustules

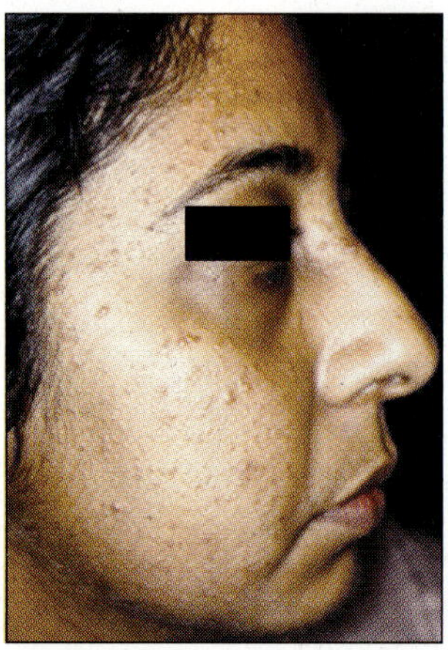

Fig. 15.6 Acne vulgaris: pustules and comedones

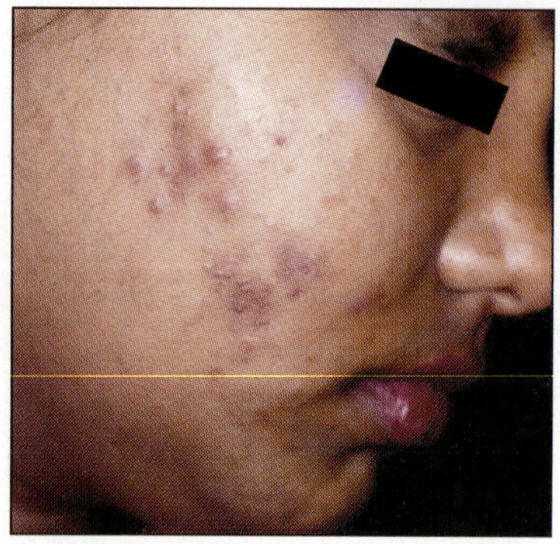

Fig. 15.7 Acne vulgaris: pustules

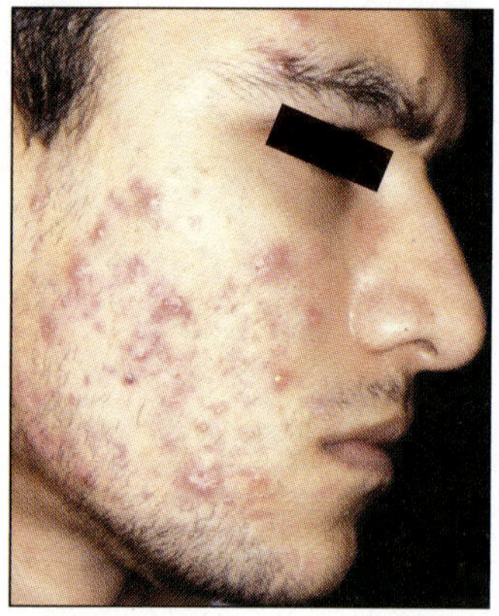

Fig. 15.8 Acne vulgaris: nodules

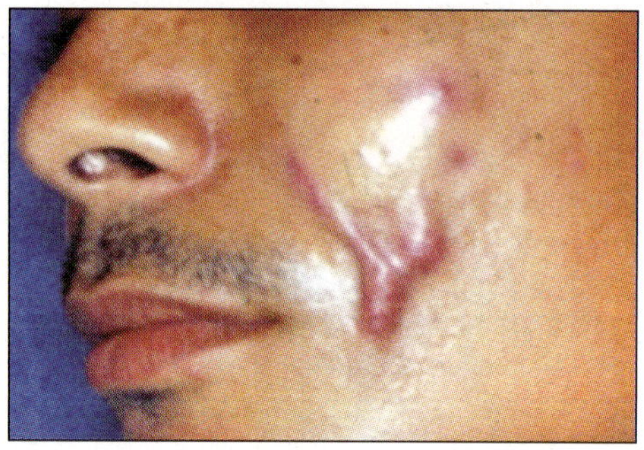

Fig. 15.9 Acne vulgaris: cystic

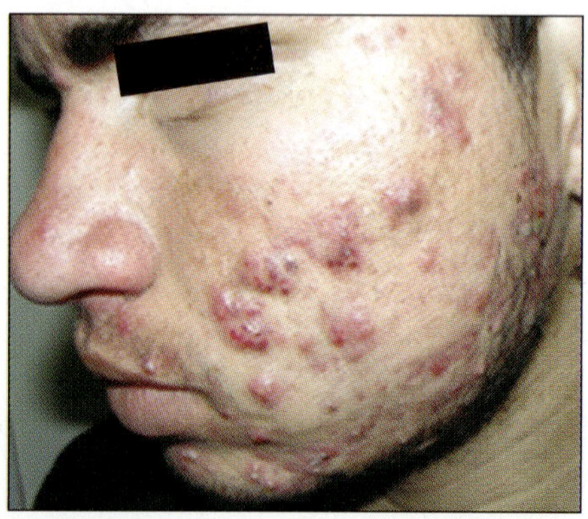

Fig. 15.10 Acne vulgaris: cystic lesion—face

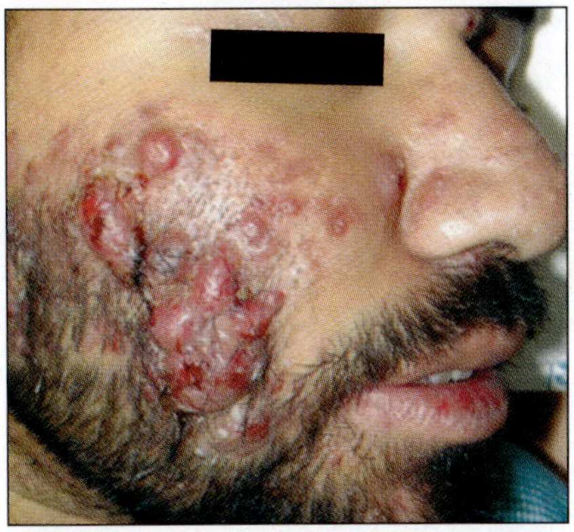

Fig. 15.11 Acne vulgaris: cystic lesion—face

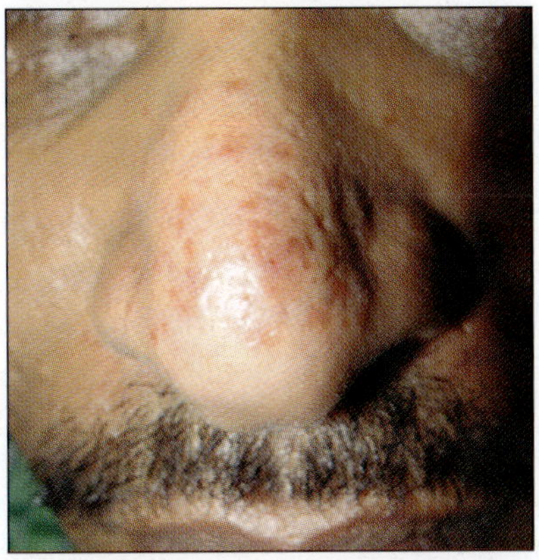

Fig. 15.12 Acne vulgaris: cystic lesion—nose

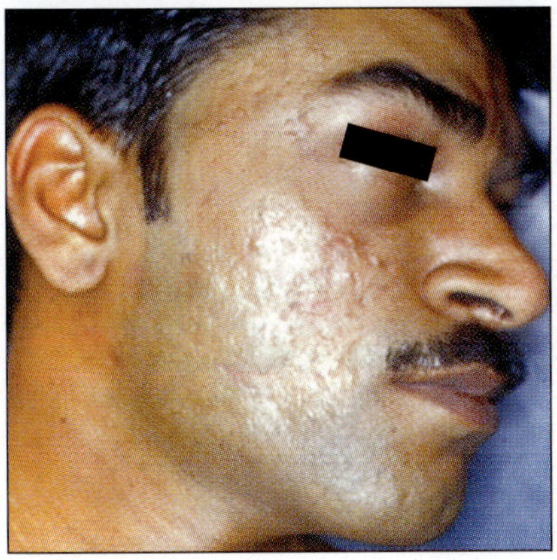

Fig. 15.13 Acne vulgaris: scars

- Papulo-pustules (Fig. 15.5), pustules (Figs 15.6 and 15.7), nodules (Figs 15.8, 15.20) or excoriations (Figs 15.18 and 15.19) or large cysts (Fig. 15.9–15.12) may occur.

Sites

- Usually appears on the cheeks, forehead, chin, nose and the temporal regions.
- In severe cases, shoulders, back and central part of the chest may also be involved.
- Occasionally, lesions are on the buttocks also, or only on the back.

Complications

Healing may result in the formation of scars of varying sizes and shapes on the face. They are as follows:

- Superficial pits may follow comedones or papules; which tend to fade with time.
- Irregular deep scars (Fig. 15.13) follow large, inflammatory, nodular or cystic lesions.
- Sometimes, hypertrophic scars, and even keloids, may result (Fig. 15.14).

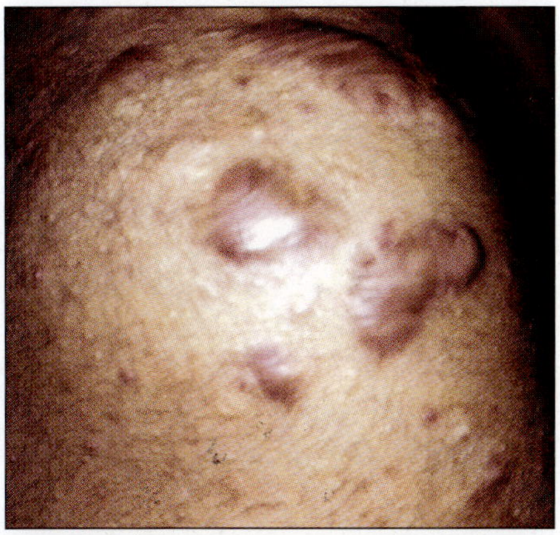

Fig. 15.14 Acne vulgaris: keloid

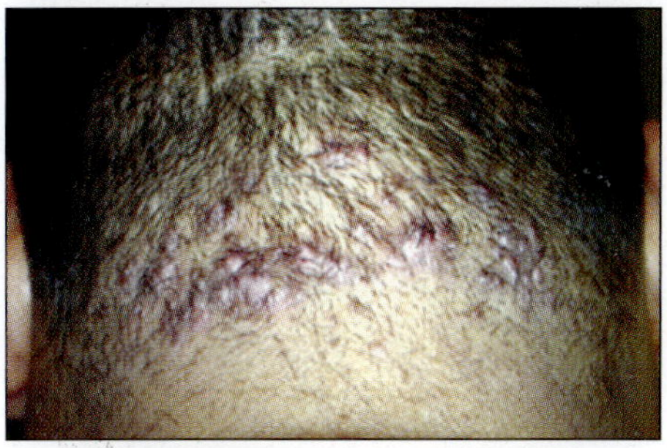

Fig. 15.15 Acne cheloidalis

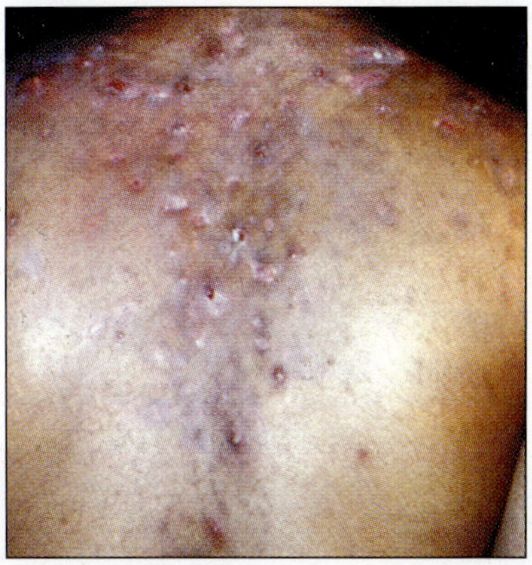

Fig. 15.16 Acne vulgaris: back

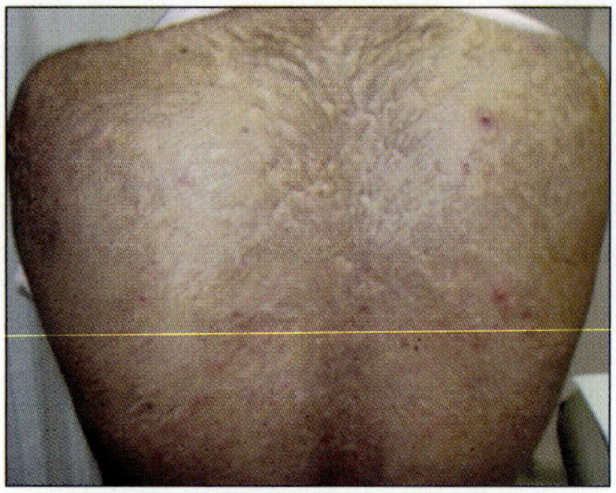
Fig. 15.17 Acne on back: treated

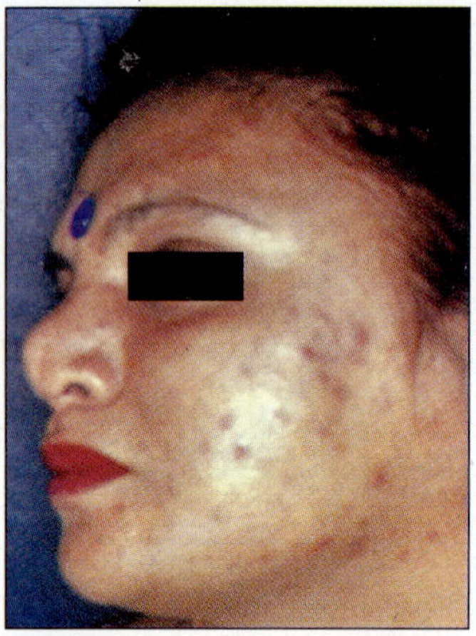
Fig. 15.18 Acne excoriativa

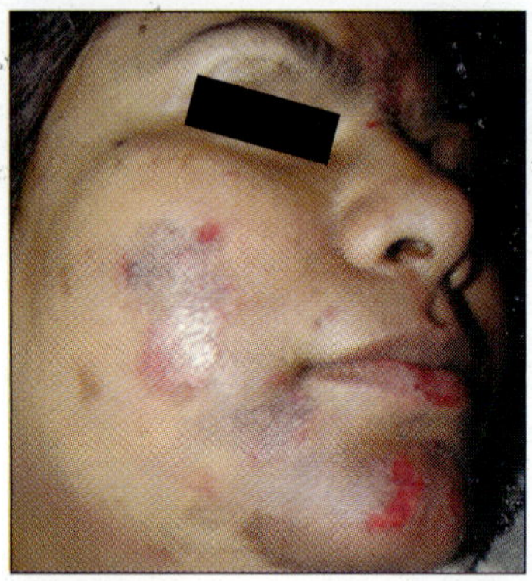
Fig. 15.19 Acne excoriativa

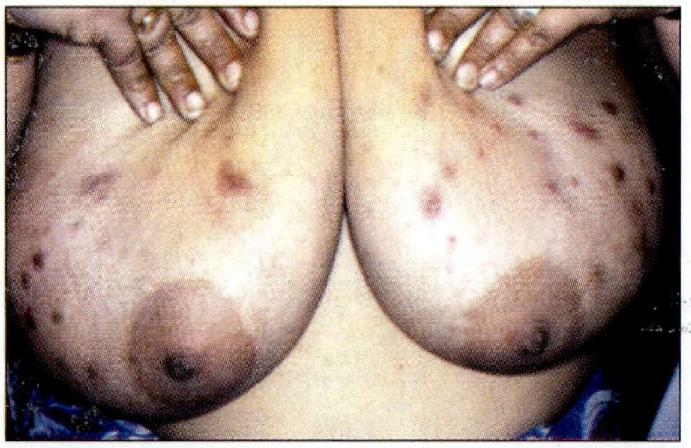
Fig. 15.20 Acne vulgaris on breasts

Treatment

General Measures

- Acne is a self-limiting disease.
- Rapid cure cannot be promised.
- Strictly stop using hair oil as well as any greasy makeup on the face, as these have been found to aggravate the acne.
- Clean the skin with ordinary toilet soap and wash the hair thoroughly with shampoos.
- No restriction of any diet is recommended in acne as sebaceous glands are secretory and not excretory glands.

Topical Applications

- Sulphur precipitate: 10% in calamine lotion.
- Erythromycin: 2%.
- Clindamycin: 1%.
- Azelaic acid.

Predominantly comedonic lesions

- Adapalene: 0.01% and retinoic acid: 0.025 to 0.05% cream, used at night to avoid phototoxic reaction. Adapalene also affects the cellular growth and is an anti-inflammatory.
- Benzoyl peroxide: 5–10% gel is a powerful antimicrobial and an anti-inflammatory agent.
- Most of the time, topical applications are sufficient to control the lesion. However, severe acne need appropriate systemic antibiotics, e.g., tetracycline, doxycycline, co-trimoxazole, erythromycin, minocycline and azithromycin in full therapeutic doses for 4–6 weeks, or till all the inflammatory lesions disappear.
- Such courses may be repeated whenever needed. Treatment with topical applications should be continued even if there is no lesion, till the patient is out of acne age.
- Cystic lesions sometimes require incision to drain out the pus in addition to the above treatment.
- Resistant acne may be treated with oral isotretinoin (a retinoid) in a dose of 0.5–1 mg/kg body weight daily for 4–6 months.

Isotretinoin

Mechanism of Action

- It reduces the sebum production by shrinking the sebaceous glands.
- Reduces the bacterial population.
- Decreases the ductal keratinisation.
- Also exhibits anti-inflammatory action.

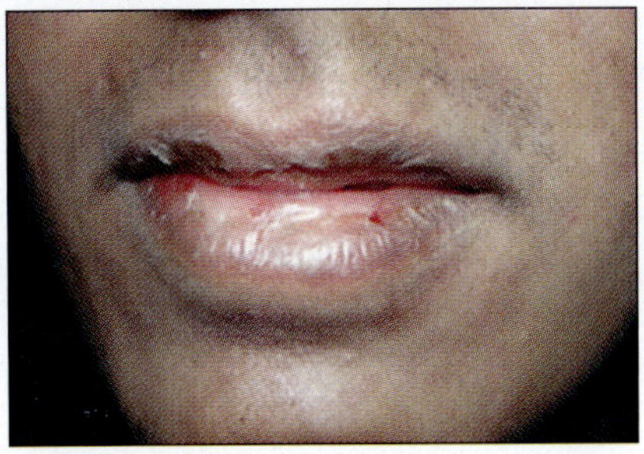

Fig. 15.21 Scaling lip with isotretinoin

Side Effects

- Drying and cracking of lips (Fig. 15.21).
- Hepatotoxicity, i.e., small rise in liver enzymes.
- Rise in triglycerides and cholesterol.
- Bone toxicity like osteoporosis.
- Teratogenicity.

Contraception must be practiced during, and one month after stopping the drug by all women in reproductive age.

Antiandrogens

Mechanism of Action

They reduce the sebum production and may be used in resistant cases of acne in women. Common antiandrogens being used are:

- Cyproterone acetate : 2 mg, daily.
- Estrogen ethinyl oestradial : 35 mcg, daily.
- Spironolactone : 50–100 mg, daily.

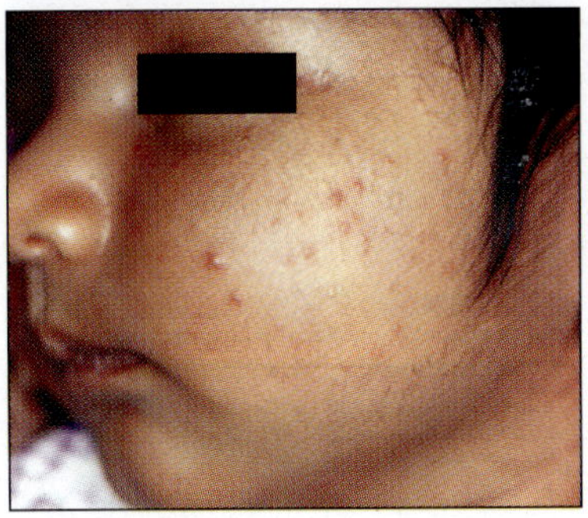

Fig. 15.22 Acne neonatorum

Acne Neonatorum

Synonym

Acne in infancy. These are acne occurring during the first 2 years of life.

Etiology

- Obscure.
- Hereditary predisposition:
- Frequent family history of acne.
- Increased susceptibility of affected infant to subsequent development of severe acne at adolescence.

Two groups are seen:

i) Onset under 3 months.
ii) Onset between 3 months and 2 years of age.

Clinical features

- Lesions may be present at birth or appear any time during first 2 years.
- Scattered comedones are seen on the cheek (Fig. 15.22).
- Papules, pustules and occasionally, nodules and cysts are present.
- Lesion is always confined to face.

Treatment

- No treatment is needed in mild cases,
- For severe cases, the same measures are indicated as in adolescent acne.

Acneform Eruptions

Certain drugs and chemicals (Table 15.2) can produce lesions resembling acne in a predisposed individual. These lesions are known as acneform eruptions (Fig. 15.23).

Table 15.2 Causes of acneform eruptions

Systemic corticosteroids.
Androgens.
Isonicotinic acid hydrazide.
Rifampicin.
Phenobarbitone.
Trimethadione.
Phenytoin/dilantin sodium.
High doses of vitamin D.
Iodides and bromides.
Lithium and actinomycin D.

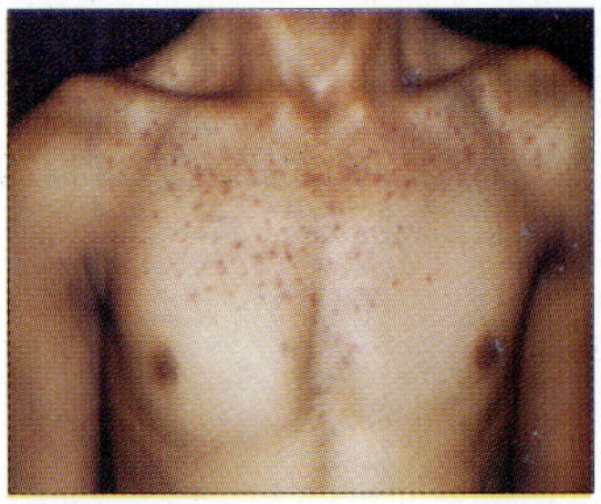

Fig. 15.23 Acneform eruption

Clinical Features

- The lesions are usually non-inflammatory papules.

- Comedones are not seen.
- Iodides and bromides generally produce highly inflammatory, cystic lesions.

Sites

The eruptions are generally more widespread and commonly involve the back, forehead, chest and shoulders.

Treatment

- Withdraw the causative agents.
- Institution of topical applications used for acne vulgaris.

Oil Acne

- A variety of chemicals and mineral oils are known to induce acne on external application (Table 15.3).
- Industrial workers exposed to mineral oils can develop acne.

Clinical Features

Primarily open comedones (Fig. 15.24) and cystic lesions are seen all-over the body including the hairy areas of legs and forearms.

Treatment

- Avoidance of contact with the causative agents.
- Thorough cleaning of the area after the day's work.
- Topical application of tretinoic acid 0.05% at night, till all the lesions disappear
- Systemic antibiotics for cystic lesions.

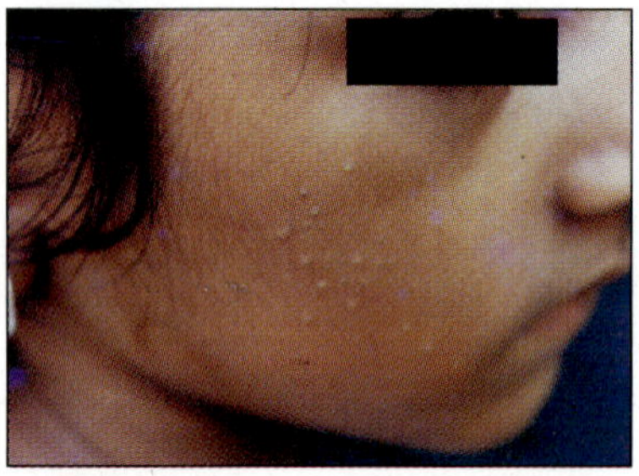

Fig. 15.24 Oil acne

Table 15.3 Causes of oil acne

• Crude petrolatum.
• Heavy coal tar distillates.
• Cosmetics containing:
i) Lanolin.
ii) Petrolatum.
iii) Vegetable oils.
iv) Topical corticosteroids.

Chemical Peeling

It is a procedure, where a chemical agent of a particular strength is applied on the skin, which causes a controlled destruction of the skin layers leading to regeneration and remodeling with improvement of texture and surface abnormalities

It causes destruction at required depth followed by remodeling without scarring

Different types of peeling include the following:

- Glycolic acid peel.
- Salicylic acid peel.
- Trichloroacetic acid peel.
- Tretinoic acid peel.

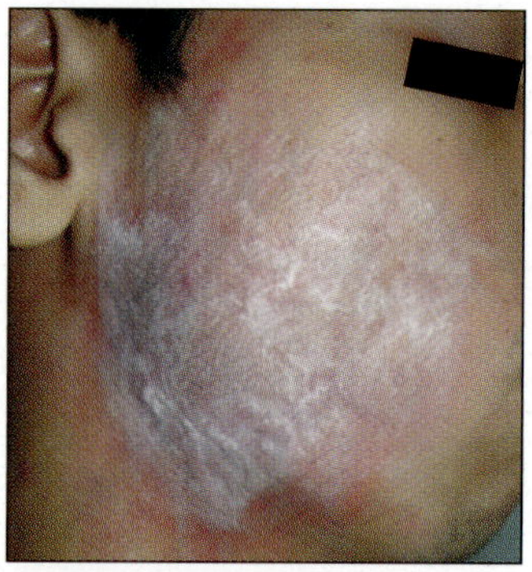

Fig. 15.25 Acne scar: salicylic acid peeling

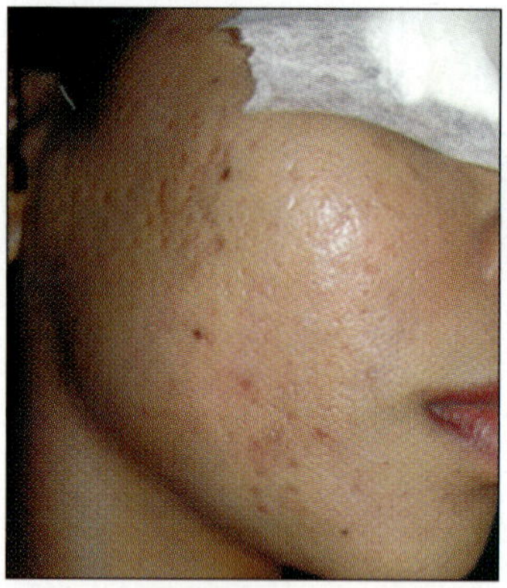

Fig. 15.26 Acne scar: after peeling

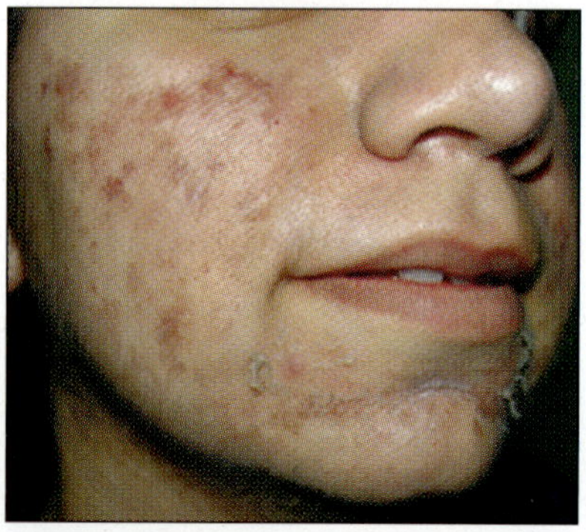

Fig. 15.27 Scaling: after peeling

- Phenol peel.
- Jessner's peel.

Rosacea

Rosacea is a chronic skin disorder characterised by persistent erythematous and telangiectatic lesions interrupted by acute episodes of erythema.

Age

Mainly in middle-age, can be seen in younger individuals.

Sex

Females predominantly, but can also be seen in males.

Etiology

Precipitating factors are as follows:
- Emotional stress.
- Ingestion of hot, spicy foods or beverage.

Clinical Features

- Recurrent episodes of transient erythema and hot flushes, initially.
- Later on, erythema becomes persistent with telangiectasia and erythematous papules.

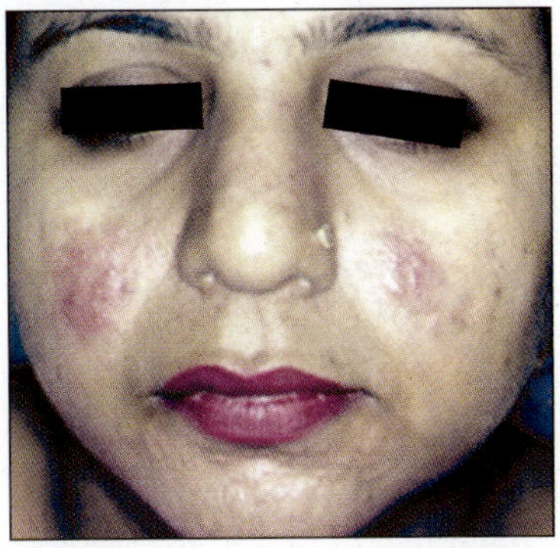

Fig. 15.28 Rosacea

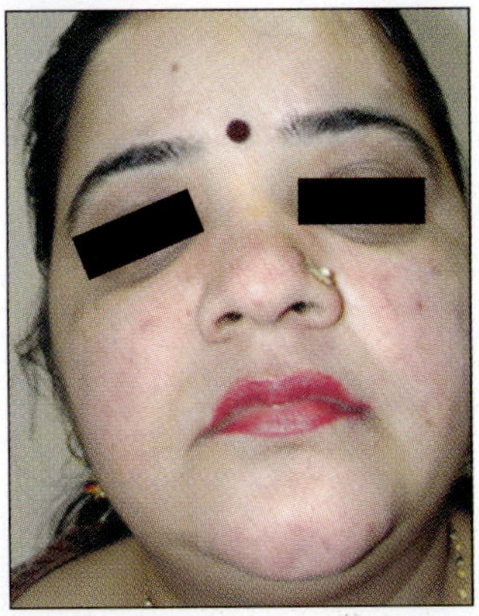

Fig. 15.29 Rosacea

Sites

- Lesions are usually confined to blush area of the face like nose, cheeks, chin (Fig. 15.28–15.30) and forehead (Table 15.4).
- Occasionally seen at other sites.
- It may be seen on any part of the body.

Course

The episodes can continue for several years if not treated properly.

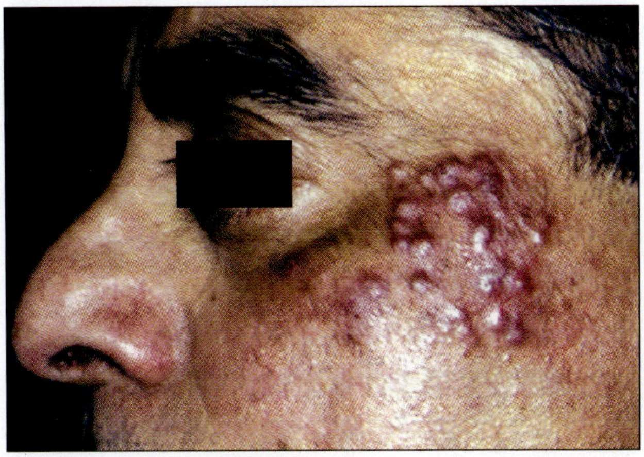

Fig. 15.30 Rosacea: temple

With appropriate treatment, the lesions should stop recurring within 6–12 months.

Table 15.4 Difference between rosacea and acne vulgaris

Rosacea	Acne vulgaris
Middle aged women.	Adolescent patient.
Lesions on face (cheeks, nose, forehead).	Face, upper trunk, chest, shoulders and back.
Comedones absent; erythema papules and telangiectasia prominent.	Presence of comedones with papules, nodules, pustules, cysts and scars.

Treatment

- Patient should be explained about the temporary nature of the episodes.
- Situations known to precipitate the episodes should be avoided.
- Avoid hot spicy foods and beverage.
- Local application of calamine lotion, with or without sulphur precipitate, helps in reducing the erythema and telangiectasia.
- Repeated course of oral antibiotics for 4–6 weeks at a time whenever there is recurrence, leads to permanent remission.
- Topical corticosteroids should be avoided.

CHAPTER 16

Diseases of the Sweat Glands

SWEAT GLANDS

Sweat glands are found all over the body except for the mucous membranes. They are in abundance on the palms and soles. The main function of sweat glands is to regulate the body temperature by evaporation of sweat from the skin surface.

Embryology

- Sweat glands are specialised down growth of the epidermis. They develop around the fourth month of intra-uterine life.
- No new sweat glands develop after birth.

Anatomy

The gland consists of a secretory coil in between the lower dermis and subcutaneous tissue, and a duct leading through the dermis to become the intra-epidermal sweat duct unit.

Functions

The main function of sweat glands is regulation of body temperature. It depends on an intact sympathetic nerve supply, usually cholinergic.

There are three modes of sweating:

Thermogenic Sweating

- When the sweat glands get stimulated through the heat regulating centre in the hypothalamus, they secret sweat to maintain the body temperature.
- It occurs from all over the body, especially, and more profusely from the upper trunk and the face.

Mental Sweating

- Occurs in response to emotional stimuli like mental tension, emotional stress, etc.
- It is usually seen on palms, soles, axillae and to a lesser extent, on the other parts of the body.

Gustatory Sweating

- Hot and spicy food can stimulate sweating.
- It is generally profuse on the forehead, scalp, lips and nose.

DISEASES RELATED TO SWEAT GLANDS

Miliaria

This is due to an obstruction in the sweat duct.

Depending upon the level of obstruction, three types of miliaria are seen:

- Miliaria crystallina.
- Miliaria rubra.
- Miliaria profunda.

Miliaria Crystallina

- Seen in patients having high fever with profuse sweating.
- It occurs due to the obstruction of sweat ducts just below the stratum corneum.

Clinical Features

- Multiple asymptomatic, thin walled, tiny vesicles filled with clear fluid, mainly on the trunk (Fig. 16.1).
- Lesions are very small, erythematous papules and papulo-vesicles aggregating into large, ill-defined patches (Fig. 16.2).
- No inflammation on the skin.
- In a short time, the vesicles rupture on their own with superficial desquamation.

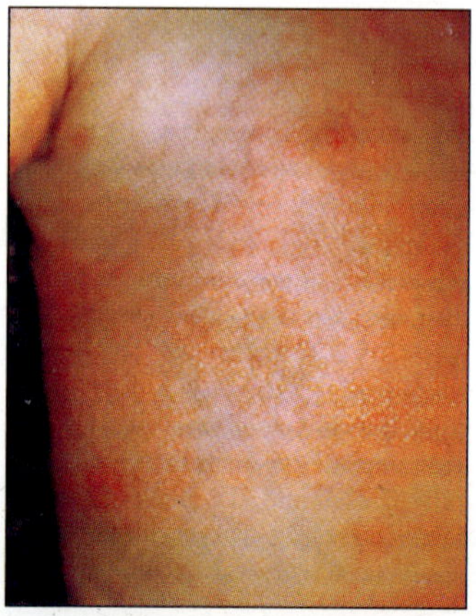

Fig. 16.1 Miliaria crystallina

Treatment

It does not require any treatment.

Miliaria Rubra

Synonym

Prickly heat.

Pathogenesis

- Occurs due to obstruction of the intra-epidermal part of the sweat ducts.
- The obstruction causes swelling of keratin resulting in the occlusion of sweat ducts leading to accumulation of sweat.
- The accumulation of sweat leads to rupture of sweat ducts with leakage of sweat into the surrounding structures causing the formation of lesions.

Predisposing Factor

This condition is mainly seen in the following cases:

- Industrial workers.
- Children.
- Occlusive therapy with polythene.
- Sweating in hot and humid climates.

Clinical Features

- Intense discomfort.
- Unbearable pricking sensation and severe itching.
- Occasionally, the lesions may be infected with pyogenic organisms.

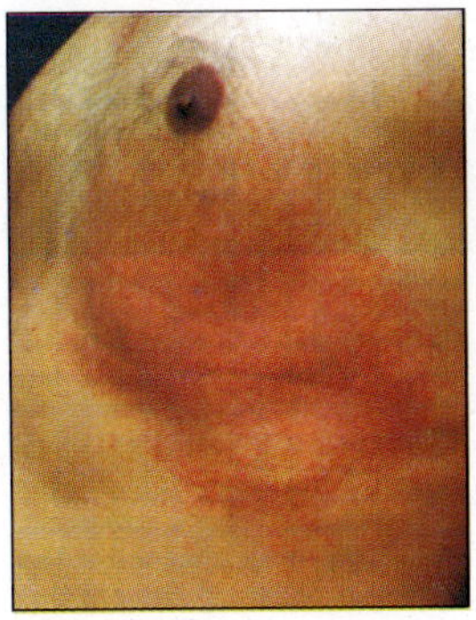

Fig. 16.2 Miliaria rubra

Sites

- Very frequently on the neck, trunk, groin and axillae.
- Can be seen on any part of the body.

Treatment

- Further sweating should be avoided by avoiding the exposure to environmental heat.
- Frequent bathing with cold water.
- Application of soothing lotion, like calamine lotion, 2–3 times daily.
- Oral vitamin C: 500 mg, twice daily.
- If itching is severe, antihistamine may be given 1–2 times, daily.
- For secondary infection, topical or systemic antibiotics are prescribed.

Miliaria Profunda

- This is due to the rupture of sweat ducts at dermo-epidermal junction.
- This usually follows the repeated attacks of miliaria rubra.

Clinical Features

Asymptomatic, pale and firm papules, 1–3 mm in size.

Sites

The lesions usually appear on the trunk.

Treatment

This condition does not require any treatment.

Hyperhidrosis of Palms and Soles

Etiology

- Emotional activity normally increases mild sweating from the palms and soles (Fig. 16.3).
- In some individuals, sweating is so profuse that it interferes with the routine activities and leads to foul smell in the feet.
- Most of these patients are emotionally tense.
- They start worrying for prolonged periods over small things of daily life.

Treatment

- Assurance and explanation about the nature of the disease.

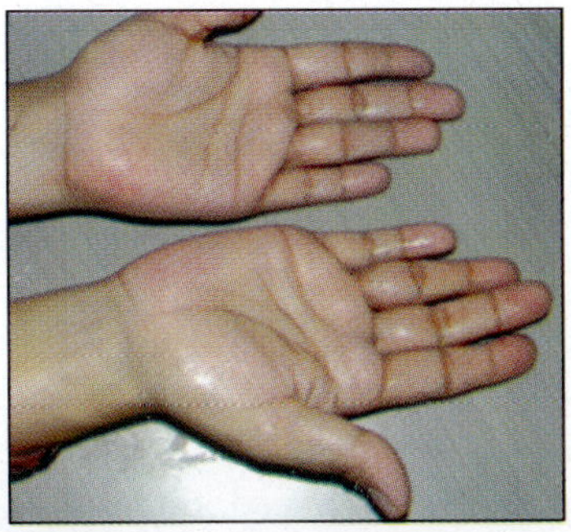

Fig. 16.3 Hyperhidrosis

- Advice to adopt a mature and philosophical attitude towards the problems of life.
- Usually, hyperhidrosis disappears when patient learns to relax during the periods of stress.

Anhidrosis

This condition is the absence of sweating from the skin surface in the presence of proper stimuli.

Etiology

Anhidrosis may be due to the following reasons:

Abnormality of Sweat Glands

An abnormality of the sweat glands, e.g., congenital absence of the sweat glands seen in anhidrotic ectodermal dysplasia.

Interruption of Sweat Reflexes

Interruption of the sweat reflexes due to damage of the nerve fibres.

Damage of Sweat Glands

Damage or even necrosis of the sweat glands may be caused due to certain drugs or chemicals.

Anhidrotic Ectodermal Dysplasia

Clinical Features

Anhidrosis may be complete or partial. The clinical features are presented in Table 16.1.

Table 16.1 Clinical features of anhidrotic ectodermal dysplasia

Present since birth. Inherited as an autosomal dominant character. May be associated with conical or sparse teeth. Depression of bridge of the nose.

Anhidrotic ectodermal dysplasia may also be caused due to the **damaged nerve fibres** in certain diseases (Table 16.2).

Table 16.2 Diseases causing anhidrosis due to damage to nerve fibres

• Mechanical injuries. • Surgical operations. • Syringomyelia. • Leprosy. • Diabetes mellitus. • Other causes of autonomic neuropathy.

- Anhidrosis is **usually unilateral**.
- It is localised to the distribution of nerves.
- Anhidrosis may be caused due to **chemicals or drugs** (Table 16.3).
- Anhidrosis is almost complete.
- It occurs later in life.
- In summer, anhidrosis causes extreme degree of discomfort.
- Generalised erythema, even hyperpyrexia.
- Incomplete absence of sweat glands in the patient may result in compensatory hyperhidrosis.
- Even miliaria at sites of remaining sweat glands.
- Localised area of loss of sweating may not be noticed even by the patient.

Table 16.3 Drugs responsible for anhidrosis

• Phenolic compounds. • Barbiturates. • Anticholinergic drugs.

Treatment

Table 16.4 Treatment of anhidrosis: At a glance

• Avoid hot environment and excessive physical exertion. • Clothes of synthetic material should be avoided.
Anhidrosis due to chemicals or drugs • Usually recover with systemic corticosteroids equivalent to • 15–20 mg daily of prednisolone for 2–3 months.
Congenital anhidrosis Promote heat loss from the body with: • Air-conditioning. • Baths with cold water. • Frequent ingestion of cold water or foods. • Sprinkling of cold water on the skin.

Diseases of the Apocrine Sweat Glands

Anatomy

Apocrine glands have two parts, viz., a secretory coil that lies at the junction of dermis and subcutaneous tissue and a duct which connect into the mid portion of the hair follicle.

Table 16.5 Apocrine sweat glands

• Axillae. • Perianal region. • Areola of the breasts. • Mammary glands and glands in the external auditory meatus are modified apocrine glands

Embryology

- Develop as part of pilosebaceous follicles in the fourth to fifth month of intra-uterine life.
- They are undeveloped in childhood.
- Start to enlarge near puberty.

Activity

- Apocrine glands secrete very small quantities of an odourless oily fluid.

- On the skin surface, bacterial decomposition of the fluid liberates fatty acids.

Chromhidrosis

When the secretion is coloured, it is called chromhidrosis. It is usually due to the decomposition of secretion by chromogenic bacteria, especially *Corynebacteria*. The pigment is usually a **lipofucin**.

Function

Axillary glands are important for body odour.

Fox–Fordyce Disease

Etiology

It occurs due to retention of apocrine sweat leading to inflammatory changes.

Clinical Features

This disease occurs mainly in women after puberty.

In the Early Stage

The patient complains of severe itching in:

- Axillae.
- Anogenital region.
- Around the nipple of the breasts.

Later On

- Skin-coloured or slightly pigmented dome-shaped follicular papules develop at all or a few sites of itching (Fig. 16.4).
- Itching is usually provoked by all those emotional stimuli which normally produce aprocrine secretion.

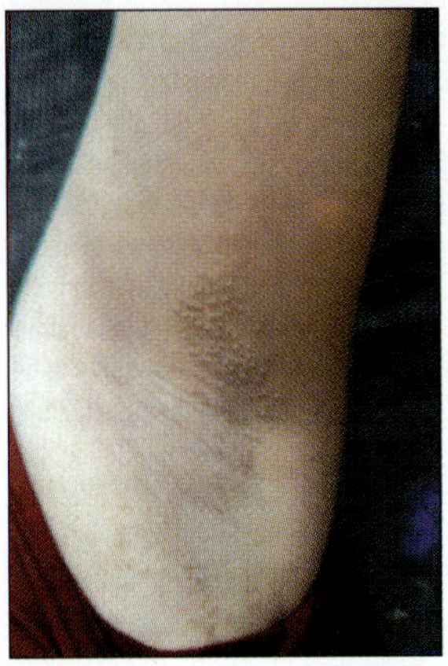

Fig. 16.4 Fox–Fordyce disease

Course

- The disease is usually chronic and persists till menopause.
- Remission may occur in pregnancy.

Treatment

- Usually unsatisfactory.
- Topical corticosteroids or retinoic acid may help in some cases.
- Some patients are benefitted with oral contraceptives.
- Some with severe itching may require surgical excision of the affected areas along with the subcutaneous tissue and apocrine glands.

Hidradenitis Suppurativa

It is a chronic infective condition of apocrine glands.

Etiology

Unknown.

Clinical Features

- Itching or vague discomfort follows small, firm subcutaneous nodules.
- Initially, there is pain without any constitutional symptoms.
- Later on, deep abscesses extend to the skin surface and rupture leading to the formation of sinuses (Figs 16.5–16.7).

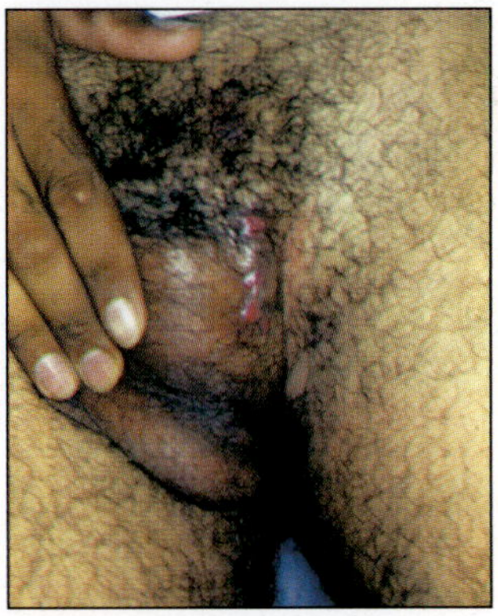

Fig. 16.5 Hydradenitis suppurativa: groin

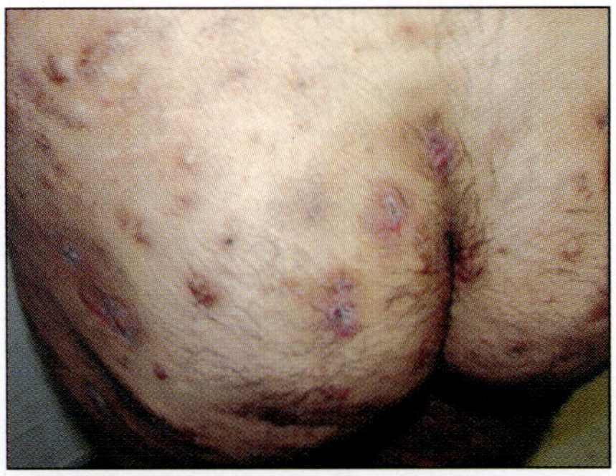

Fig. 16.6 Hidradenitis supurativa: buttocks

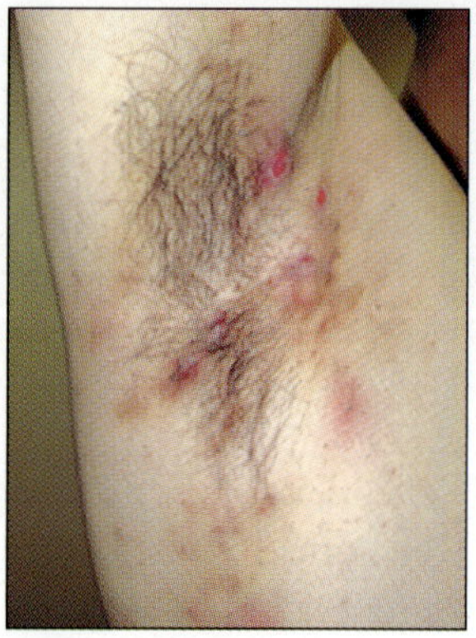

Fig. 16.7 Hydradenitis suppurativa: axilla

Sites

Axillae and anogenital region.

Treatment

- Cosmetics, especially antiperspirants and talcum powder, should be stopped.
- The area should be cleaned regularly with soap and water.
- Secondary infection should be treated with adequate dose of suitable antibiotics for 4–6 weeks.
- In **acute phase**, systemic corticosteroids, in a dose of 20–30 mg prednisolone, daily.
- Retinoids, both isotretinoin 1 mg/kg body weight per day or etretinate 0.5 mg/kg body weight, daily for 4–6 months.
- **Refractory cases** are treated with deep and wide excision of affected area with silastic foam dressing or skin grafting.

Chapter 17

Diseases of the Nails

HUMAN NAIL

The human nail is formed by invagination of epidermis on the dorsum of the distal phalanx of each digit. Human nail is a vestigial organ, its only function is to provide strength and protection to the tips of the fingers and toes.

Structure

The nail consists of the following components:

Nail Plate

It is made up of hard keratin and is produced by the nail matrix.

Nail Matrix

It consists of rapidly dividing cells which are filled with keratin. It is responsible for producing the nail plate. Matrix of the finger nail grows four times faster than the toe nail, i.e., about 3 mm a month.

Nail Bed

It is the tissue to which the nail plate gets attached.

Nail Fold

It is a fold of hard skin overlapping the base and sides of the nail.

Nail Cuticle

It is the skin present immediately around the finger nail.

Embryology

- Nails are visible in a nine-week-old embryo.
- The nail plate is almost completely formed by the twentieth week of intra-uterine life.

Growth

- Nails grow continuously throughout life.
- The growth of nails is fastest in childhood and it decreases with age.
- Normally, the finger nails grow 2–5 mm per month.
- The toenails grow at a rate one-third to half of the finger nail.

DISORDERS OF NAILS

Disorders seen in nails may be localised and limited to nails only or may be a part of the generalised skin or systemic disorder. Common nail disorders are presented in Table 17.1.

Table 17.1 Common nail disorders

- Ingrowing toenail.
- Beau's lines.
- Pterygium unguis.
- Koilonychia.

Ingrowing Toenail

Etiology

Due to compression of toe(s) from the sides, because of ill-fitting footwear (Fig. 17.1).

Penetration is usually caused by spicules of the nail at the edges of the nail plate.

Great toe is commonly involved.

Clinical features

Penetration of the lateral nail-fold by the edge of nail plate causes the following problems:

- Pain, redness and swelling.
- Sepsis, and later, granulation tissue (Fig. 17.2).

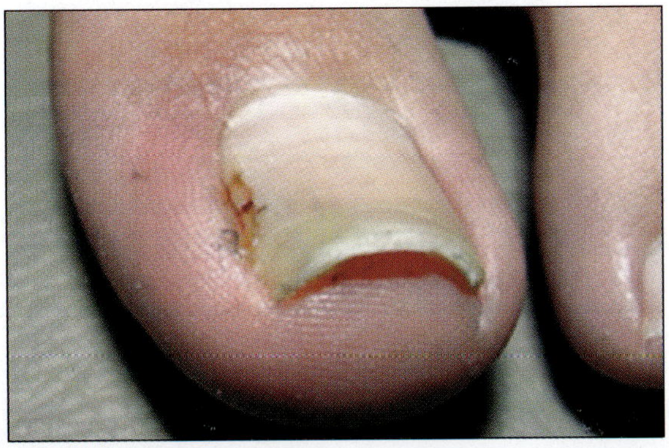

Fig. 17.1 Ingrowing big toenail

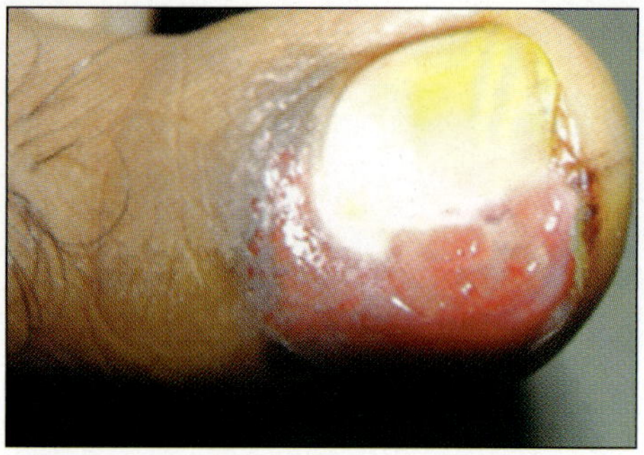

Fig. 17.2 Granulation tissue in ingrowing toe nail

Treatment

- Patient should wear shoes with sufficiently wide toe spaces.
- The nails should be cut straight across.
- Nail should be allowed to grow till its edges are clear from the toe before it is cut. This prevents the formation of further marginal spicules.
- Control of infection with appropriate systemic antibiotics.
- Granulation tissue requires destruction with trichloroacetic acid: 30–50%, silver nitrate or phenol.
- In extreme cases, avulsion of the nail may be required if the conservative methods fail.

Beau's Lines

- These are the transverse depressions on the nails
- (Fig. 17.3) that appear due to temporary interference with nail formation.
- Growth of the nails gets temporarily depressed.
- Return to normal during recovery from the disease.

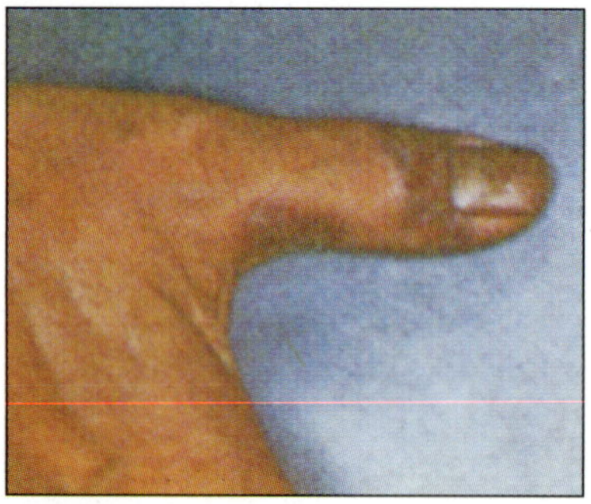

Fig 17.3 Beau's lines

Etiology

- Traumatic injury on the nail matrix.
- Dermatitis of the adjacent skin.

Treatment

- Needs no special treatment.
- Nails grow normally once the disease process is controlled.

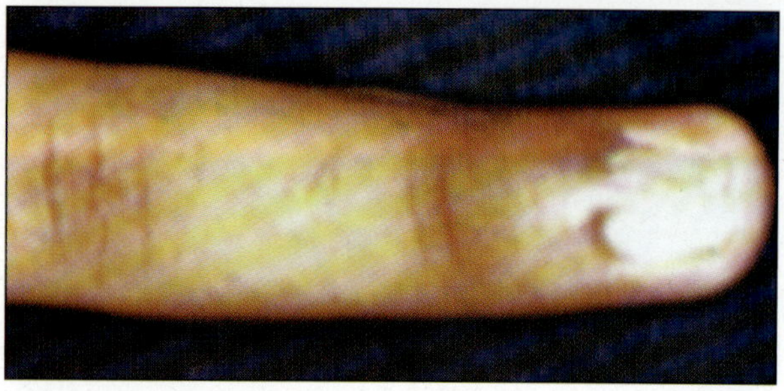

Fig 17.4 Pterygium unguis

Pterygium Unguis

Pterigium unguis occurs when an adhesion forms between the epidermis of the dorsal nail fold and the nail bed causing partial destruction of the nail plate (Fig. 17.4).

Etiology

- Lichen planus.
- Impaired circulation.
- Developmental defect.

Treatment

Treatment of the causative disease.

Koilonychia

Etiology

Commonly seen in hypochromic anaemia.

Clinical Features

- Nails become flat or concave (Fig. 17.5).
- Nails are usually thin and brittle.

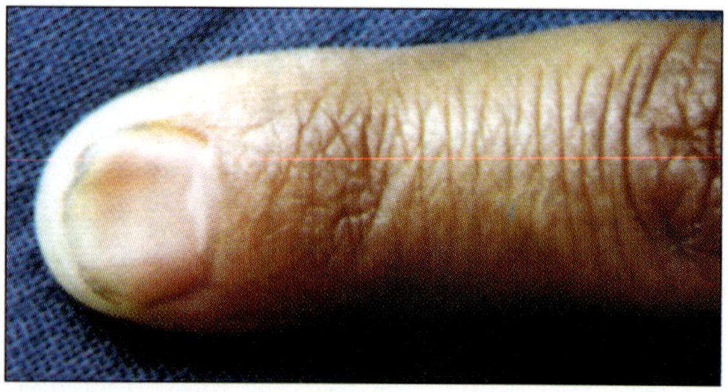

Fig 17.5 Koilonychia

Treatment

- Improvement is seen after treatment of the underlying disease.

- Recovery is slow and the nail takes longer time to return to normal.

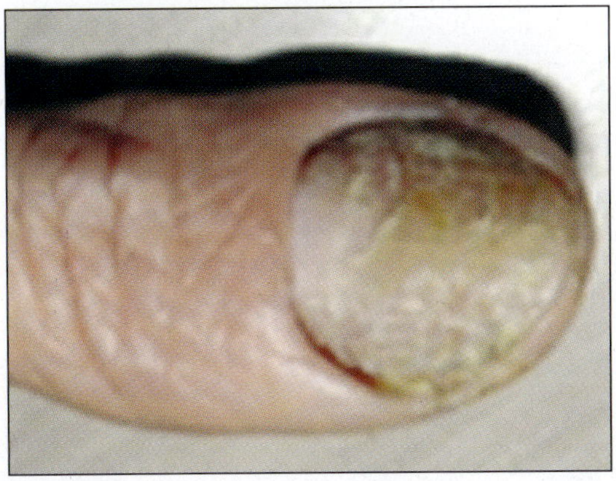

Fig 17.6 Nail changes in chronic paronychia

Paronychia

This is due to the involvement of posterior nail plate fold with *Candida albicans*. Sometimes, it is due to chronic inflammation of the posterior nail fold.

Clinical Features

- Nail changes occur due to paronychia (Fig. 17.6).
- Due to the posterior nail fold involvement and inflammation, multiple Beau's lines occur on the nails.

Treatment

- Avoidance of wetting of nail fold.
- Continuous application of anti-fungals and anti-inflammatory corticosteroid creams.

CHAPTER 18

Disorders of Pigmentation

PIGMENTATION OF SKIN

Colour of the skin depends on the oxidised and reduced forms of melanin, haemoglobin and carotenoids found in the keratin and subcutaneous fat. Differences in skin colour are related with the number, size, shape, distribution and degradation of melanosomes produced by melanocytes. Melanosomes contain melanin and are present in the basal layer of the epidermis. Each melanocyte is surrounded by a group of keratinocytes. The whole structure is known as **epidermal melanin unit**.

Formation of Melanin

The melanin is produced (Table 18.1) from an amino acid called tyrosine through a series of complex reactions. Tyrosine converts into **dihydroxyphenylamine** (DOPA) under the action of a copper-containing enzyme called tyrosinase. DOPA is further converted into dopaquinone by tyrosinase. Both these reactions require oxygen, are stimulated by sunlight and oxidising agents and are inhibited by reducing agents. Later on, through a series of non-enzymatic chemical reactions, dopaquinone gets converted to melanin. Melanin is transferred from the melanocytes to the surrounding keratinocytes. Pigment is ultimately lost through exfoliation of keratinocytes from the surface of epidermis.

DISORDERS OF PIGMENTATION

Etiology

Etiology for the disorders of pigmentation is presented in Table 18.2.

Table 18.2 Disturbances leading to disorders of pigmentation

Disturbances in the following:
- Formation of melanin.
- Transfer of melanin.
- Loss from the skin.
- Incontinence of melanin in the dermis (Table 18.4).
- Deposition of various extraneous pigments, e.g., due to drugs (Table 18.3).

Tanning

Tanning is the increase in the melanin pigmentation of skin after exposure to sunlight or ultra-violet light. Tanning is of two types—**immediate pigment darkening** (IPD) and delayed tanning.

Immediate Pigment Darkening

- In **immediate pigment darkening** (IPD) there is alteration in the distribution of melanosomes in melanocytes induced by both, the long wave (320–380 nm), as well as visible light (400–700 nm).
- The reaction is instantaneous and reaches a maximum 1–2 hours after exposure to sunlight.
- It slowly decreases during the next 3–24 hours on going to dark.

Table 18.3 Drugs causing hyperpigmentation

Drugs	Type of hyperpigmentation
Clofazimine	Dark pigmentation, especially of leprosy lesions.
Psoralens	Brown pigmentation.
Minocycline	Blue-black deposits in healing acne lesions. Discoloration of shins and mucosae.
Bleomycin	Generalised hyperpigmentation.
Busulphan	Generalised hyperpigmentation.

Delayed Tanning

- This occurs due to the formation of new melanosomes, i.e., neomelanogenesis. The melanocytes often increase in number and size.

Table 18.1 Formation of melanin

Tyrosine —Tyrosinase (0) Slow→ DOPA —Tyrosinase (0) Fast→ DOPA quinone → Eumelanine / Melanin / Phaeomelanin

Table 18.4 Differences in epidermal and dermal pigmentation

Epidermal pigmentation	Dermal pigmentation
Brown.	Slate grey.
Inceased by wood's lamp.	Not increased by wood's lamp.
Due to increase in the number of melanocytes or melanin in the epidermis.	Due to the presence of melanin in the dermis.

- Occurs 48–72 hours after exposure to light.
- DOPA reaction is markedly increased.

Chloasma

Synonym

Melasma.

Etiology

Estrogens play a role as the condition mainly affects the pregnant women in their first trimester, or the women who are on oral contraceptives.

Clinical Features

- Asymptomatic, superficial, brownish pigmentation mainly seen in women.
- In some patients, it becomes more prominent after exposure to the sun.

Sites

- On the bridge of the nose, both cheeks (Figs 18.1 – 18.4), upper lip and forehead.
- The lesions are usually bilateral and often symmetrical.

Precipitating factors for chloasma are presented in Table 18.5.

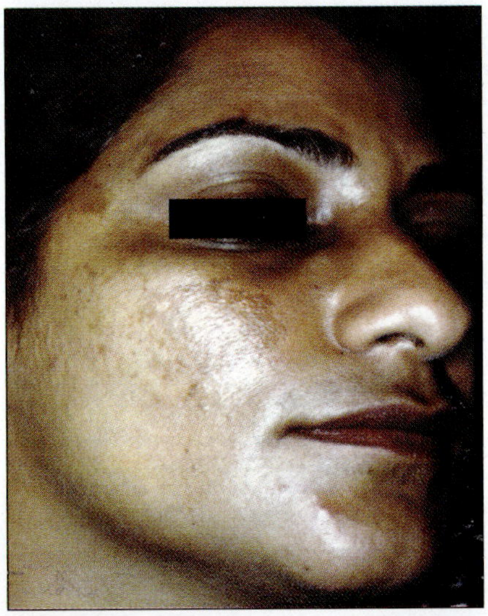

Fig. 18.1 Chloasma

Table 18.5 Precipitating factors for chloasma

- Pregnancy.
- Contraceptive pills.
- Hydantoin.
- Disturbed menstrual cycle.
- Persistent anaemia.
- Chronic gastrointestinal infestations.
- Excessive bleeding.
- Liver disorders.

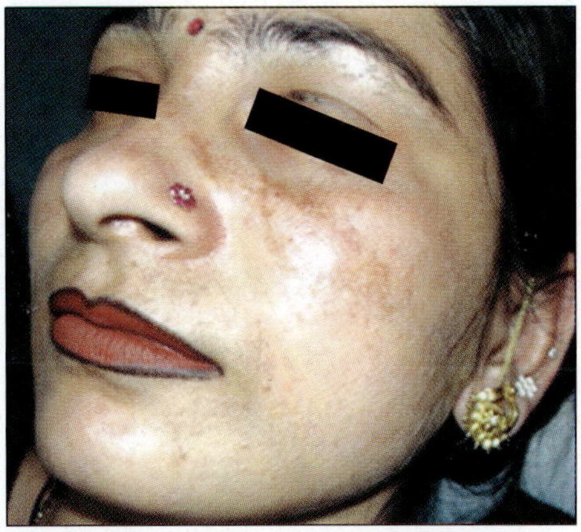

Fig. 18.2 Chloasma

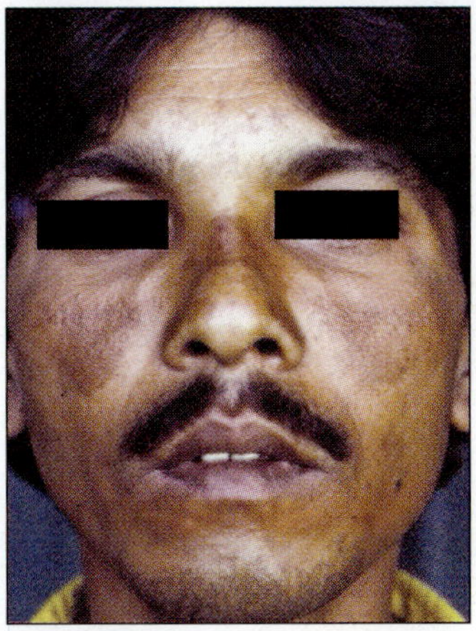

Fig. 18.3 Chloasma: male

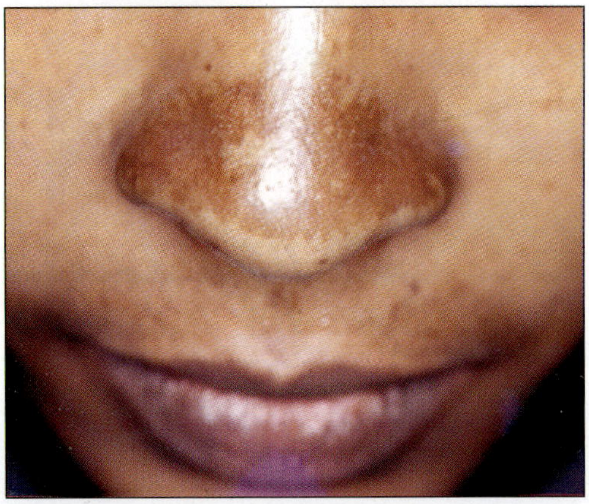

Fig. 18.4 Chloasma: bridge of the nose

Treatment

Treat the following underlying causes:
- Endocrine disorders.
- Anaemia.
- Gastrointestinal infestations.
- Liver disorder.

The following medication helps in treating this condition:
- Local massage of 2–5% hydroquinone with or without tretinoic acid 0.025–0.05% cream at night.
- Other agents include azelaic acid and glycolic acid.
- For **resistant lesions**, chemical peeling is done by using 20% alpha-hydroxy acid or 20–50% glycolic acid etc.
- Photosensitive lesions are to be protected with sunscreen.

Melanoderma Toxica

Etiology

Unknown

Clinical Features

- Asymptomatic, multiple, pin-point, brownish, hyperpigmented macules and areas are present on major parts of the face (Fig. 18.5), neck, chest and arms.
- Sometimes itching and erythema with pigmentation is seen.
- Small pigmented macules (mainly follicular) are present on the legs and forearms.
- New lesions keep on appearing for a few weeks to months.

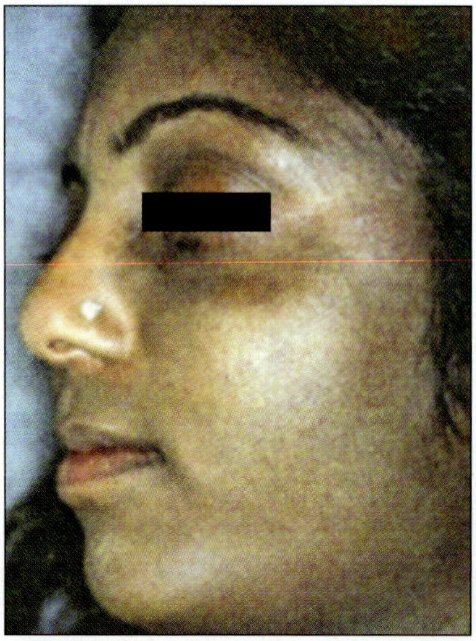

Fig. 18.5 Melanoderma toxica

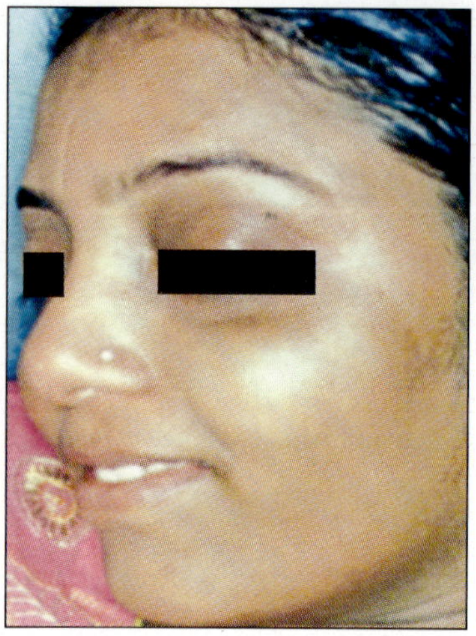

Fig. 18.6 Melanoderma toxica: after treatment

Treatment

- The lesions disappear spontaneously over a period of several months to few years.
- Systemic corticosteroids are given, in active phase of the disease in a dose of 15–20 mg prednisolone daily. It takes about 6–8 weeks for new lesions to stop appearing when the corticosteroids should be slowly tapered and stopped.
- Hyperpigmentation in most of the cases disappears in the due course. Local massage of hydroquinone 2–5% along with retinoic acid at night helps in fast disappearance of the lesions (Fig. 18.6).

Berloque Dermatitis

Etiology

Here the phototoxicity results from the effect of long wave ultraviolet radiation (320–400 nm) on bergamot oil or 5 methoxypsorlen (the photoactive component in bergamot oil).

Bergamot oil is found in the following items of day-to-day use:

i) Perfumes.
ii) Cosmetics.
iii) Oils used for hair or skin.

Clinical Features

- Deep brown pigmentation seen on the affected areas.
- Lesions are present as minute punctate spots if the perfume was used as a spray.
- If perfume was applied with the hand or cotton balls, lesions are seen as irregular smudges.

- Linear streaks with drop-like appearance are seen if the perfume flows down from the area of application.
- In cases of hair oil, the pigmentation is more prominently seen around the forehead, ears and side of face.
- Upper-central part of the back in women, not covered by the clothing, is also affected.

Treatment

- Pigmentation fades spontaneously after a few months, if further exposure to the causative agents is avoided.
- Duration can be shortened with the local massage of hydroquinone 2–5% with retinoic acid 0.025–0.05% at night.

Phytophotodermatitis

Etiology

It is an inflammatory and pigmentary reaction of the skin towards sunlight in the presence of chemicals 'furocoumarins' found in some plants.

Clinical Features

- History of contact with plants containing furocoumarins and simultaneous exposure to sunlight.

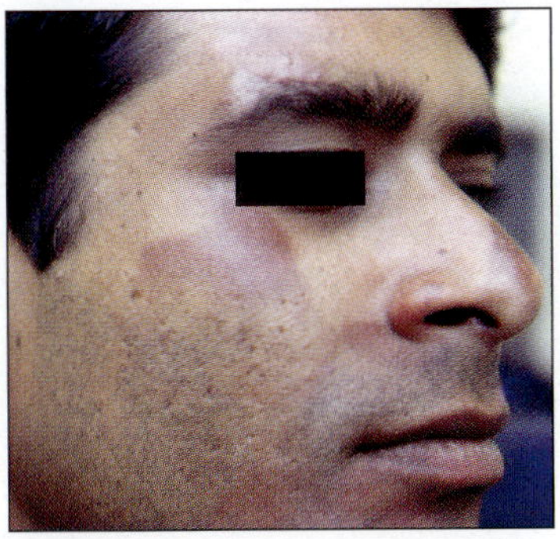

Fig. 18.7 Post inflammatory hyperpigmentation

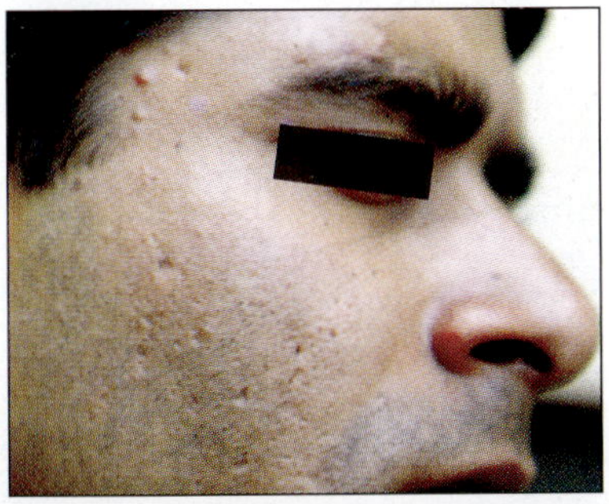

Fig. 18.8 Post inflammatory hyperpigmentation: after treatment

- Hyperpigmentation is seen in cases with mild reaction (Figs 18.7–18.11).
- Blister or bullae on the exposed area may occur if the reaction is severe.
- Shape and size of the lesions depend upon the types of the offending agents.

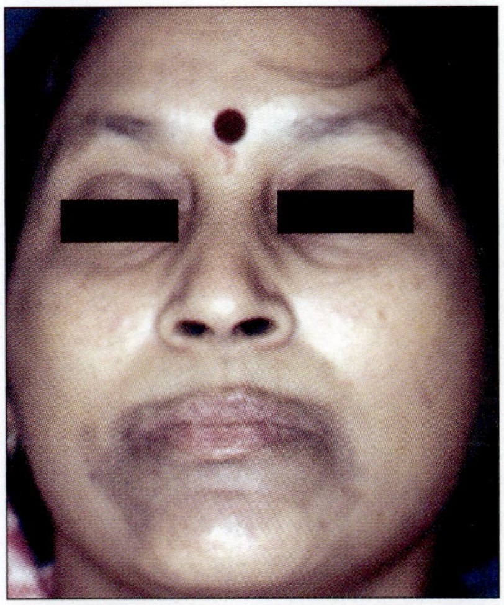

Fig. 18.9 Perioral pigmentation

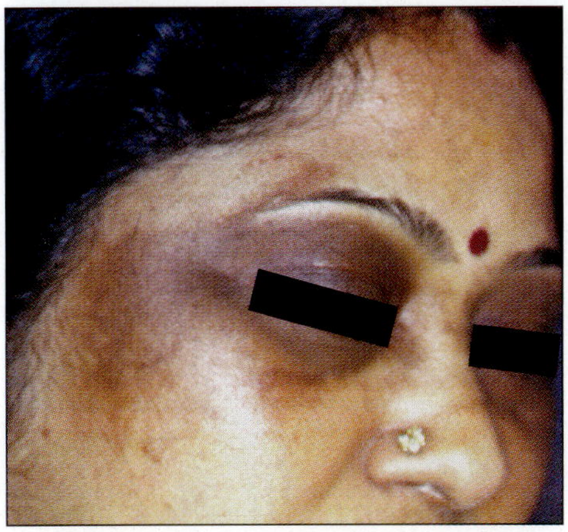

Fig. 18.10 Periorbital pigmentation

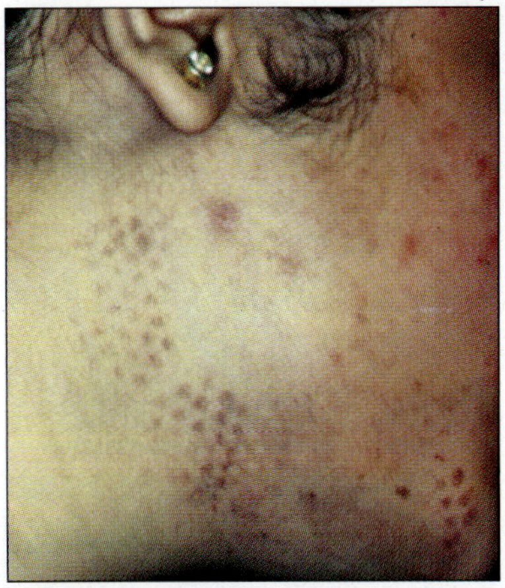

Fig. 18.11 Post inflammatory hyperpigmentation: after laser

Treatment

- Find out the causative agent and avoid further exposures to the same and other similar agents.
- Skin should be protected from sunlight.
- Severe reaction should be controlled with oral corticosteroids in a dose of 15–20 mg prednisolone, daily for 4–5 days.
- Old lesions disappear spontaneously in due course. The hyperpigmentation may take several months to clear.
- Local application of hydroquinone 2–5% and retinoic acid 0.025–0.05% at night clear the hyperpigmentation faster.

Vitiligo

Etiology

The disease occurs due to stoppage of melanin formation by the melanocytes.

Autoimmune Mechanism

Lesions of vitiligo associated with autoimmue disease are caused by autoimmune mechanisms where auto-antibodies destroy the melanocytes resulting in depigmentation.

Neurogenic Mechanism

Segmental vitiligo (Fig. 18.12) is very difficult to differentiate from naevus achromicus, except that it appears later and is supposed to be due to neurogenic stimuli.

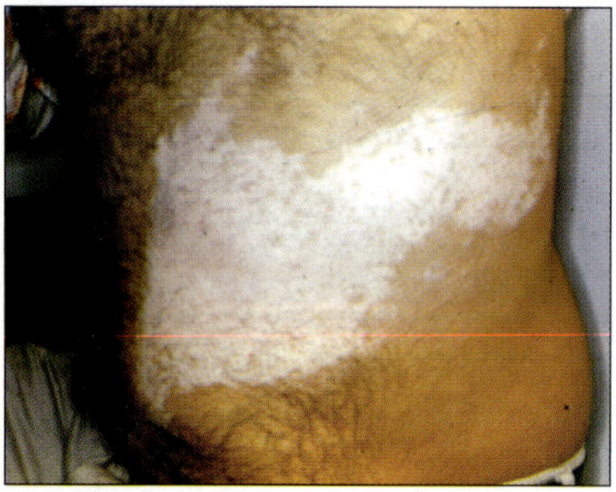

Fig. 18.12 Vitiligo: segmental on abdomen

Melanocytes self destruction is due to a defect in the natural protective mechanism which removes toxic melanin precursors.

In a large number of cases, the cause still remains unknown.

Clinical Features

The lesions appear any time after birth.

- Asymptomatic depigmented macules are seen.
- Macules vary in size and shape, as well as in colour. In some lesions, the hair are also white called **leucotrichia** (Fig. 18.19).
- Margins of the lesions are usually well-defined and occasionally hyperpigmented. Sometimes the depigmented centre is surrounded by a hypopigmented rim, which in turn has normal pigmented skin around it (trichrome).

Sites

Anywhere on the body including mucous membranes of lips and genitalia (Figs 18.13–18.25, 18.27–18.31 and 18.35).

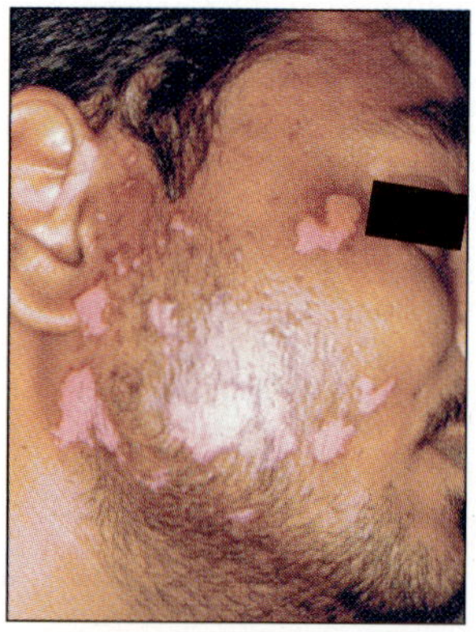

Fig. 18.13 Vitiligo: face

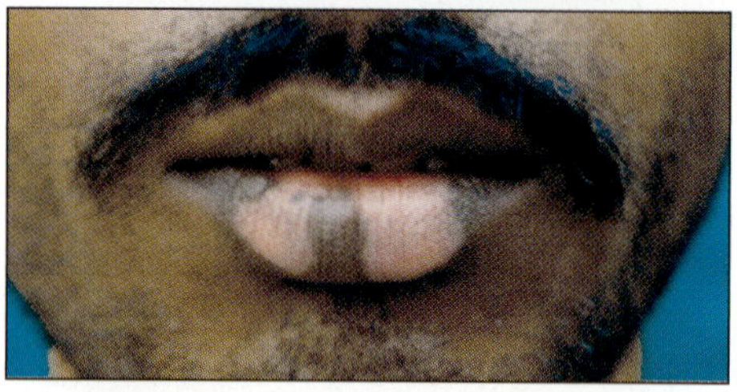

Fig. 18.14 Vitiligo: lips

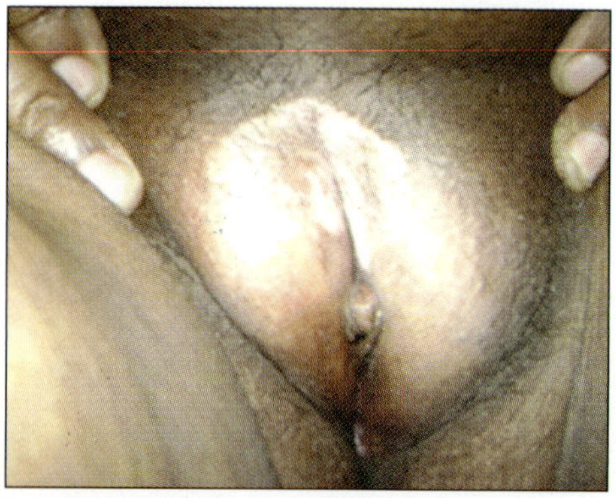

Fig. 18.15 Vitiligo: vagina

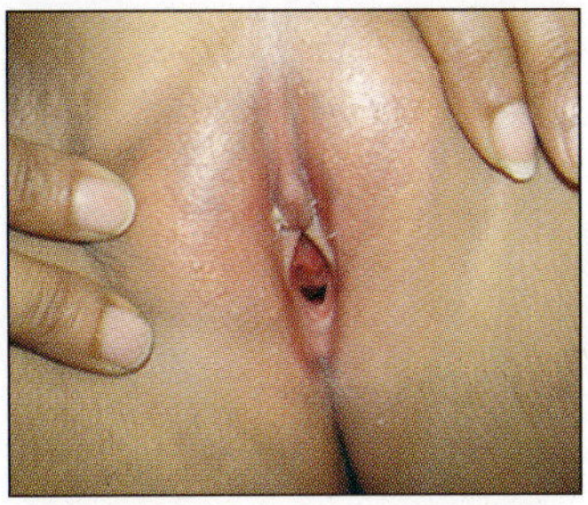

Fig. 18.16 Vitiligo: vagina

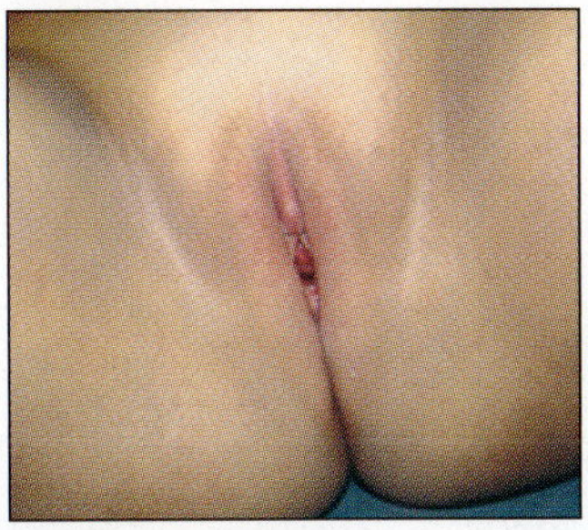

Fig. 18.17 Vitiligo: vagina treated

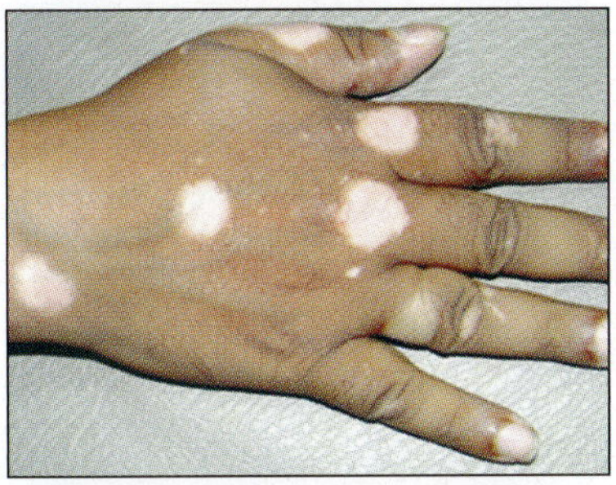

Fig. 18.18 Vitiligo: dorsum of hand

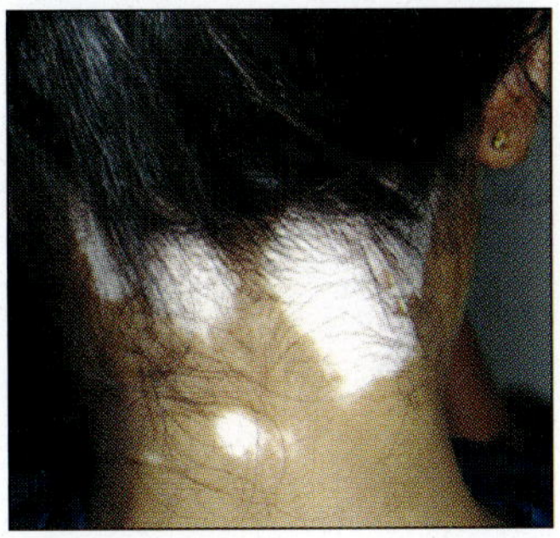

Fig. 18.19 Vitiligo: back of neck

Histopathology

There is marked reduction or even absence of melanocytes and melanin in the epidermis.

Histochemical

There is lack of DOPA-positive melanocytes in the basal layer of epidermis.

Degenerating melanocytes are seen especially at the margins of vitiligo in few cases.

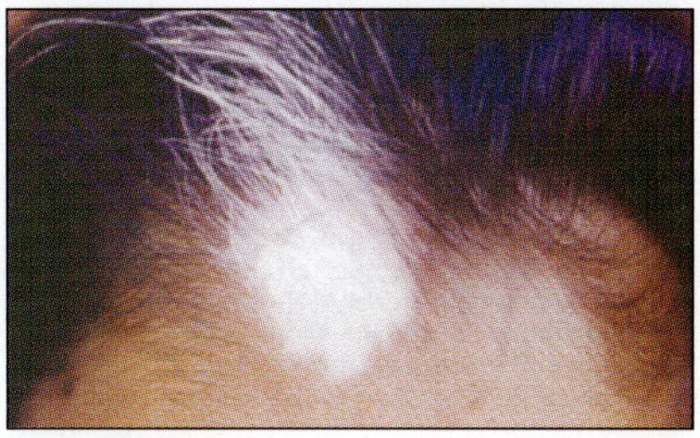

Fig. 18.20 Leucotrichia

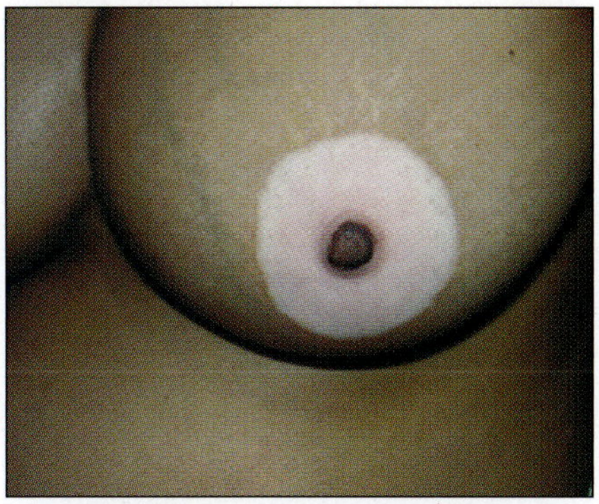

Fig. 18.21 Vitiligo: nipple

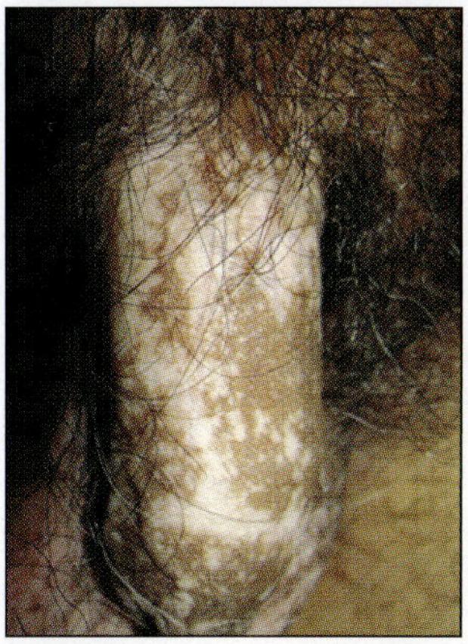

Fig. 18.22 Vitiligo: penis

Course

The course of this disorder is variable—static to progressive, or very fast. The repigmentation is usually perifollicular.

Table 18.6 Causes of vitiligo

- Transmitted by an autosomal dominant gene with irregular penetration.
- 10–30% of the patients have some relative having vitiligo.
- Vitiligo seen on the flanks of some ladies who wear tight string petticoats are due to prolonged pressure.
- Lesions occur very frequently on knees, elbows, ankles, knuckles and other areas of skin subjected to repeated trauma
- Linear lesions are seen at the site of scratching (Koebner's phenomenon)
- Repeated trauma, even a minor one, may produce depigmentation.

Table 18.7 Diseases associated with vitiligo

- Hyper and hypothyroidism.
- Pernicious anaemia.
- Addison's disease.
- Diabetes mellitus.
- Malignant melanoma.
- Halo naevus.

Treatment

Response to the treatment is slow:

- Pigmentation of the lesions usually starts around the hair follicles.
- Lesions in the hairy area show early and quick response.
- Repigmentation also starts at the margins of the lesion.
- There is no scientific basis for any dietary restrictions, e.g., avoidance of citrus fruits and vitamin C.

General

- Vitiligo is an absolutely harmless disease, except for its cosmetic implications.

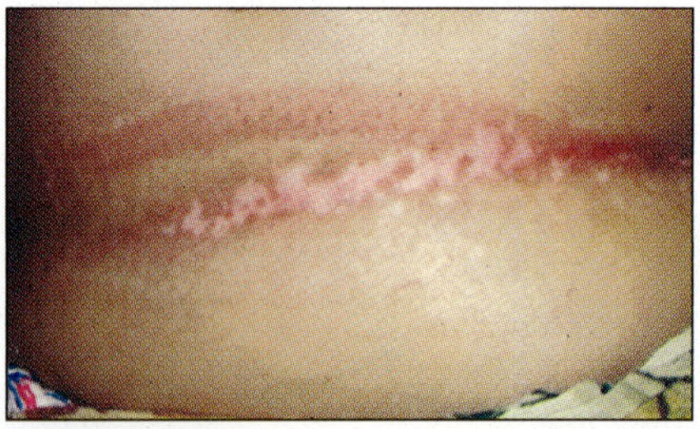

Fig. 18.23 Vitiligo: waist

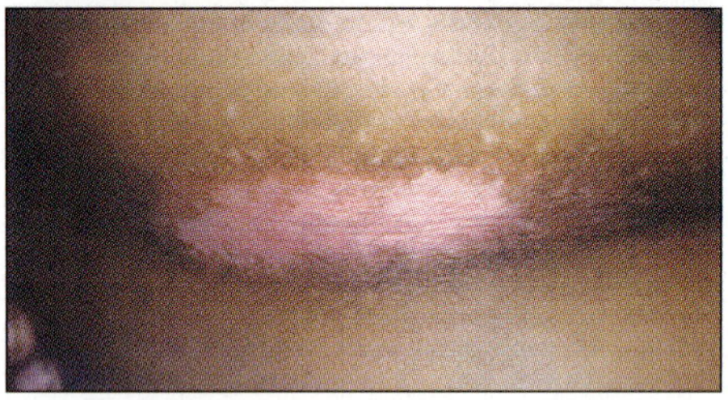

Fig. 18.24 Vitiligo waist: on treatment

- A patient of vitiligo can be as efficient physically, mentally and sexually as any other individual.

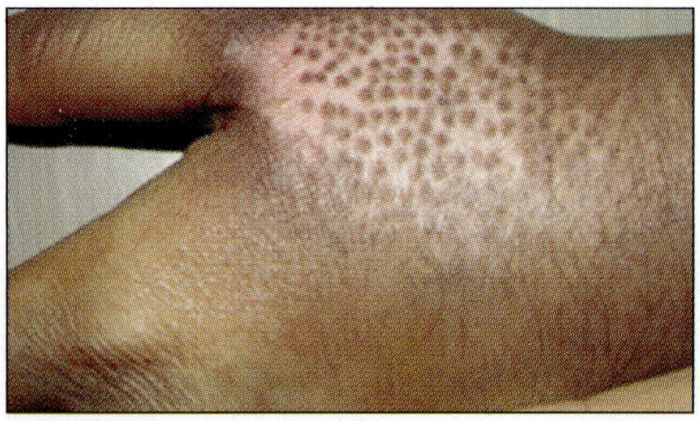

Fig. 18.25 Vitiligo: on treatment

- Any known factors causing vitiligo like pressure, trauma, etc. should be removed or minimised as far as possible (Fig 18.23 and 18.24).
- Nails should be trimmed and filed.

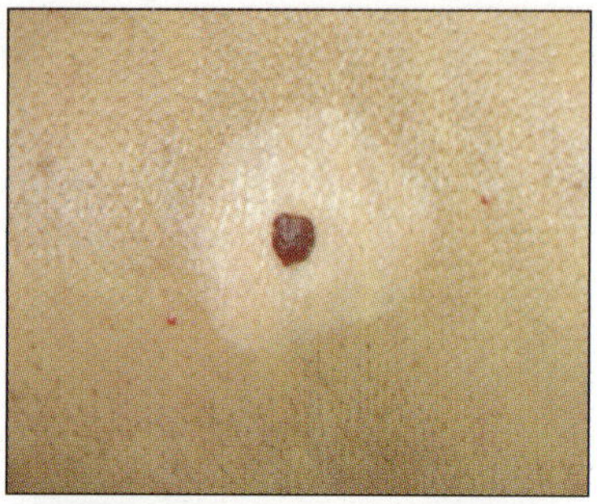

Fig. 18.26 Halo naevus

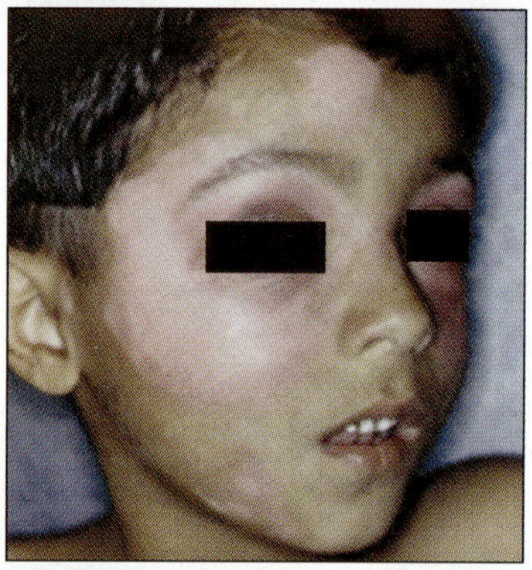

Fig. 18.27 Vitiligo face with erythema

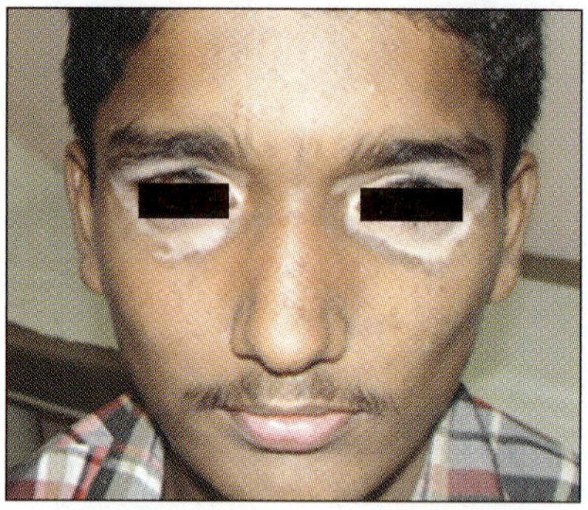

Fig. 18.28 Vitiligo: periorbital

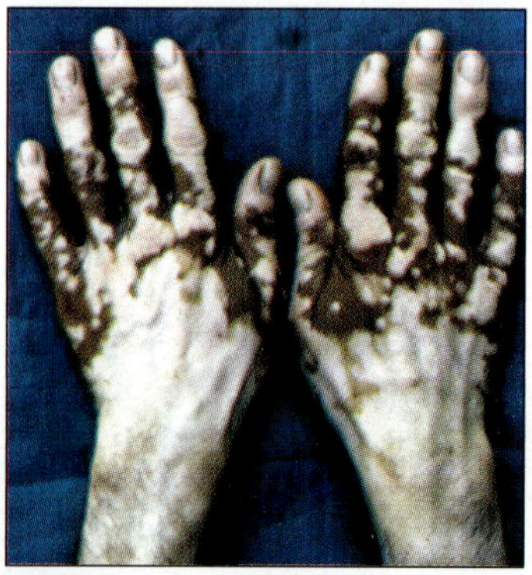

Fig. 18.29 Vitiligo: acral

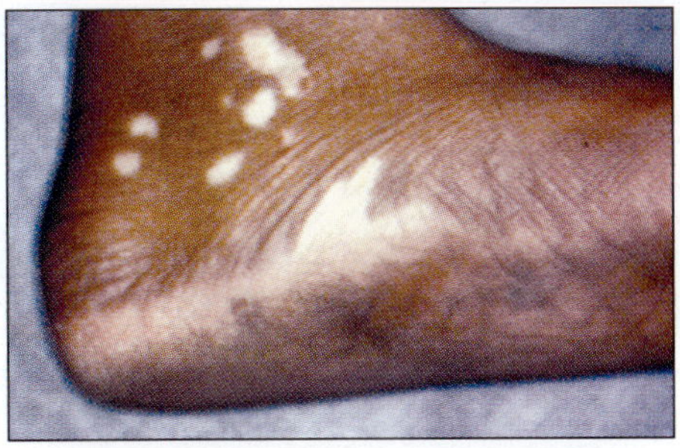

Fig. 18.30 Vitiligo: ankle

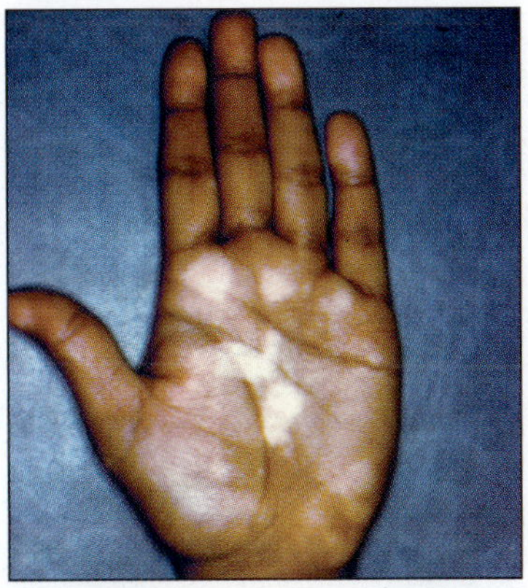

Fig. 18.31 Vitiligo: palm

Medical

Medical management of vitiligo is presented in Table 18.8.

Table 18.8 Medical treatment of vitiligo

- Psoralens or its derivative: 10–20 mg, orally
- Psoralens topical application followed by one of the following treatments:
  i) Exposure to ultravoilet-A from an artificial source (PUVA).
  ii) Sunlight (PUVASOL) after 2–4 hours.
- Exposure to sunlight between 10 A.M. to 2 P.M. when the UVA is maximum.

Slow Spreading Disease

For the slow spreading disease, levamisol, 50–150 mg, on two consecutive days is given orally every week.

Fast Spreading Disease

For the fast spreading disease, oral corticosteroids equivalent to betamethasone 2.5–5 mg, given on two consecutive days, every week, has been found very effective.

Other Drugs

- Topical corticosteroids and placental extracts.
- For lesions that have stopped improving further and are static, camouflage with an appropriate shade of cream for temporary concealing of the lesions is done.

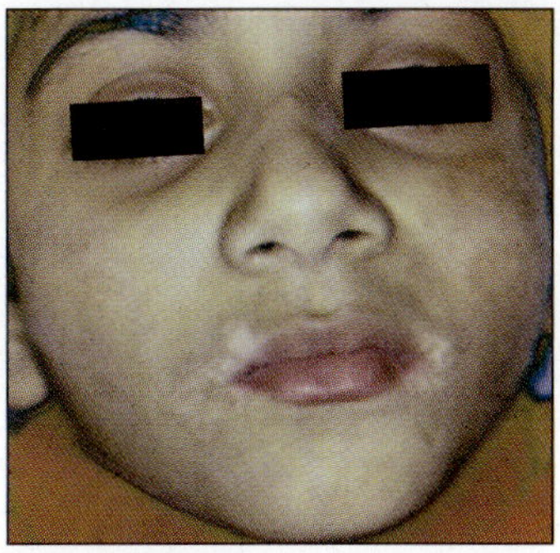

Fig. 18.32 Vitiligo: after herpes simplex

Response to Treatment

The response to treatment is very poor and incomplete in the following conditions:

- Extensive vitiligo.
- Lesions with leucotrichia of long duration.
- Lesions located on non-hairy areas like palms, soles, fingertips or mucosae.

Surgery

- In vitiligo with halo naevi, excision of the pigmented mole(s) initiates the repigmentation in the lesions (Fig. 18.26).
- Dermabrading the depigmented area and covering it (Fig. 18.33) with the following:
  i) Split thickness graft.
  ii) Suction blister graft.
  iii) Melanocyte graft.

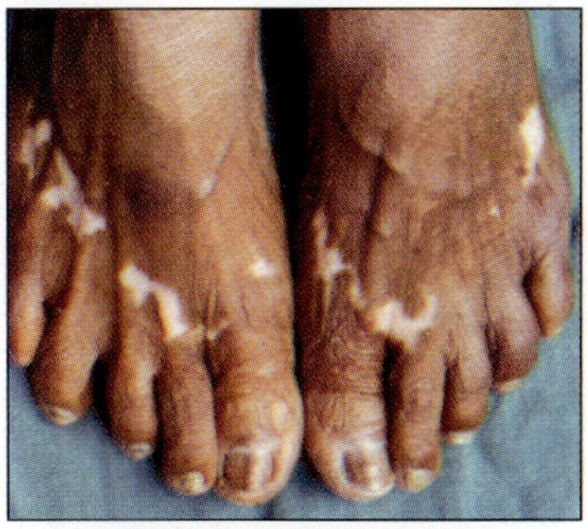

Fig. 18.33 Acquired vitiligo due to chappal

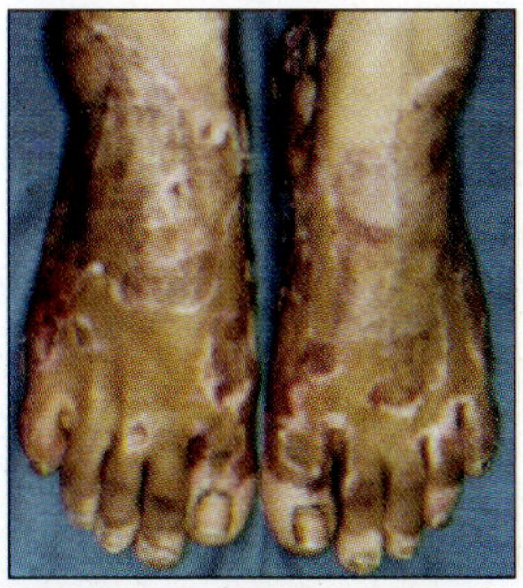

Fig. 18.34 Pigmentation on vitiligo 6 weeks after graft

The graft is taken from another area of the body preferably antero-lateral aspect of the thighs. Multiple punches of normal skin can be grafted in different areas of depigmented lesions

Acquired Vitiligo

Synonym: Leucoderma

Etiology

Caused by the action of **monobenzyl ether of hydroquinone** (MBH) or substituted phenols:

- P-tertiary butyl phenol.
- P-tertiary amyl phenol.

These are used as accelerators and anti-oxidants in the manufacturing of rubber and plastic.

Clinical Features

Vitiligo-like lesions are seen on the following areas:

- Dorsum of the feet corresponding to the straps of the slippers or shoes (Fig. 18.34).
- Hands due to plastic or rubber gloves.
- Forehead where the plastic bindi is applied.
- Breast corresponding to the area in contact with the purse (usually tucked in the blouse).
- On both breasts if the patient wears rubber-padded brassieres.
- Many of these patients might develop allergic contact dermatitis at the site prior to the development of depigmentation.

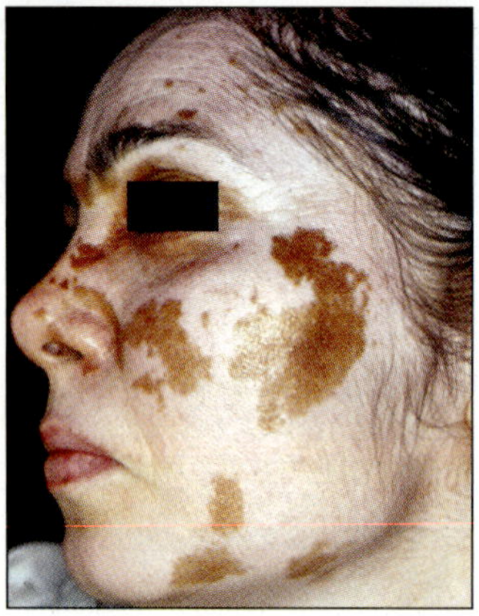

Fig. 18.35 Pigmentation of face in generalised vitiligo

Treatment

- The area of depigmentation may or may not repigment even after removal of the causative agents and adequate treatment.
- Systemic treatment for leucoderma is the same as of vitiligo.

Tattooing

This is a method of camouflaging (Fig. 18.36).

Method

- Opaque dye either of a black colour or a mixture of red, yellow, black and brown is deposited in the superficial dermis to compensate for the absence of melanin.
- The dyes should not react with the tissues.
- Tattooing should be used as a last resort, an alternative to the surgery.
- Disease should be inactive.

Limitation

One can still make out that the skin in this region is not normal.

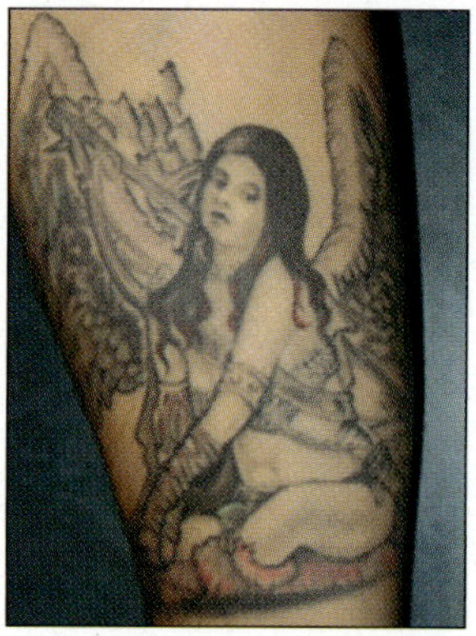

Fig. 18.36 Tattoo

Albinism

This is a heterogeneous group of disorders with the following variations:

- Complete absence of melanin pigment in the skin, hair and eyes, or in the eyes alone.

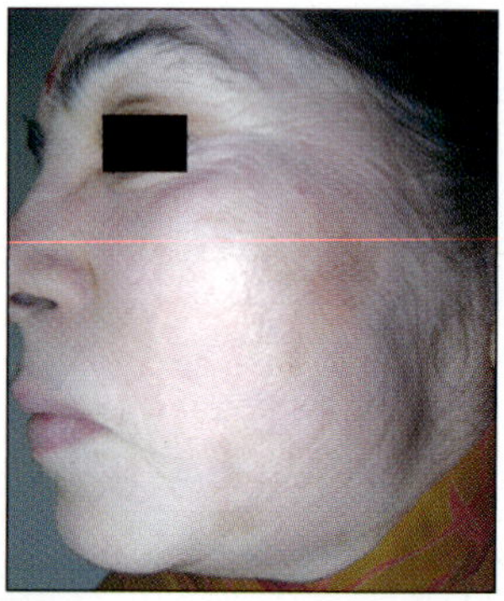

Fig. 18.37 Albinism

- In **oculocutaneous albinism** (OCA), both skin and eyes are involved.

- In **ocular albinism** (OA), the lesion is limited to eyes only.
- There are ten types of oculocutaneous and four types of ocular albinism.
- OCA is transmitted as an autosomal recessive characteristic, except for the one which is transmitted as X-linked recessive characteristic.
- Patients have normal numbers of melanocytes, but they are unable to produce the melanin because of defective melanosomes,
- Some types are tyrosinase are positive, while others are negative.

Clinical Features

- The whole skin including the hair is completely white, with eyes showing prominent red reflex especially in tyrosinase-negative types (Figs 18.37 and 18.38).

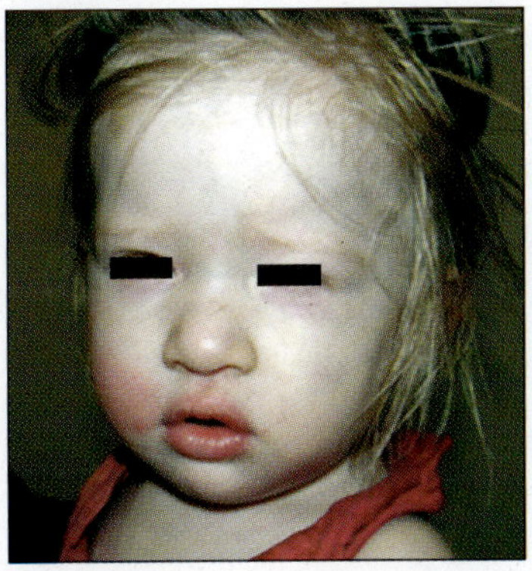

Fig. 18.38 Albino Child

- Both types show moderate to severe photophobia and nystagmus, which become more prominent in bright light.

Changes are present at birth and remain throughout life.

- Tyrosinase-positive patients develop some pigment in the skin, hair and iris with increasing age.
- The patients may tan and develop dark brown freckles, especially in the sun exposed areas.

X-linked Ocular Albinism

- Only eye symptoms are present.
- Skin and hair show normal pigmentation.
- In yellow mutant type of albinism, the hair turns yellow-red in colour by the age of one year.
- Increased sensitivity to sunlight is present.

Complications

There is an increased tendency to develop the following complications:

- Actinic keratoses.
- Squamous cell carcinoma.
- Occasionally, even melanomas.

Treatment

- No treatment is available.
- Skin should be protected from sunlight by covering maximum body surface with clothes.
- Application of local sunscreen.
- Patients should be advised to work mostly indoors.
- Regular check-up for pre-malignant and malignant lesions is to be done.

Chapter 19

Allergic Disorders

ALLERGIC REACTIONS

An individual is exposed to a large variety of agents in the environment, e.g., food, physical agents like heat, cold, sunlight, etc., drugs prescribed by the doctor for different diseases, clothes, jewellery, cosmetics, a variety of inhalants which are breathed in unknowingly, a large number of micro-organisms, parasites, plants and animals. Though each one of these is capable of causing allergic reactions in some specific individuals, generally they do not produce any harmful effects. Occasionally, the body reacts in an abnormal manner and starts forming antibodies or sensitised lymphocytes against such substances.

Common observations about the allergic disorders and their clinical manifestations are summarised in Tables 19.1 and 19.2.

Table 19.1 Common observations about allergy

- Allergy or sensitivity is seen more frequently to the substances which are more commonly used.
- Some substances produce more frequent allergic reactions than the others, and thus are more potent antigens.
- Some individuals are more prone to develop allergic reactions.
- Once an individual develops allergy to a particular substance, every subsequent exposure to that substance would result in recurrence of the allergic reaction unless the exposure is inadequate.
- If further exposure to causative or its chemically related substances is prevented, the allergic reaction would improve even without any treatment, unless it has been complicated by secondary infection or changes.

Table 19.2 Factors affecting the clinical manifestations of allergy

- The nature of the antigen.
- Its mode of entry into the body.
- The target tissue organ.

ALLERGIC DERMATOSES

Various allergic dermatoses seen in day-to-day practice are presented in Table 19.3.

Table 19.3 Common allergic dermatoses

- Urticaria.
- Contact dermatitis.
- Drug allergy.
- Atopic dermatitis.

Urticaria

Clinical Features

- Manifests as a sudden appearance of itchy wheals (Figs 19.1–19.5).
- The lesions vary in size and shapes from very small circular lesions to very large irregular areas.
- They can be located on any part, or nearly all over the body.
- The wheals disappear within 24 hours even without any treatment, though fresh ones may continue to appear.

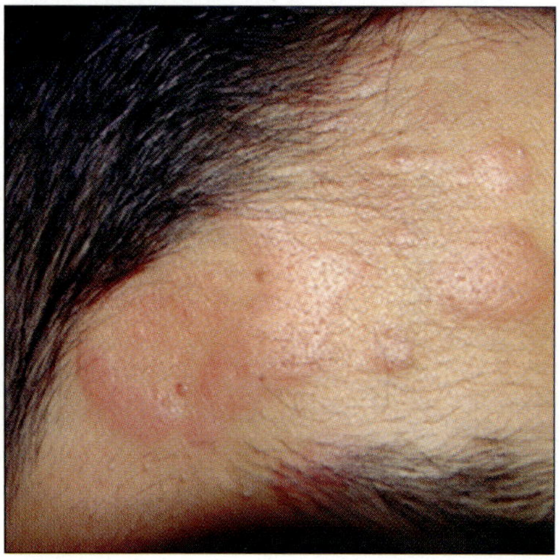

Fig. 19.1 Urticaria

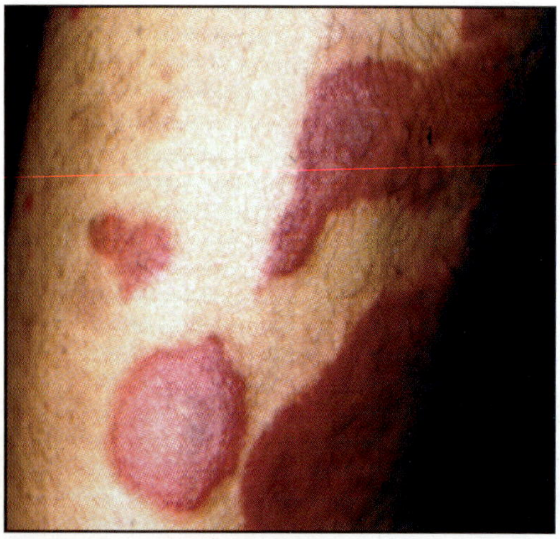

Fig. 19.2 Urticarial wheal

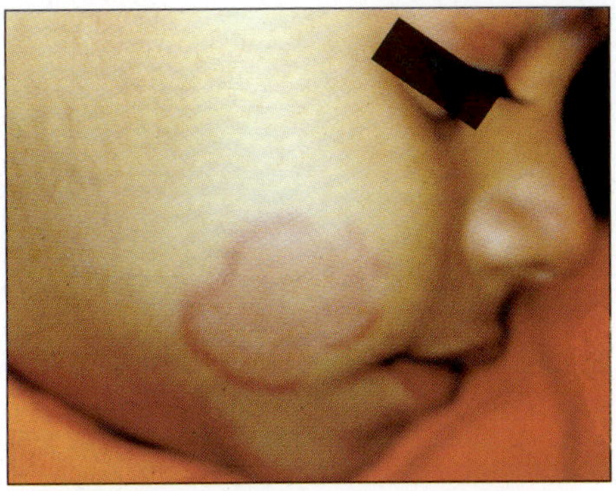

Fig. 19.3 Urticaria: face (child)

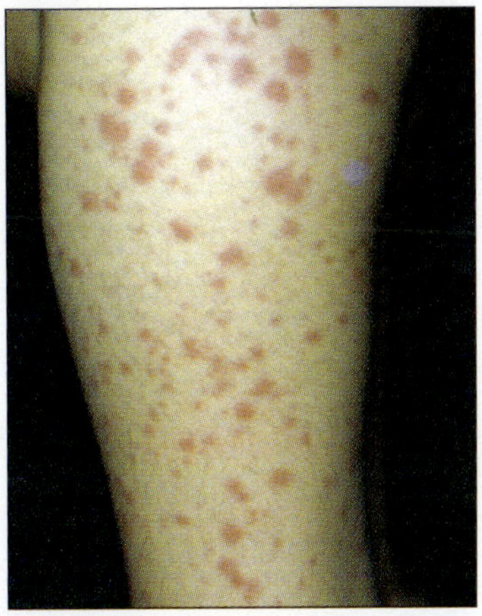

Fig. 19.4 Urticaria: small wheal (leg)

- Severe attacks may be associated with abdominal pain, nausea, vomiting and headache with high fever (especially in children). In adults, fever is infrequent.
- All the responses are mediated by histamine.
- Most cases of urticaria are type I hypersensitivity reactions (Table 19.4).

Table 19.4 Type I hypersensitivity

- Mediated by IgE antibodies fixed on the surface of mast cells and basophils.
- As a result of antigen–antibody reaction on the mast cell, degranulation of mast cells occurs.
- This leads to the release of histamine which causes itching, vasodilatation and increased permeability of blood vessels resulting in the formation of wheals.
- Sometimes urticaria is due to Type III hyper- sensitivity reaction (Table 19.5) and is mediated by IgG antibodies.

Table 19.5 Type III hypersensitivity

- Mediated by IgG antibodies.
- Form immune complexes with antigens.
- This leads to the release of vasoactive substances from complement components which release histamine with the formation of wheals.
- Such types of urticaria are usually associated with arthritis, arthralgias, albuminuria and fever even in adults.

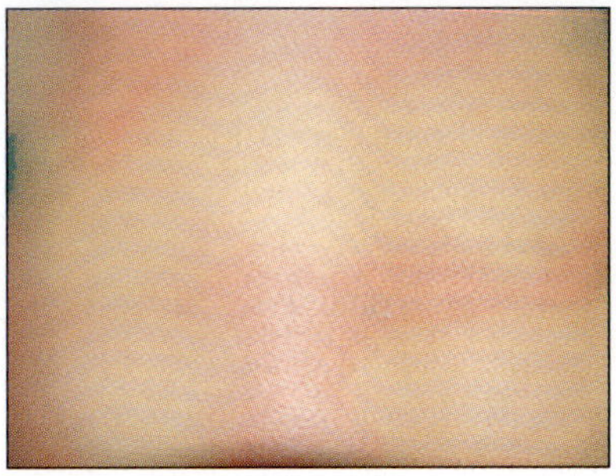

Fig. 19.5 Urticaria: back

Etiology

Various causes of urticaria are summarised in (Table 19.6).

Cold Urticaria

Cold urticaria occurrs due to cold. It can be familial or acquired.

Table 19.6 Causes of urticaria

Drugs By allergic reactions • Salicylates • Penicillins • Sulphonamides • Tetracyclines	By non-allergic mechanism causing direct degranulation of the mast cells • Salicylates • Polymyxin B • Morphine and • Curare
Foods	Meat, fish, eggs, milk, wheat, rice, pulses, nuts, potato, or anything which contains sufficient amount of protein.
Inhalants	Pollen, fungal spores, fragments of insects, human and animal dander present in the dust.
Septic foci	Present anywhere in the body like tonsils, paranasal sinuses, teeth, bones, kidneys, gall-bladder, etc.
Gastrointestinal parasites: Many of the parasites, when they pass through the skin and/or lungs during their larval stage, may produce urticaria.There is no proof yet that adult parasite of gastrointestinal tract cause urticaria. **Physical causes:** Cold, heat, pressure.	
Other causes of urticaria: • Viral and fungal infections. • Autoimmune disorders. • Malignant diseases.	

Table 19.7 Differences between urticarial vasculitis and urticaria

Urticarial vasculitis	Uricaria
Lesions last longer than 72 hours.	Evanescent.
Subside with scaling, bruising and hyperpigmentation.	Subsides without residual changes.
May be associated with abdominal pain and arthritis.	Only occasionally associated with abdominal pain.

Familial Cold Urticaria

- Positive family history.
- Its occurrence is very rare.

- Presenting symptoms are a huge swelling with fever and leucocytosis.
- It appears on exposure to cold.

Acquired Cold Urticaria

Usually occurs in otherwise healthy individuals. However in some cases, it occurs due to cryoglobulins associated with the following conditions:

- Lymphoma.
- Collagen vascular diseases.
- Secondary syphilis etc.

The precipitating factors for cold urticaria are summarised in Table 19.8.

Table 19.8 Conditions causing precipitation of acquired cold urticaria

- Cold water bath.
- Washing hands with cold water.
- Exposure to cold, early in the morning or late in the evening.
- Exposure to winds after getting drenched in the rain.
- Sitting under the fan while sweating.
- Intake of ice cold food or drink.
- Touching or holding cold objects.
- Going to hill station.
- Entering into an air-conditioned room.

Cholinergic Urticaria

Etiology

Urticaria occurs due to acetylcholine, a chemical agent produced in the skin itself whenever the sweat glands get stimulated. Thus, any stimulus which produces sweating will precipitate urticaria in such patients. These stimuli may include heat of kitchen, fire, ovens, stoves, room heater, sunlight, physical exertion such as running, cycling, playing or any activity which can induce sweating, eating hot foods or beverages, eating spicy foods or any emotional upset which makes the individual sweat.

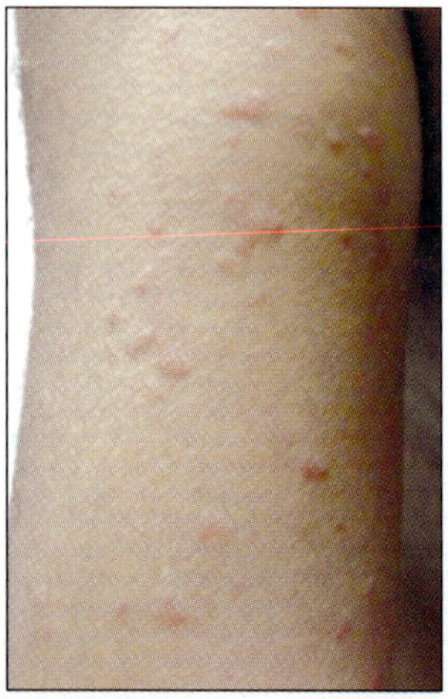

Fig. 19.6 Cholinergic urticaria

Clinical Features

Urticarial wheals in such patients are small and scattered (Fig. 19.6).

Diagnosis

Exaggerated responses are seen to intradermal injections of carbachol or to exercise.

Treatment

- The patient should avoid the corresponding hot stimuli.
- A regular use of antihistamines would also keep the attacks under control.

Solar Urticaria

Solar urticaria occurs only due to sunlight and not to heat from any other sources. The lesions may be limited to sun-exposed areas.

Pressure Urticaria

Pressure urticaria occurs due to a prolonged pressure as from the following sources:

- Tight belt.
- Straps of brassieres.
- Elastic band of socks.
- Sitting or putting arms on a hard surface for prolonged periods.

In such cases, urticaria develops only when the pressure is taken off from the site(s).

Dermographism

- This urticaria literally means 'writing on the skin'.
- In a majority of normal individuals, when the skin is stroked firmly with a blunt object, it results in the **triple response of Lewis**.
- Some patients develop urticarial wheal even on a light stroke on their skin.

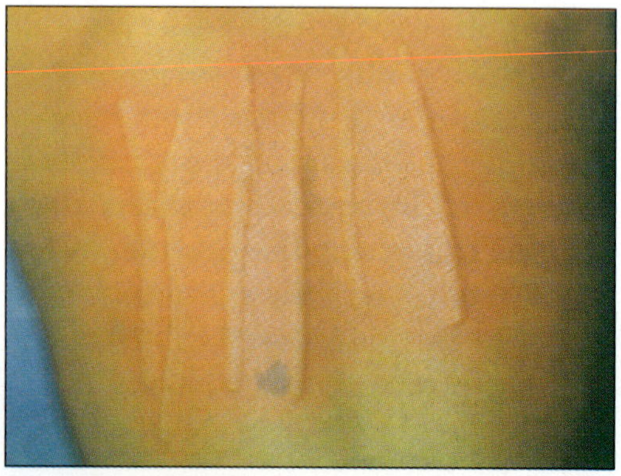

Fig. 19.7 Dermographism

- Lesions in such cases correspond to the stroked area and the impression is usually linear in shape (Fig. 19.7).

Angioedema

It is a variant of urticaria in which the oedema occurs deeper and involves the subcutaneous tissues.

Etiology

Causative factors are the same as urticaria.

Clinical Feature

- The lesions are larger and take 1–7 days to disappear and do not itch.
- Lesions are usually seen on the face (Figs. 19.8–19.10), hands or forearms as areas of swelling. However, they may be present anywhere on the body.

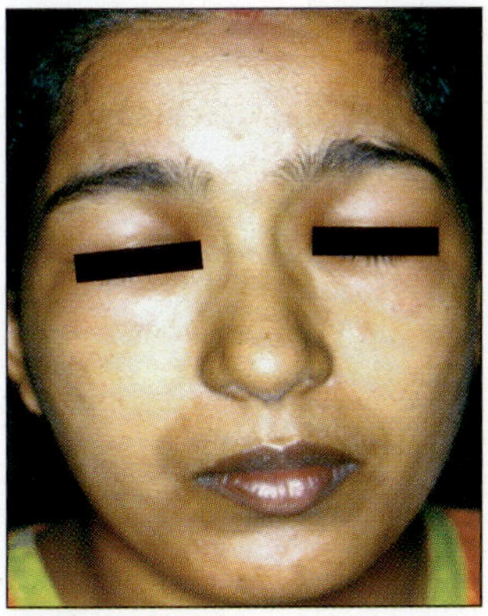

Fig. 19.8 Angioedema: swelling of eyes

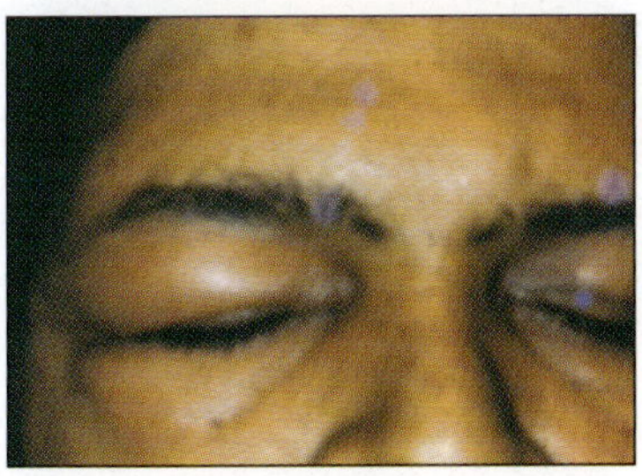

Fig. 19.9 Angioedema: intense swelling of eyes

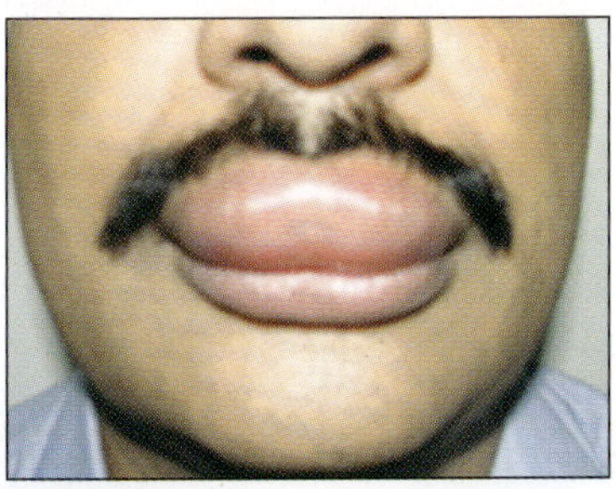

Fig. 19.10 Angioedema: lip

- If the lesions involve lips and tongue, oedema may extend to the larynx leading to the obstruction of air passages. This may even result in death. Such cases must be treated immediately as an emergency.

Treatment of Urticaria

- A detailed history is very important to trace the cause.
- Stool examination for parasites or their cysts confirm their presence in the gastrointestinal tract. This should be treated with appropriate medicines.

Urticaria due to Food

- May occur regularly after a single or each meal.
- Frequency may vary from one or two attacks in a week to several attacks in a day.
- When suspected to be due to a specific food item, urticaria disappears within 48 hours after stoppage of the causative food (**diet elimination test**).
- Recurrence of urticaria by giving a particular food is known as **provocation test.**

Treatment

Stop eating the particular offending item of food in all its forms.

Urticaria due to Inhalants

- May be seasonal or throughout the year.
- It improves spontaneously when the patients is shifted to some other place where the particular antigen is absent or its amount is lesser.
- Diagnosis is confirmed by breathing through an ordinary cloth mask for 48 hours to see if the urticaria disappears.

Treatment

- These patients should avoid the places where the antigen is in plenty.
- Use nasal filter to prevent the antigen from entering the inhaled air.

Urticaria due to Cold

Appearance of urticaria on the skin of these patients by exposure to cold or cryostimulation test or ice-filled test tube will confirm the diagnosis. Oral antihistamines are given until urticaria disappears along with the avoidance of cold.

Urticaria due to Drugs

- This is usually of short duration and disappears soon after the drug is withdrawn.
- Occurs at irregular intervals depending upon the frequency of drug intake.
- Confirmed by oral provocation tests.
- Avoidance of the causative and related drugs is best to prevent recurrences.

Urticaria due to Septic Foci

- Usually disappears either by surgical removal of the foci or by giving a course of antibiotics for 1–2 weeks.
- Almost all varieties of urticaria are controlled by antihistamines.

Contact Dermatitis

Contact dermatitis develops due to allergic reactions to locally applied substances. It is mediated by delayed hypersensitivity reaction through T cells (Table 19.9).

Contact Antigen

The substance which produces dermatitis through allergic mechanism is called **antigen** or **contact antigen**.

Cauterising Agents

These are the strong acids and alkalies which can char the skin within a few minutes of contact.

Primary Irritants

These are the agents which can produce dermatitis following their first contact with the skin through non-allergic mechanisms (Figs. 19.11–19.14).

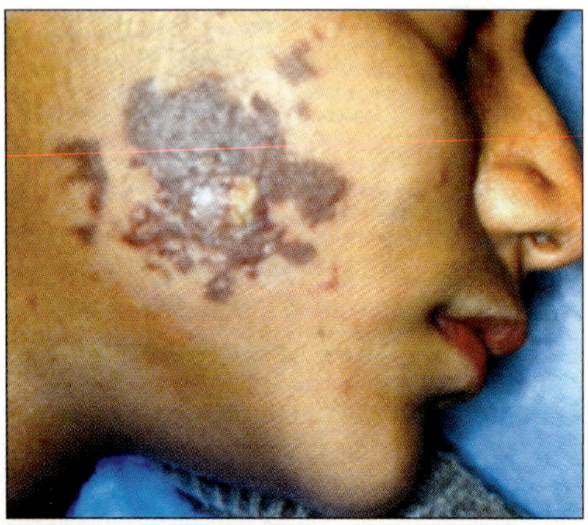

Fig. 19.11 Irritant dermatitis: face

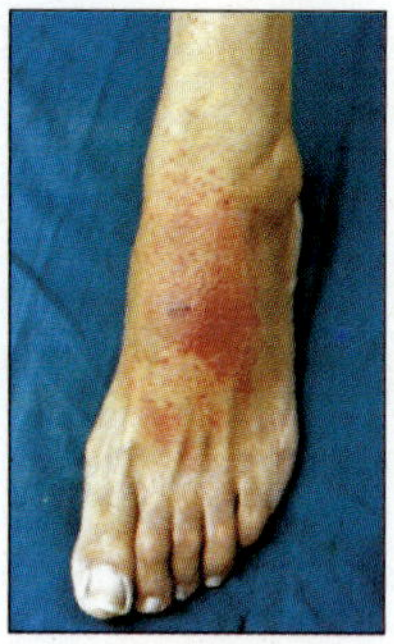

Fig. 19.12 Irritant dermatitis: foot

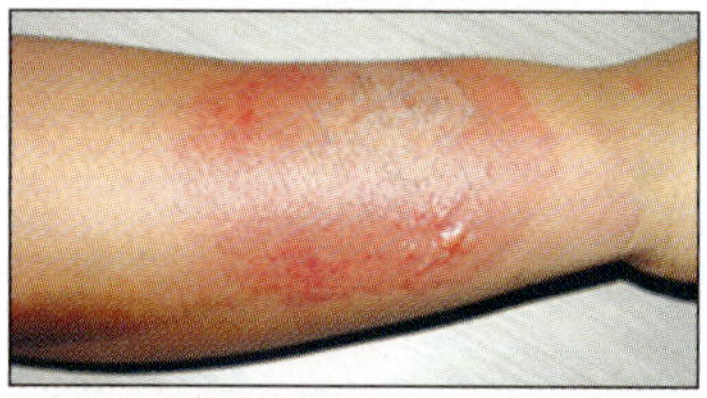

Fig. 19.13 Irritant dermtitis: arm

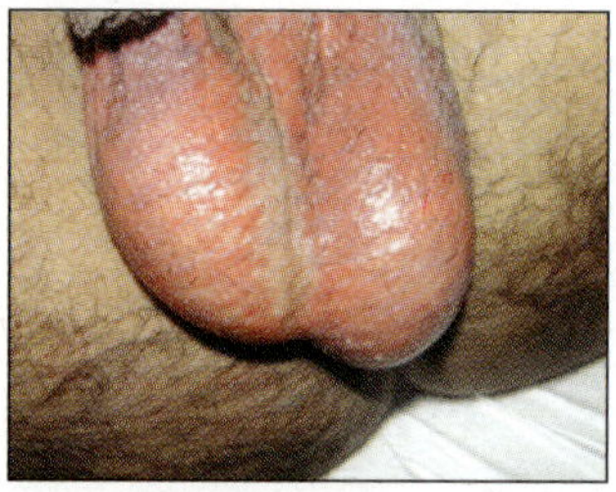

Fig. 19.14 Irritant dermatitis: scrotum

Table 19.9 Substances causing contact dermatitis

1. **Clothes, accessories and jewellery**
   Clothes, shoes, caps, hats, brassieres, socks, spectacles, wrist-watches, watch straps and various items of jewellery, etc.
2. **Cosmetics**
   Hair oils, hair dyes, shaving creams, toothpastes, lipsticks, sindoor, kajal, nail polish, etc.
3. **Drugs**
   Antibacterials, antifungals, etc. used as local applications on skin, eyes, ears or the orifices.
4. Substances coming in contact during professional activities, hobbies, social responsibilities, etc.
   - Some vegetables and fruits, chemicals and tools employed in factories and industries.
   - Inks, pens, pencils, chalks, plants, weeds, fertilizers, insecticides, etc.
   - Some agents present in the air, e.g., plant components and industrial pollutants.

Clinical Features

- Dermatitis occurs only in those areas which get exposed to the antigen
- Thus, there is a specific pattern of distribution of the lesions which is characteristic for different causative antigens (Figs 19.15–19.35).
- Causative agents are recognised in a majority of the cases by the distribution of the lesions.

- Sometimes the antigens get unintentionally applied to unconventional areas like nail polish getting applied on the neck or face.
- Once the individual gets sensitised, his whole skin is capable of reacting to the antigen.

Depending upon the degree of individual's hypersensitivity and nature of the substance, lesions representing a dermatitic reaction may be classified as follows:

- Acute.
- Subacute.
- Chronic.

Acute Reaction

Acute reaction is usually caused by liquids and volatile substances. The clinical features are as follows:

- Severe itching.
- Oedema.
- Erythema.
- Papules.
- Papulo-vesicles.

Subacute Reaction

Solid agents cause subacute reactions with:

- Itching.
- Erythematous scaly lesions.
- The lesions on palms and soles are usually erythematous with fissuring.

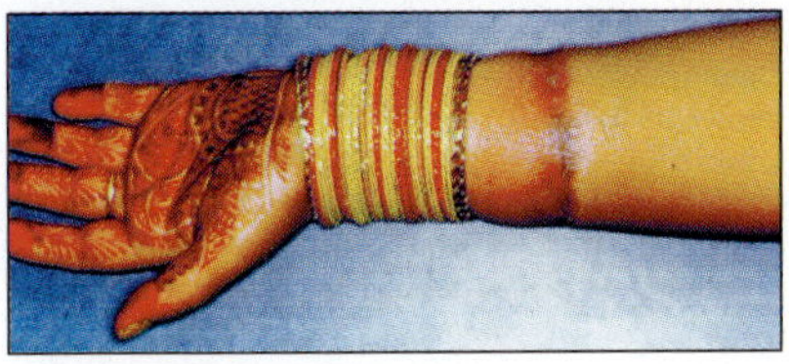

Fig. 19.15 Contact dermatitis: bangles

Investigation

The cause of contact dermatitis is confirmed by a **patch test** (Figs. 19.36–19.38) with the suspected substances along with those substances which are likely to be recommended as substitutes. The preferred site for the test is the back and parts of upper arm. Prior to the test, all drugs including the systemic corticosteroids and immunosuppressants, should be stopped. The antigen is applied on a gauze, attached to the skin by a tape and is left for 48 hours. After this, the area is inspected for the development of dermatitis reaction.

Based upon the degree of inflammation, the reaction is graded from 0 to 3+. The detailed grading is presented in Table 19.10.

Table 19.10 Grading of contact dermatitis

Grading	Interpretation
0	Negative.
?	Doubtful reaction.
+	Weak reaction.
++	Strong reaction.
+++	Extreme reaction.
NT	Not tested.
IR	Irritant reaction.

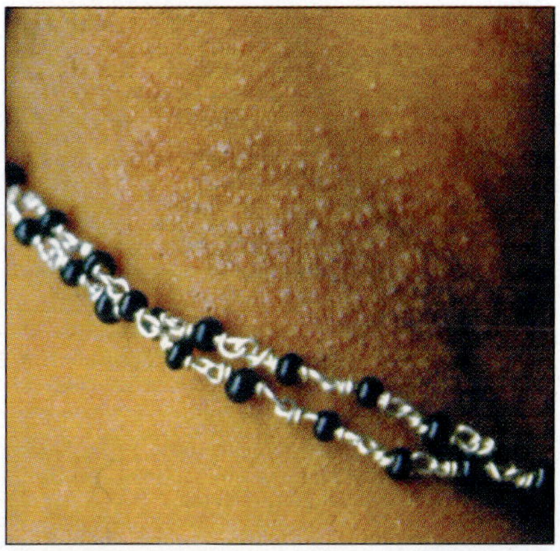

Fig. 19.16 Contact dermatitis: chain

Drug Reactions

Clinical Features

Reactions due to systemic drugs are usually sudden, generalised and bilaterally symmetrical.

Lesions vary from drug to drug and from patient to patient (Tables 19.11–19.13).

Table 19.11 Features of drug reactions

Similar to urticaria due to other causes except that the onset is:

- Severe.
- Widespread.
- Follows the administration of the drug.

Table 19.12 Various types of allergic drug reactions

- Urticaria and angioedema.
- Exanthematous eruptions.
- Erythema multiforme.
- Toxic epidermal necrolysis.
- Fixed drug eruptions.
- Erythroderma.

Table 19.13 Urticaria and angioedema due to drugs

++	Strong reaction
+++	Extreme reaction
NT	Not tested
IR	Irritant reaction

Treatment

Treatment of contact dermatitis is presented in Table 19.14.

- Topical corticosteroids clear the lesions in many cases.
- Severe cases can be treated with a short course of oral corticosteroids for 5–6 days.

Table 19.14 Treatment of contact dermatitis

- Prevention of further exposure of patients to the causative antigens.
- Dermatitis continues to worsen as long as contact with antigen continues.
- Once exposure to the antigen is stopped, the dermatitis tends to subside even without any treatment.
- Washing of the affected area with soap and water further reduces or even clears the remnant of the antigen.
- Patient should be advised to avoid contact with the causative substance(s) and use the substitutes tested safe.
- If further exposure to causative agent is not possible to avoid, one can cover the skin by clothes (physical barrier) or use barrier cream on the exposed parts.

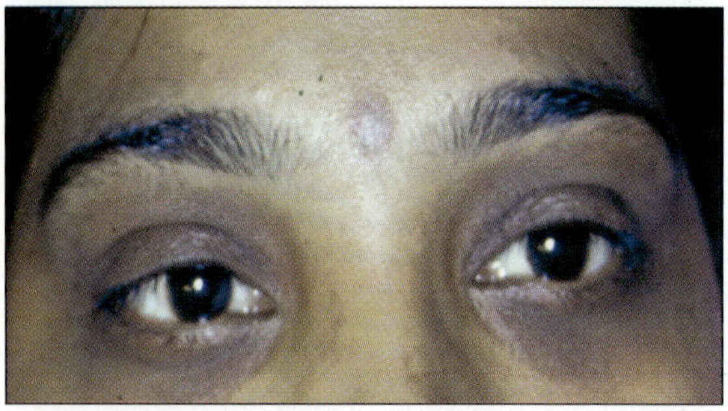

Fig. 19.17 Contact dermatitis due to bindi

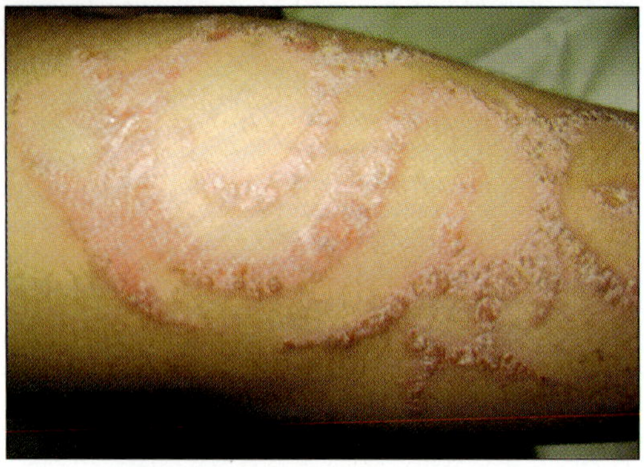

Fig. 19.18 Contact dermatitis due to tattoo

Prognosis

- The incubation period varies from a few minutes to a few hours.
- Urticaria usually disappears when the drug is withdrawn.
- Urticaria due to aspirin and penicillin may continue for 2–4 weeks after the drug is withdrawn.

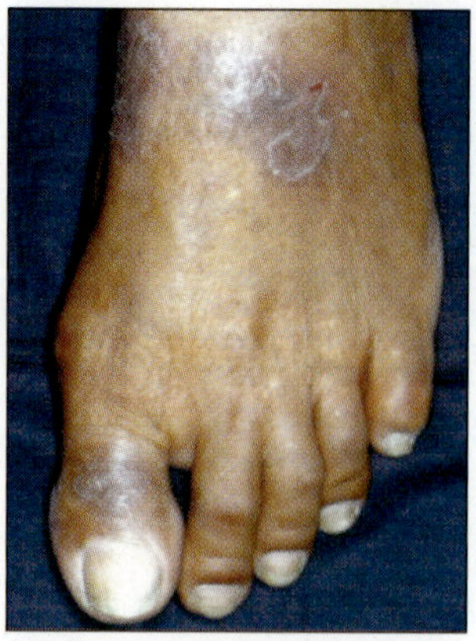

Fig. 19.19 Contact dermatitis: chappal

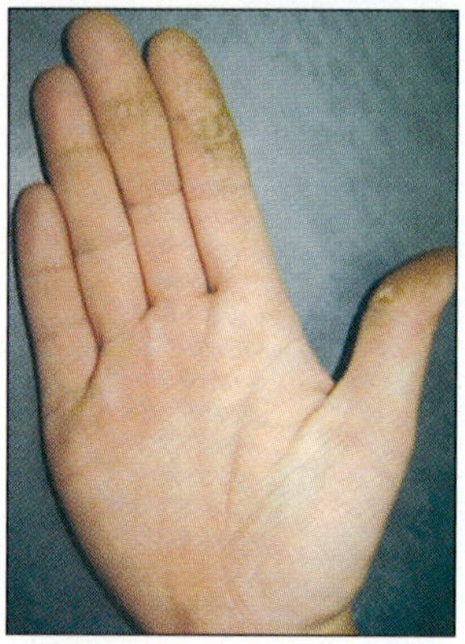

Fig. 19.20 Contact dermatitis: vegetable

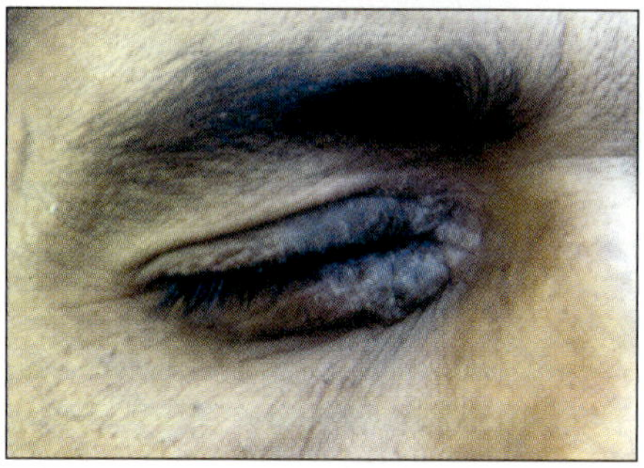

Fig. 19.21 Contact dermatitis: eye drops

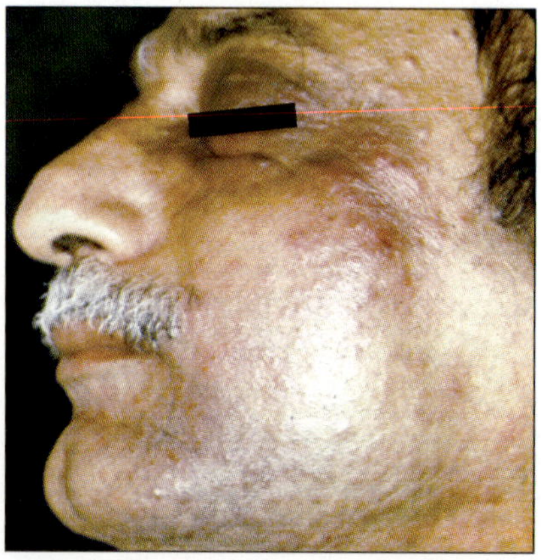

Fig. 19.22 Contact dermatitis: shaving cream

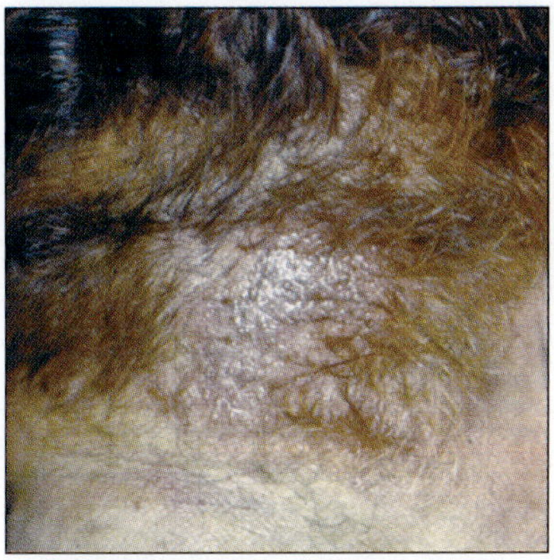

Fig. 19.23 Contact dermatitis: henna

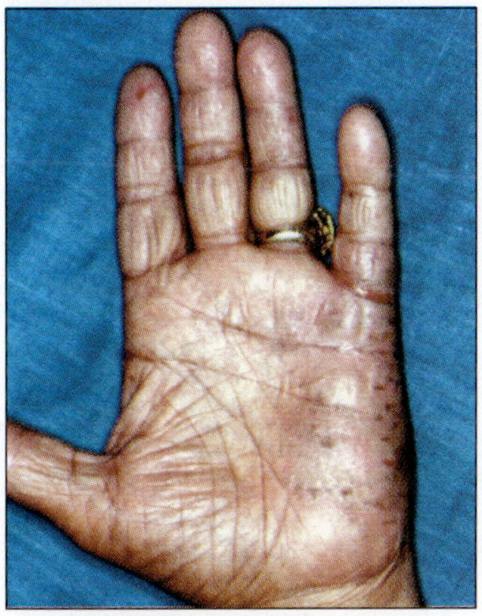

Fig. 19.24 Contact dermatitis: cleaner

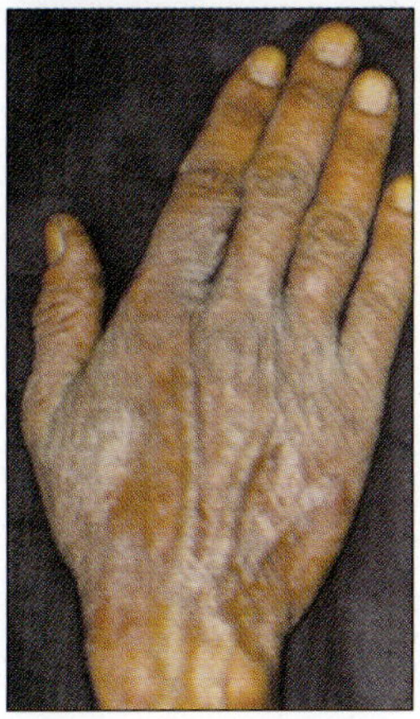

Fig. 19.25 Contact dermatitis: chandan

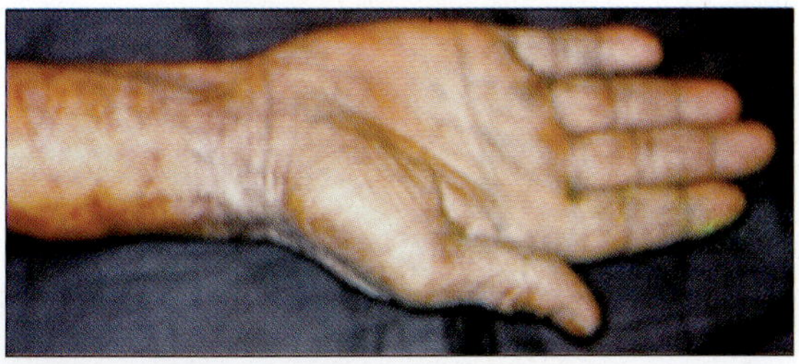

Fig. 19.26 Contact dermatitis: steering wheel

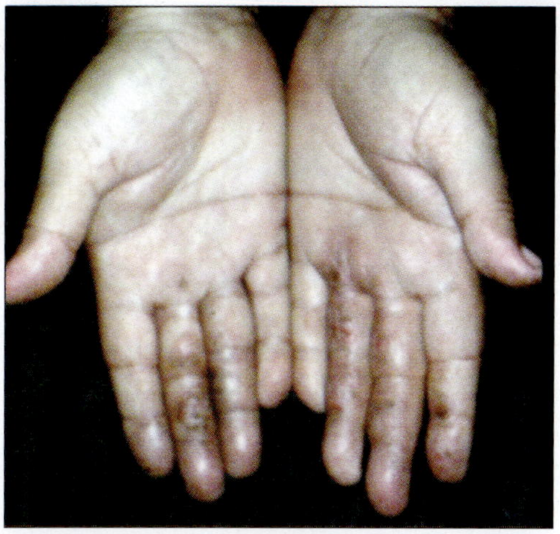

Fig. 19.27 Contact dermatitis: hand sanitiser

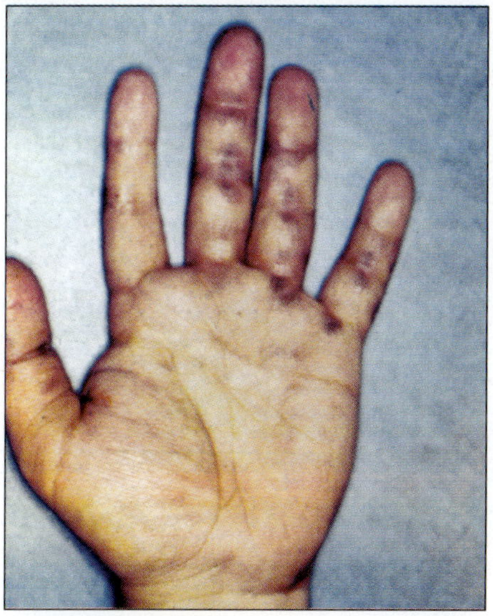

Fig. 19.28 Contact dermatitis: cement

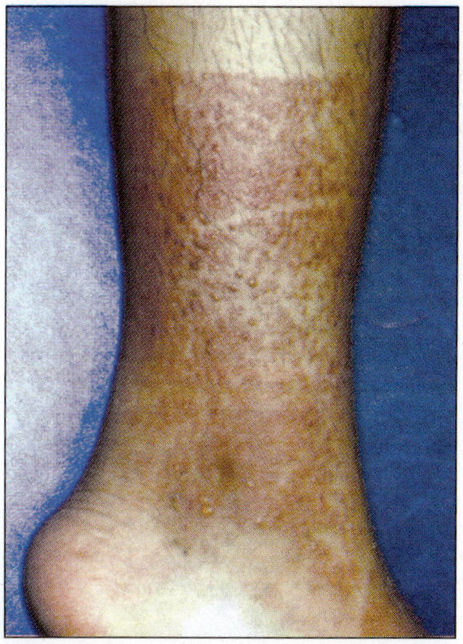

Fig. 19.29 Contact dermatitis: plaster

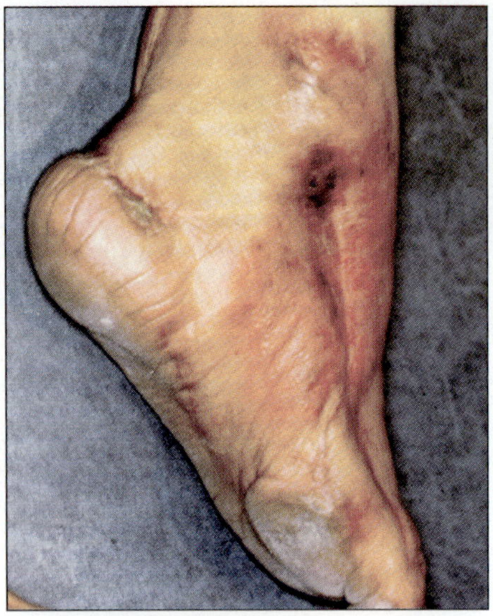

Fig. 19.30 Contact dermatitis: prosthesis

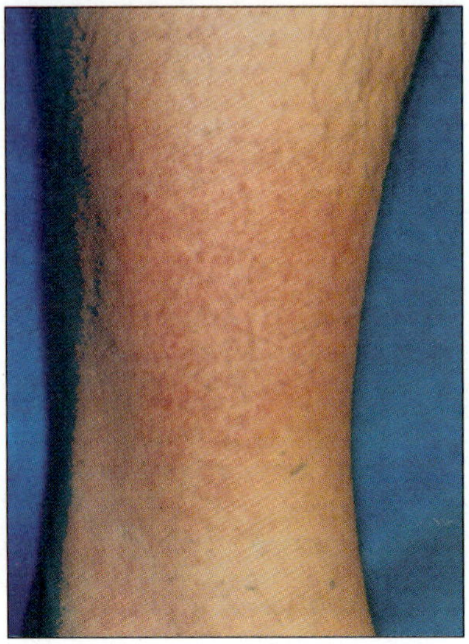

Fig. 19.31 Contact dermatitis: rubber in socks

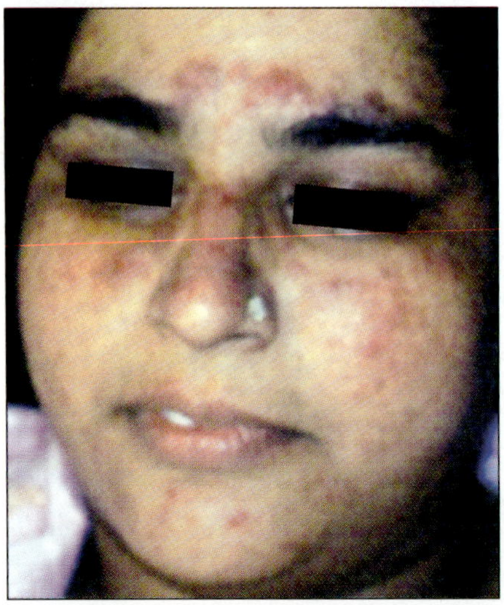

Fig. 19.32 Airborne contact dermatitis: face

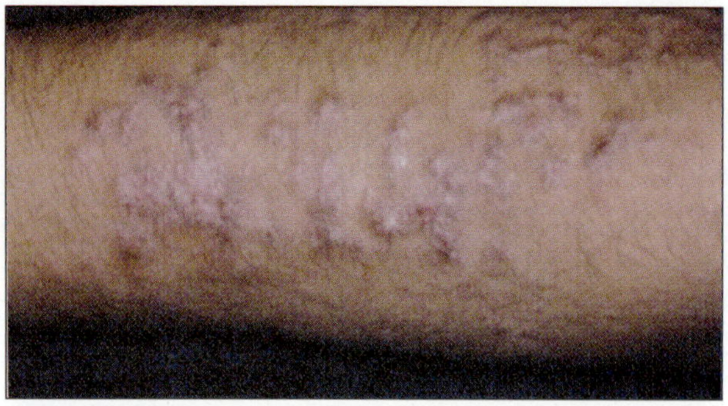

Fig. 19.33 Airborne contact dermatitis: arm

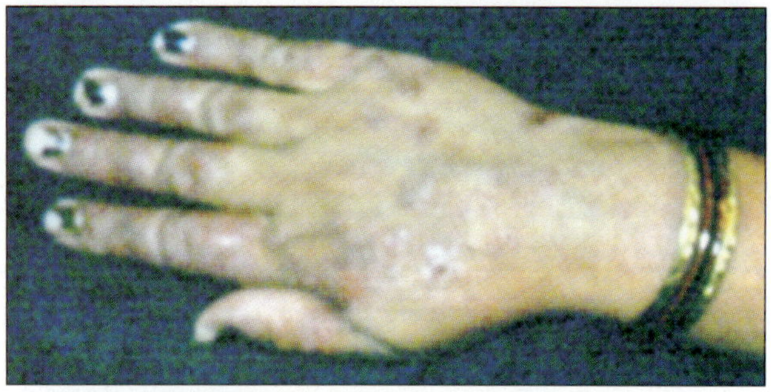

Fig. 19.34 Airborne contact dermatitis: hand

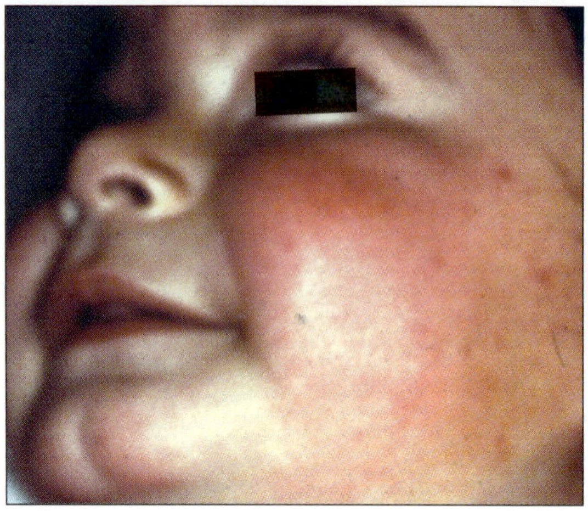

Fig. 19.35 Contact dermatitis: topical conticosteroids on face (child)

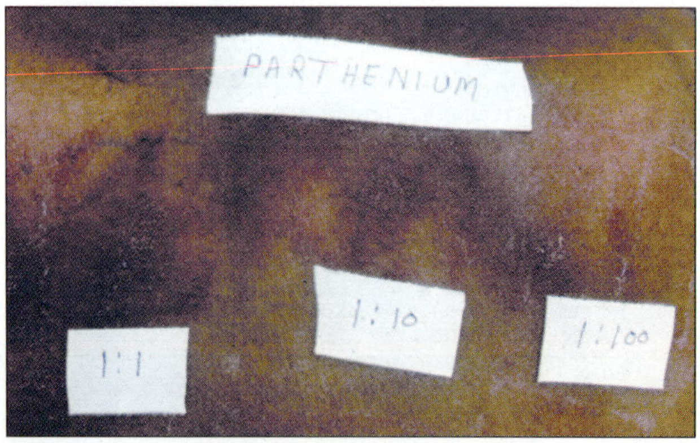

Fig. 19.36 Patch test

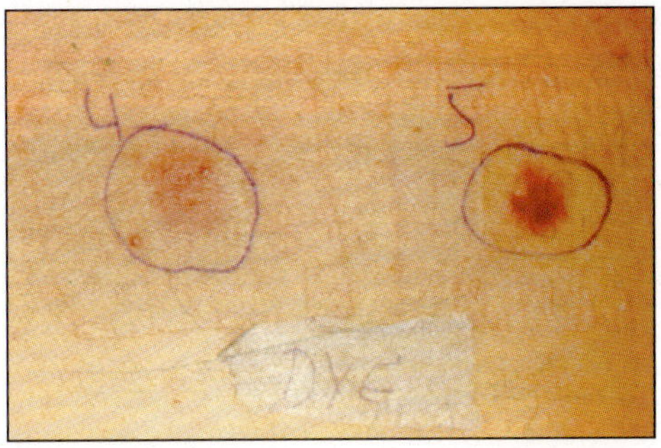

Fig. 19.37 Positive patch test

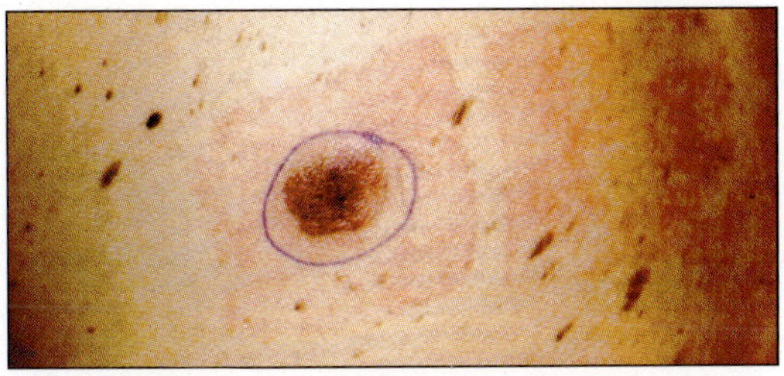

Fig. 19.38 Positive patch test to sandal wood

Exanthematous Drug Eruptions

Exanthematous eruptions include:

- Erythematous macules (Figs 19.39 and 19.40).
- Tiny papules.
- Papulo-vesicles.
- Papulo-squamous lesions.
- Purpura.
- Vesicles.
- Bullae (Fig. 19.41).

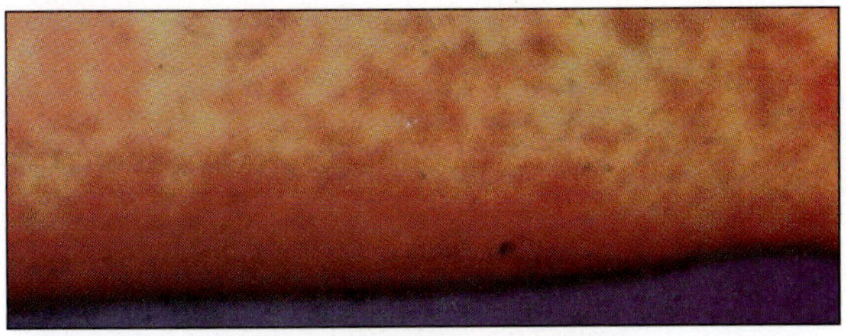

Fig. 19.39 Drug reaction: macular

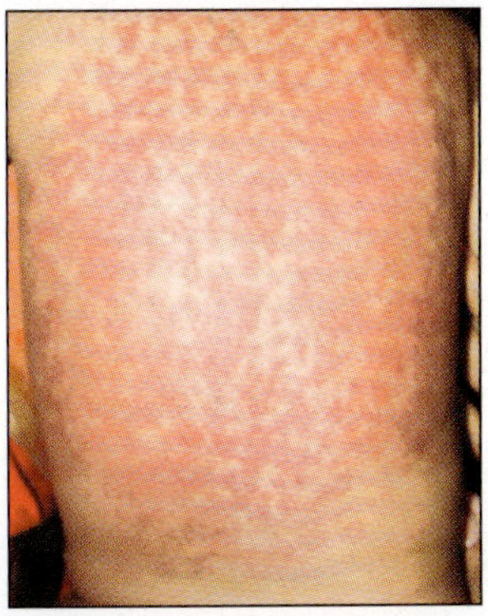

Fig. 19.40 Macular drug reaction: child

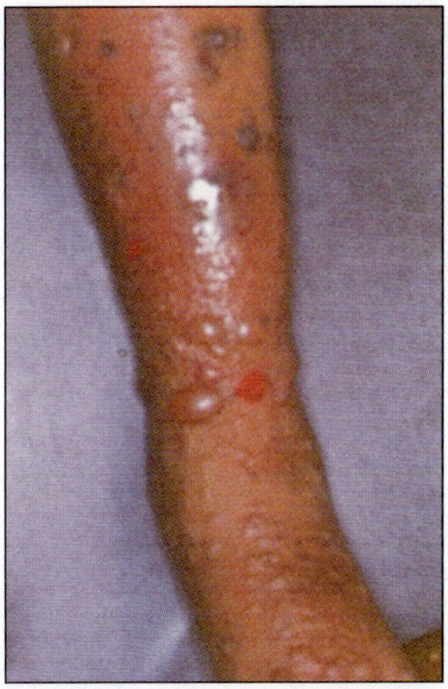

Fig. 19.41 Bullous drug reaction: homeopathic drug

Usually, these lesions appear suddenly, spread all over the body and are bilaterally symmetrical, but without fever. If these lesions are not controlled promptly with adequate treatment, they may progress to exfoliative dermatitis and may prove fatal.

Exfoliative Dermatitis

Exfoliative dermatitis is usually severe with acute onset and may be fatal.

Clinical Features

- Erythema and scaling all over the body.
- This is associated with chills and rigor.
- Sometimes, it may be a direct manifestation of the drug-reaction.
- Generally it is a complication of ill-managed exanthematous drug eruptions.

Table 19.15 Different diseases produced by drugs

- Lupus erythematosus.
- Pemphigus foliaceous.
- Lichen planus.
- Occasionally, pemphigus vulgaris.
- Pemphigus erythematosus.
- These lesions disappear slowly after the cessation of drug.

Erythema Multiforme

Clinical Features

These are circular lesions, 1–2 cm in size with dark-bluish centre surrounded by raised, erythematous periphery resembling iris of the eye or the target of a shooting range and are called **iris lesions** or **target lesions** (Figs 19.42–19.46)

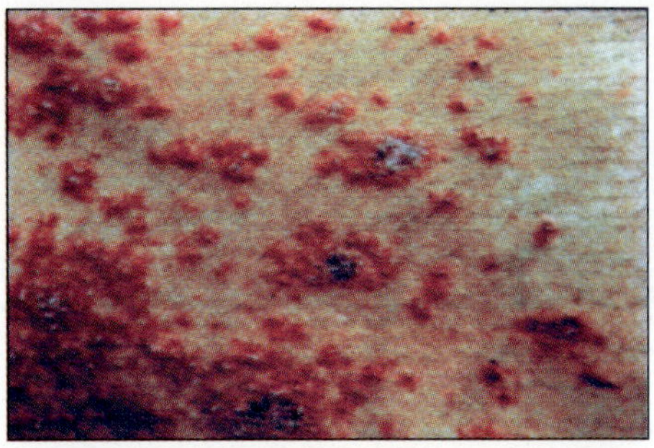

Fig. 19.42 Erythema multiforme

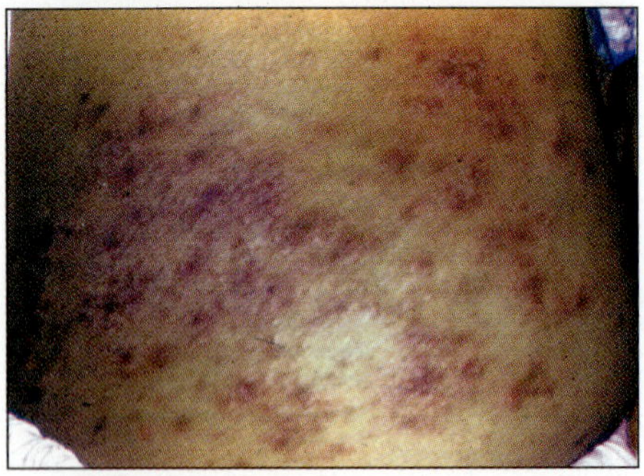

Fig. 19.43 Erythema multiforme due to ignitia (a homeopathic drug)

Etiology

- Drugs, bacteria, viruses, mycobacteria, fungi and toxins/antigens of malignancies.
- Causative agent remains unidentified in a large number of cases.
- Severity varies in different patients.

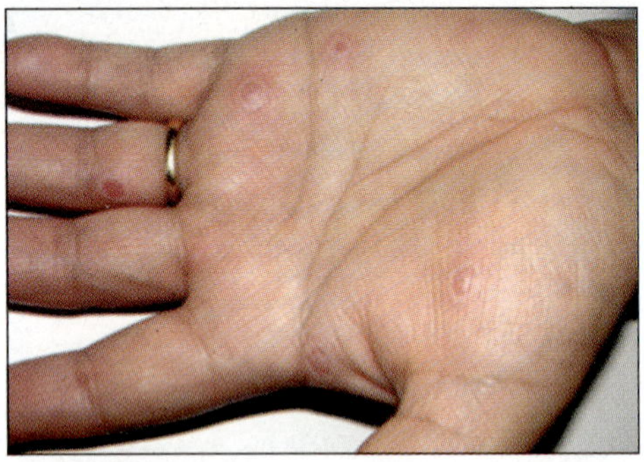

Fig. 19.44 Erythema multiforme: palm

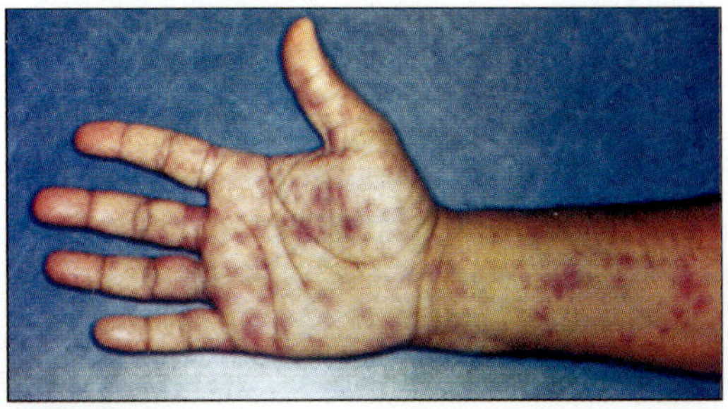

Fig. 19.45 Erythema multiforme: palm

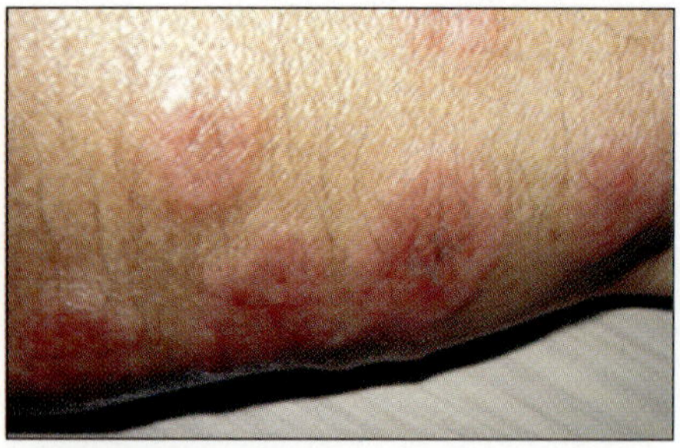

Fig. 19.46 Erythema multiforme

Bullous Erythema Multiforme

Some patients develop tense blisters at the centre of the lesions (Fig. 19.47).

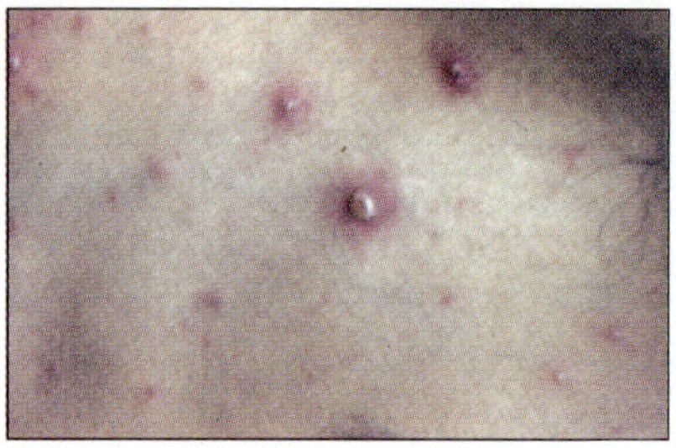

Fig. 19.47 Bullous erythema multiforme

Stevens–Johnson Syndrome

Clinical Features

It is a severe variety of drug reaction and may present as:

- Fever.
- Arthralgia/arthritis.
- Involvement of eye, oral and/or genital mucosae with ulceration and crusting.
- Severe toxaemia with or without involvement of the kidney.
- May prove fatal if not controlled rapidly with adequate treatment.

Toxic Epidermal Necrolysis

The acronym for **toxic epidermal necrolysis** is TEN.

Etiology

- Drug.
- Systemic lupus erythematosus.
- Graft vs host reaction.

Clinical Features

- Most severe form of drug reaction.
- Consists of erythematous macules varying in shape and size.
- Later on, the macules merge with each other.

- Skin lesions turn dark brown (Fig. 19.48) within the next 24 hours with necrosis of superficial layers of epidermis.
- The epidermis ultimately starts peeling off (Figs 19.49–19.53), leaving behind raw areas.
- Mucosae, especially of lips, oral cavity, genitalia and conjunctivae are often involved.
- Involvement of cornea leads to corneal opacities and blindness in a few cases.
- Patient is very vulnerable, and if neglected, may die within a few days.

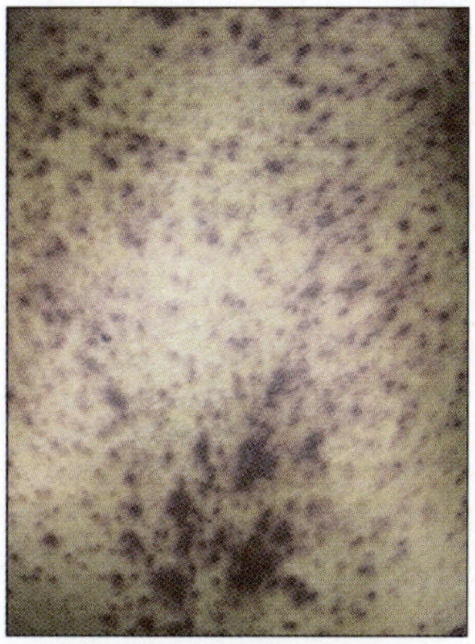

Fig. 19.48 Toxic epidermal necrolysis (TEN)

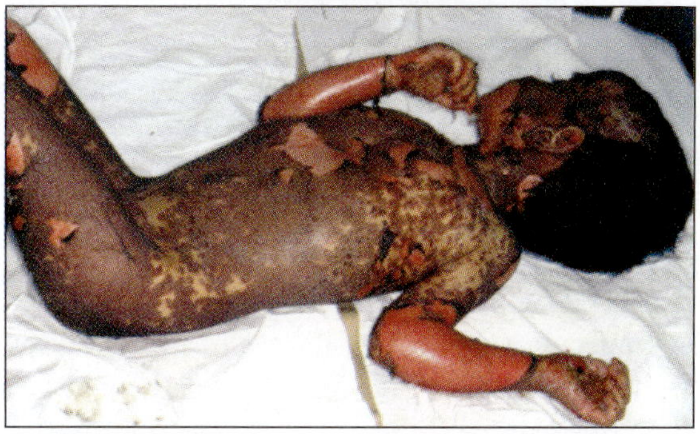

Fig. 19.49 TEN in child

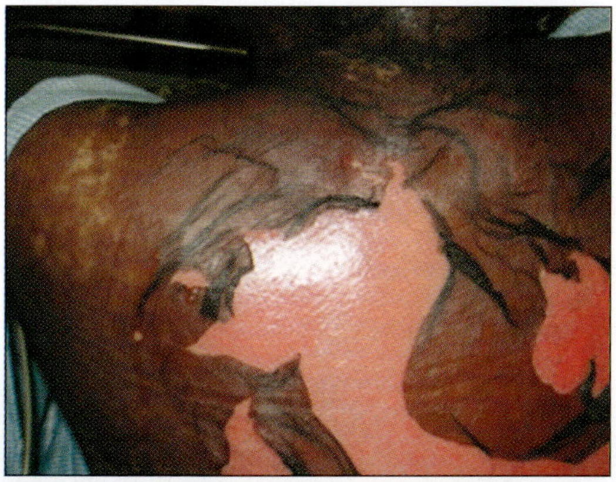

Fig. 19.50 Toxic epidermal necrolysis in adult: back

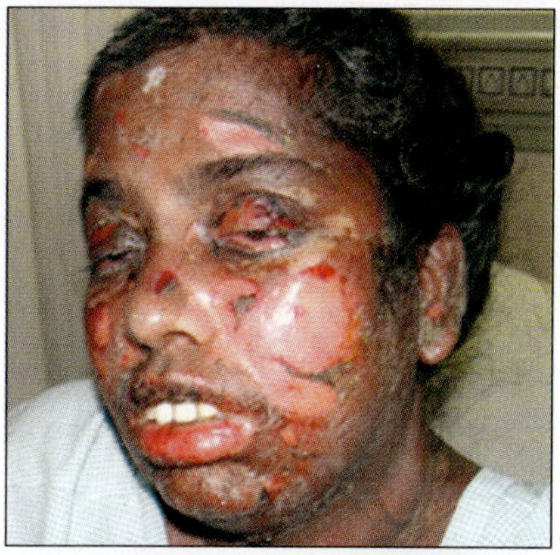

Fig. 19.51 Toxic epidermal necrolysis in adult: face

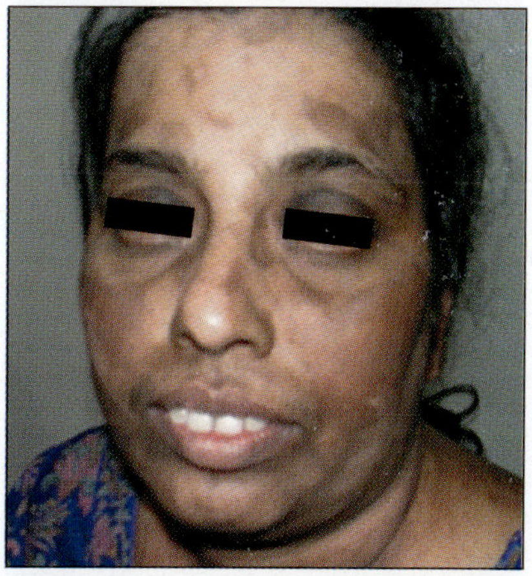

Fig. 19.52 TEN in face: after treatment

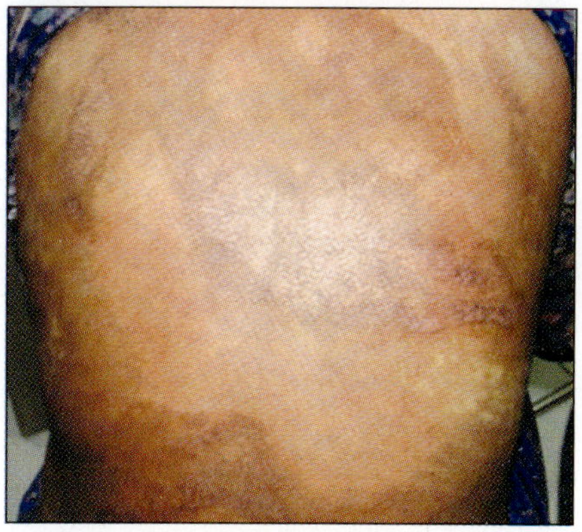

Fig. 19.53 TEN in back: after treatment

Fixed Drug Eruption

This is a special type of allergic drug reaction limited to a few spots only.

Clinical Features

- Itchy, circular, erythematous macules are seen (Figs 19.54–19.56).
- They heal in a couple of days leaving behind hyperpigmentation (Fig. 19.57).

- Whenever the same drug is administered the hyperpigmented macules get reactivated with itching and erythema.
- Lesions may be multiple.
- Blisters may develop at the centre in severe cases.

Sites

Any part of the body and mucous membranes.

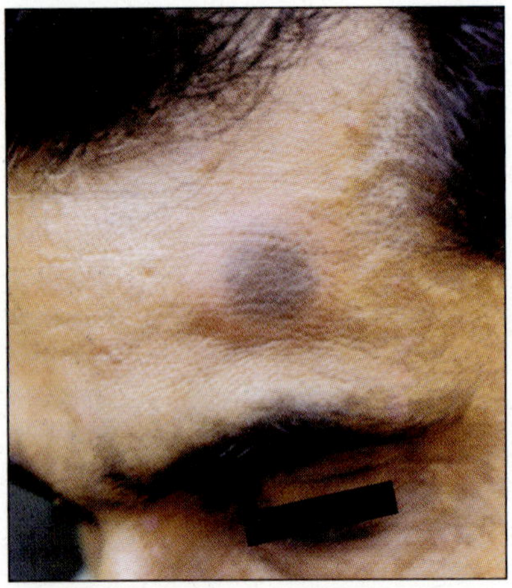

Fig. 19.54 Fixed drug eruption: forehead

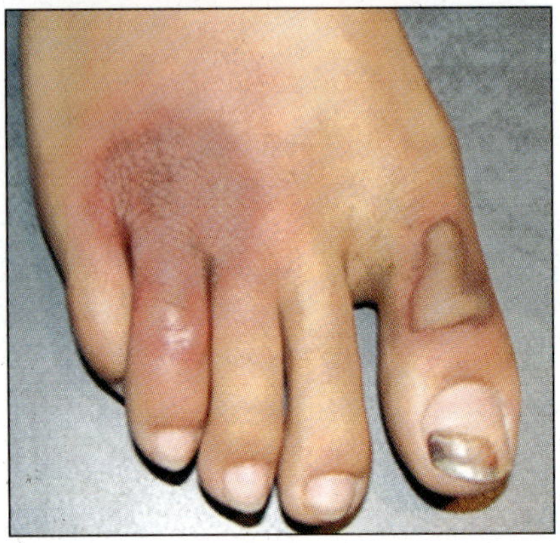

Fig. 19.55 Fixed drug eruption

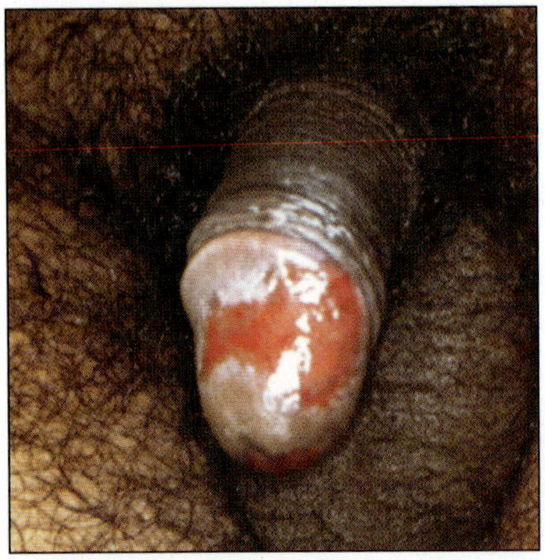

Fig. 19.56 Fixed drug eruption: glans

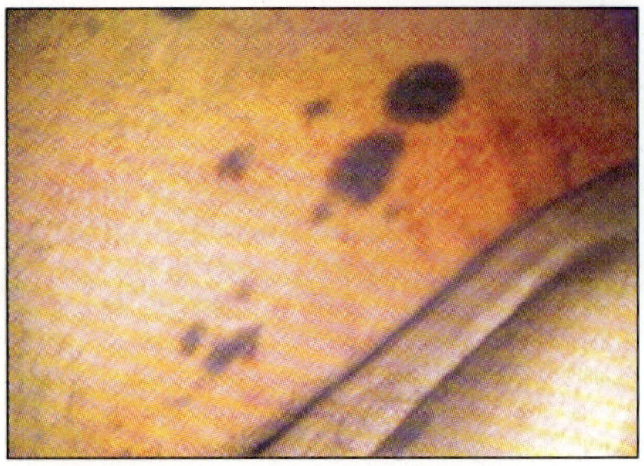

Fig. 19.57 Pigmentation on subsided FDE abdomen

Investigations for Drug Reactions

To find out the causative drug, graded dosage of the drugs are administered one by one.

Whenever any drug causes the recurrence of the reaction, it should be withdrawn and the patient is treated promptly.

Treatment of Drug Reactions

- All the drugs which the patient is taking should be stopped immediately.
- Essential drug should be substituted by a drug which has not been taken by the patient earlier.
- Urticaria should be controlled with adequate doses of antihistamine.
- Other variety of reactions should be controlled with adequate doses of systemic corticosteroids within 24 hours.
- Depending upon the severity of the reaction, dose equivalent to 30–80 mg of prednisolone per day is sufficient to control the reaction.
- In case the patient does not show any signs of recovery or continues to develop new lesions within 24 hours, corticosteroid dose can be increased by 20–40 mg prednisolone everyday, till the new lesions stop appearing and the old ones start regressing.
- After the disappearance of the reaction, corticosteroids can be withdrawn rapidly during the next few days.
- Treatment for the primary disease is restarted once the reaction has been controlled.

Atopic Dermatitis

Etiology

- Inherited as a polygenic recessive trait.
- There is an increased tendency for skin hypersensitivity reactions.
- Skin may get sensitised to various antigens in the atmosphere.

Clinical Features

- The clinical features varys with age.
- Itching is the persistent symptom.

The associated features of atopic dermatitis are presented in Table 19.16.

Infantile Eczema

- It is the atopic dermatitis occurring during the first two to six months of life.
- Lesions may continue to appear during the first two years of life.
- They consist of several itchy, erythematous papules on cheeks that become exudative and crusted (Figs 19.58 and 19.59).
- Lesions subsequently spread to the other parts of the body.
- Secondary infections with pyogenic organisms and lymphadenopathy are common.
- Some cases clear up immediately and remain free for the rest of their lives.
- Others may develop the symptoms of childhood stage eczema.

Table 19.16 Associated features of atopic dermatitis

- Atopy.
- Asthma.
- Urticaria.
- Hay fever or allergic rhinitis.
- Increased IgE antibodies.
- Depressed delayed hypersensitivity.
- Transient deficiency of IgA antibody.
- Defective phagocytic function of lymphocytes.
- Reduced chemotactic migration of polymorphonuclear leucocytes and monocytes.
- Tendency for vasoconstriction of smaller blood vessels.
- Pallor of skin, especially on the face.
- White dermographism.
- Delayed blanch with acetylcholine*.
- Reduced reaction to histamine injections and cholinergic drugs.
- Pronounced vasoconstriction on exposure to cold.
- Low finger temperature.

*Delayed blanch with acetylcholine: Instead of the usual erythematous flare, patients with atopic dermatitis show 'a delayed blanch' with an intradermal injection of acetylcholine (caused by the vasoconstriction).

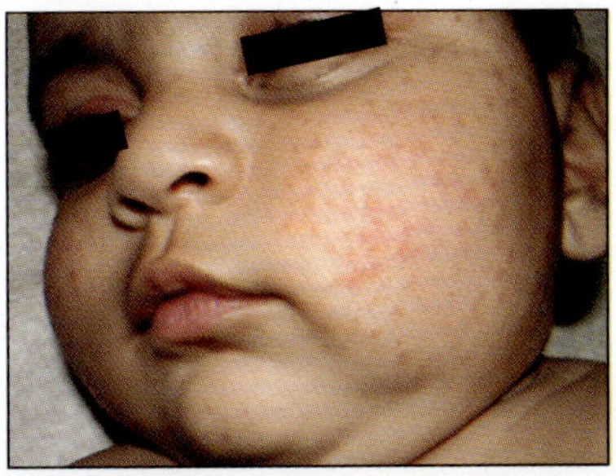

Fig. 19.58 Infantile eczema: cheek

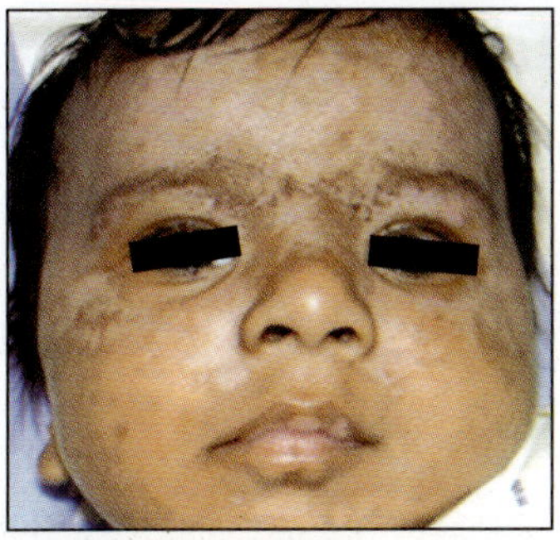

Fig. 19.59 Infantile eczema: cheek

Childhood Stage Atopic Dermatitis

- Starts from two years of age.
- The lesions predominantly involve the cubital (Fig. 19.60) and popliteal fossae (Fig. 19.61) .
- The lesions present as several itchy (mildly) erythematous papules with mild to moderate lichenification.
- The skin is dry.
- As the age advances, the lesions tend to become more dry and lichenified, and may involve the face, neck and trunk.

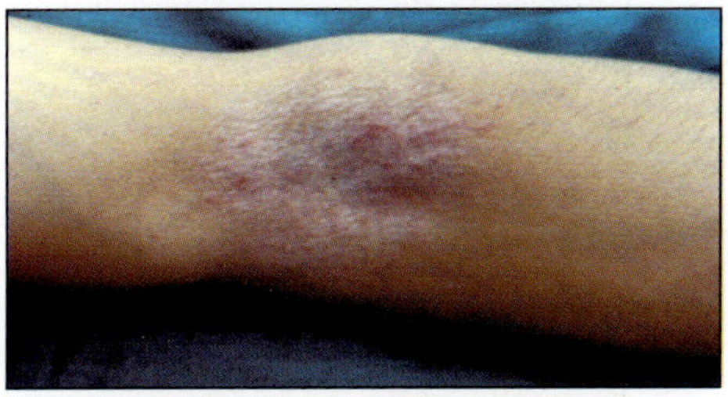

Fig. 19.60 Atopic dermartitis: cubital fossae

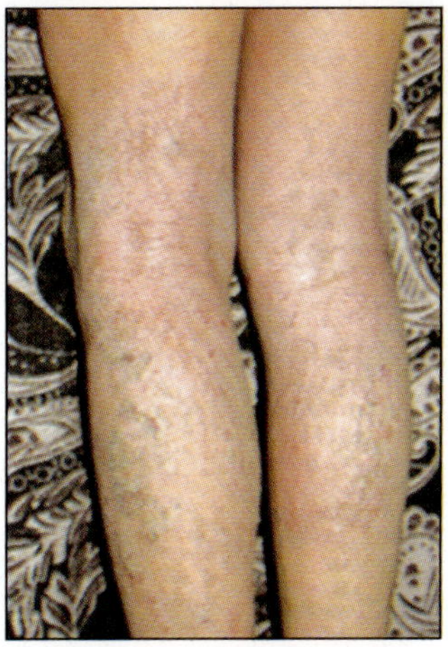

Fig. 19.61 Atopic dermatitis: popliteal fossae

Adulthood Stage Atopic Dermatitis

- In severe cases, the whole body may get involved with lichenification (Figs. 19.62 and 19.63).

- These patients are more prone to develop extensive lesions of viral warts, molluscum contagiosum, herpes simplex and pyodermas.

Treatment

- Patient should take daily bath with an ordinary toilet soap.
- Shampoo the hair daily.

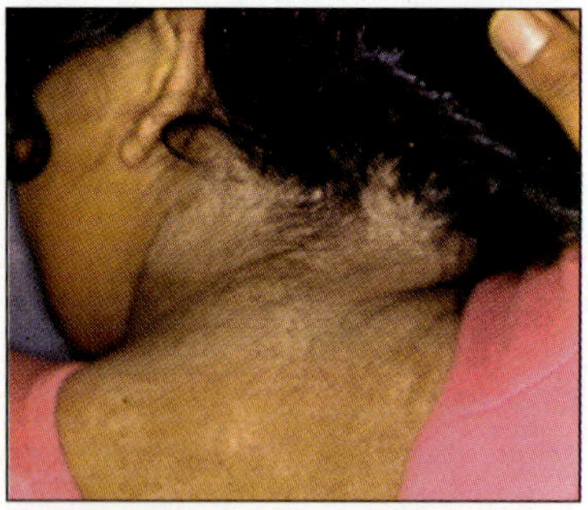

Fig. 19.62 Atopic dermatitis: back of neck

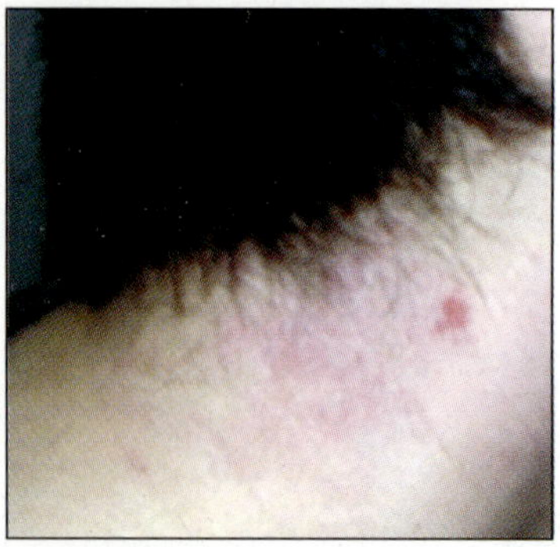

Fig. 19.63 Atopic dermatitis: back of neck

- Oil application, which interferes with the cleaning process, should be stopped even on a dry skin.
- Active lesions should be controlled with topical and/or systemic corticosteroids depending upon the severity of the lesions.
- Secondary infection should be treated with oral antibiotics.
- Severe itching should be controlled by oral antihistamines, 3–4 times daily.
- Treatment should be continued till all the signs of activity disappear. Then the drugs are withdrawn slowly. Treatment must be restarted whenever there is any recurrence.
- An attempt should be made to find out the exact cause and should be treated accordingly.

Eczema Vaccinatum

In active stage, the children are at risk of developing generalised eruptions after the smallpox vaccination.

Eczema Herpeticum

If exposed to the herpes simplex virus, the children are likely to develop generalised eruption.

Both the conditions (eczema vaccinatum and eczema herpeticum), if not controlled promptly, may turn fatal.

Chapter 20

Autoimmune Disorders

COMMON AUTOIMMUNE DISORDERS

Immunologic system of the body, as a rule, does not react to the numerous protein substances (antigens) present within the body itself. This immune tolerance to self-antigens, which is supposed to be acquired during the embryonic life, sometimes, can disappear later on due to a variety of reasons leading to production of autoantibodies to one or more autoantigens. Reaction of such antibodies with the autoantigens leads to the development of a group of diseases called autoimmune disorders (Table 20.1)

Table 20.1 Common autoimmune disorders

Pemphigus	• Pemphigus vulgaris • Pemphigus foliaceus • Pemphigus erythematosus • Pemphigus vegetans
• Bullous pemphigoid	
• Dermatitis herpetiformis	
• Benign bullous dermatosis of childhood	
• Lupus erythematosus	
• Scleroderma	
• Systemic sclerosis	
• Dermatomyositis	

Pemphigus

Pemphigus Vulgaris

The commonest variety of pemphigus is pemphigus vulgaris.

Age

Commonly seen in 20–40 years of age, although it may also occur in children and older patients.

Etiology

- Is caused by the action of IgG antibodies against the protein on the surface of epidermal cells, the intercellular substance.
- The antigen/antibody reaction leads to the separation of epidermal cells from each other, this is called **acantholysis** which results in the formation of splits between the layers of epidermis and the intraepidermal bullae.

Clinical Features

- Presents as diffusely scattered vesiculo-bullous lesions in the skin and the mucosae (Figs. 20.1–20.7).

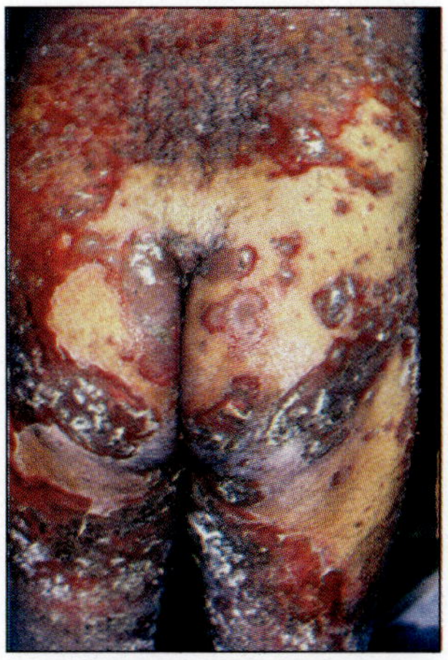

Fig. 20.1 Pemphigus vulgaris: thick crusts

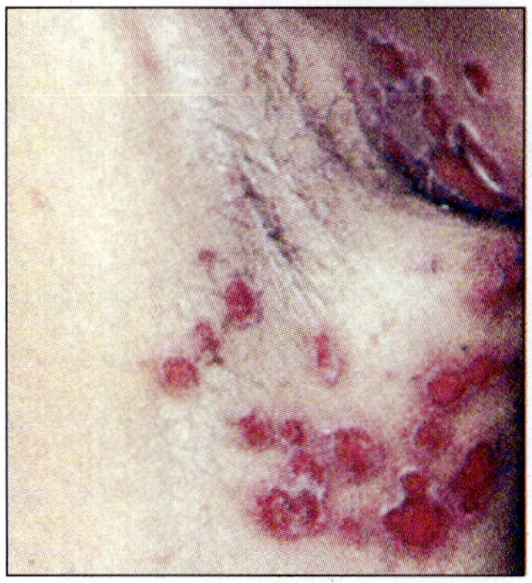

Fig. 20.2 Pemphigus vulgaris: axilla

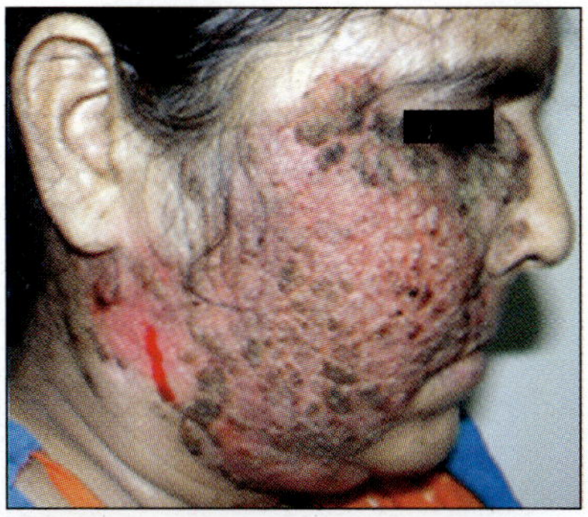

Fig. 20.3 Pempigus vulgaris: face

- The lesions are flaccid.
- The blisters rupture easily, leaving behind superficial ulcers.
- The lesions may dry-up to form crusts.
- As a rule, the ulcers heal slowly.
- If the disease is not controlled, new lesions may appear at other areas with extension of old lesions at their periphery (**bulla spread sign**).

Sites

- The lesions may occur on any part of the body (Figs. 20.5–20.7).
- Involvement of the mucous membranes is very frequent.
- Sometimes, it may be the only manifestation of the disease even for several months.
- The oral mucosa is very frequently involved (Figs. 20.6–20.7).
- Mucous membranes of nose, larynx, oesophagus, genitals or conjunctivae are less frequently involved.

Course

- Remissions and relapses at irregular periods are very common.
- When the lesions heal, they produce hyperkeratotic areas with hyperpigmentation (Fig. 20.4).

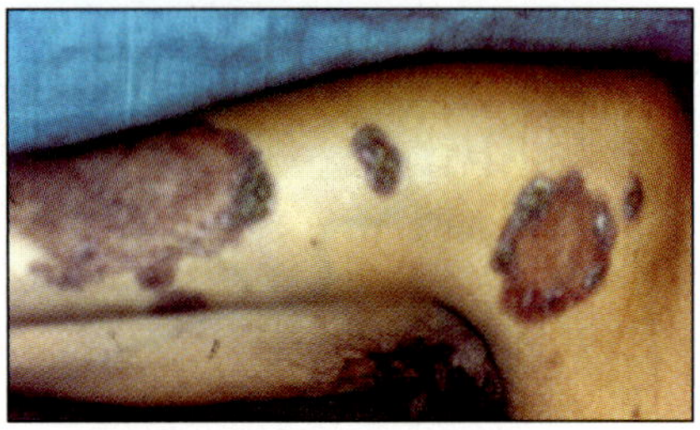

Fig. 20.4 Pemphigus vulgaris: hyperkeratotic, hyperpigmented lesion

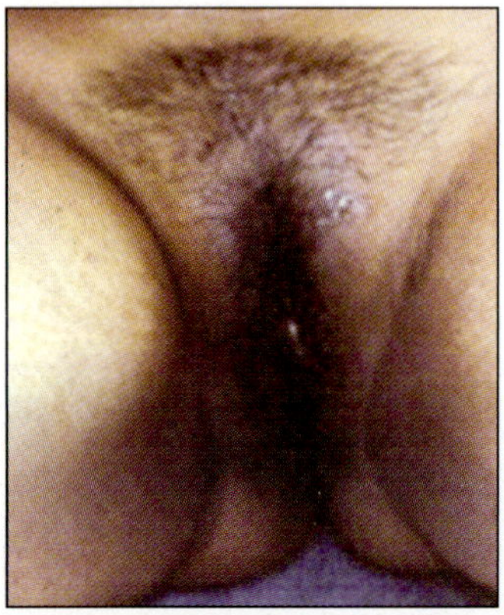

Fig. 20.5 Pemphigus vulgaris: ulcers in female genital

- Secondary infection with *candida* and/or pyogenic organisms is very common when the oral mucosa is involved.
- Oral lesions are large, superficial ulcers which do not heal for prolonged periods.

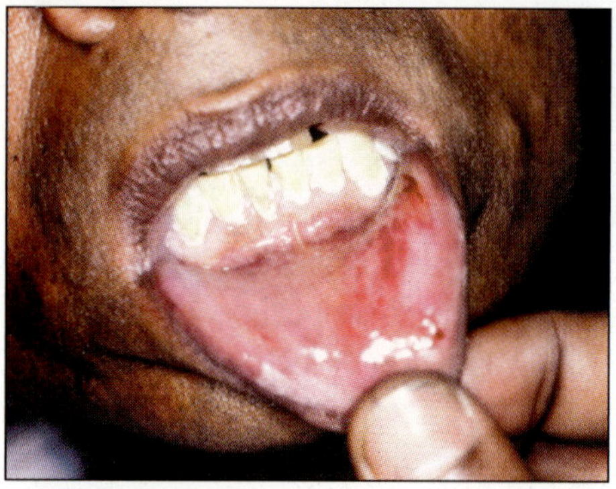

Fig. 20.6 Pemphigus vulgaris: ulcer lower lip

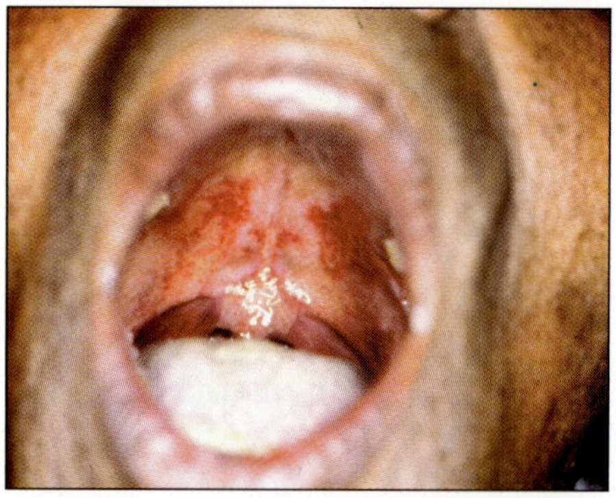

Fig. 20.7 Pemphigus vulgaris: ulcer soft palate

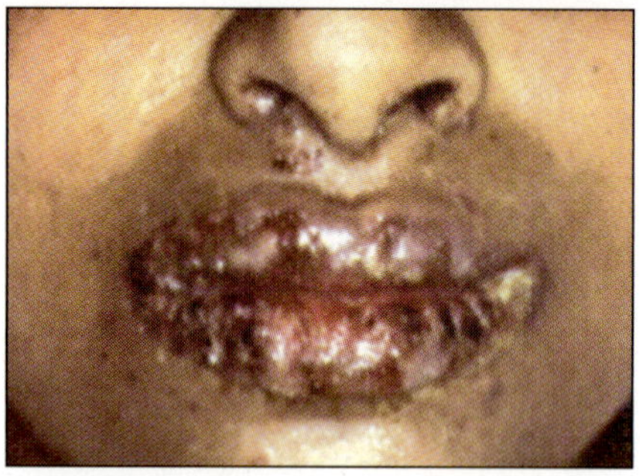

Fig. 20.8 Pemphigus foliaceous

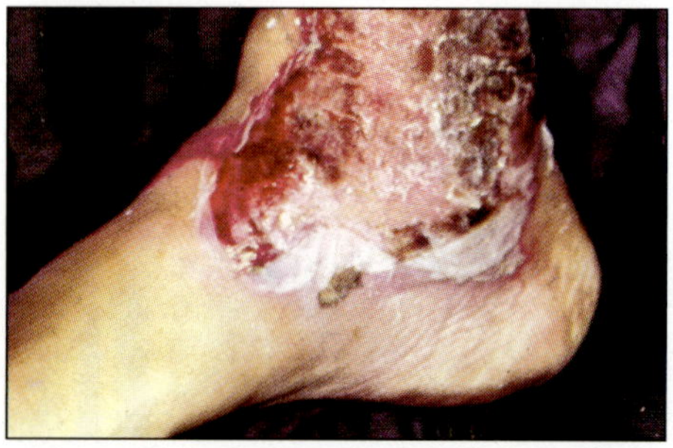

Fig. 20.9 Pemphigus foliaceous: superficial ulcers leg

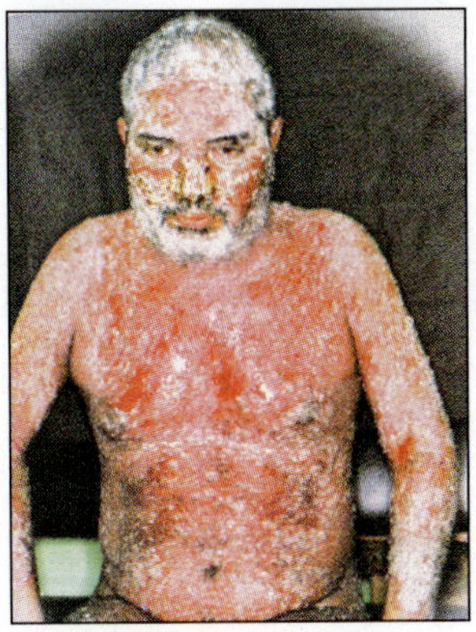

Fig. 20.10 Pemphigus foliaceous

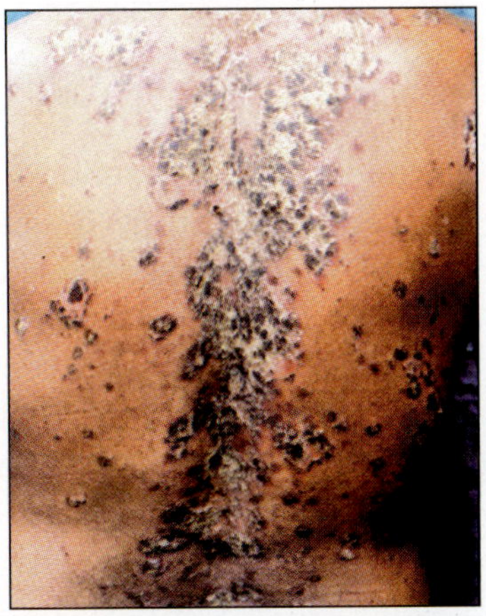

Fig. 20.11 Pemphigus foliaceous: crust on back

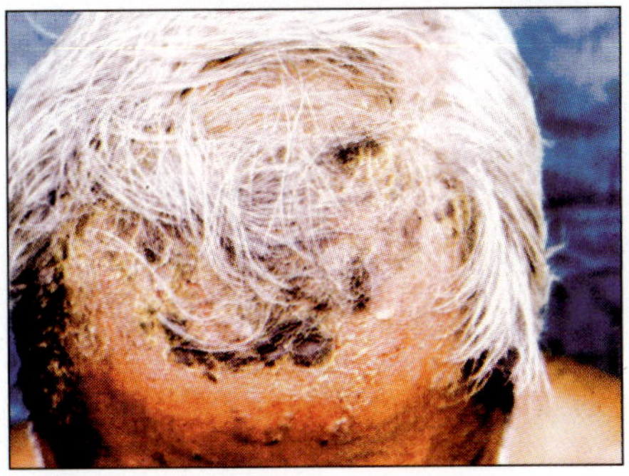

Fig. 20.12 Pemphigus foliaceous: crust (scalp)

Pemphigus Foliaceus

Clinical Features

- Ulcers occur just below the stratum corneum.
- The predominant lesions look like scales (Figs. 20.8–20.13).
- Blisters are very few and transient.
- The lesions produce a burning sensation.
- This variant is milder than pemphigus vulgaris.
- The patient is often alive for several decades before the fatal termination.
- Spontaneous cures are well known.

Sites

- Starts on the face or scalp and spreads rapidly to the rest of the body.
- Resembles exfoliative dermatitis.
- Usually, the mucous membranes are not involved.

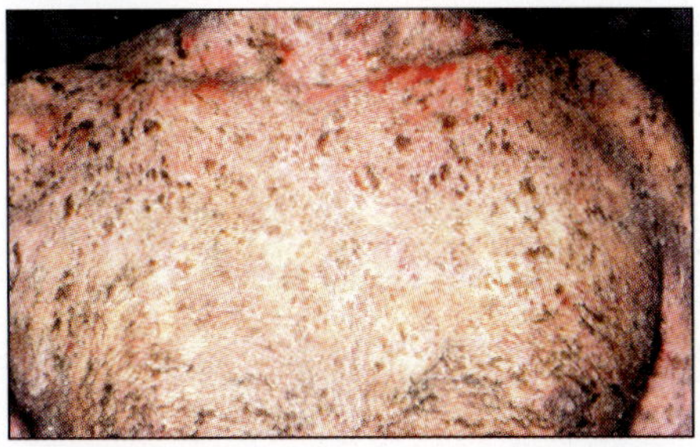

Fig. 20.13 Pemphigus foliaceous: crust upper chest

Pemphigus Erythematosus

Clinical Features

- Lesions consist of scales on an erythematous base.
- Looks like a combination of pemphigus and lupus erythematosus. However, the disease behaves like pemphigus.
- Does not show any systemic manifestations of SLE except the presence of antinuclear and basement membrane antibodies.
- It is milder than pemphigus foliaceous.

Sites

Present on the scalp and face extending to the V of chest.

Pemphigus Vegetans

Mildest form of pemphigus.

Clinical Features

- Lesions are present as vegetating growth.
- Skin folds, e.g., axillae and the groins, are commonly affected.
- Initially, it starts with blisters, but subsequently the base of the ulcer develops into vegetating growth.
- Maceration, exudation and secondary infections are frequently present.

Course

Usually mild.

Drug Induced Pemphigus

Clinical Features

- This presents 2–3 months after the patient has started taking the drug (Table 20.2).

- Develops lesions like pemphigus.
- Intercellular antibodies are found in the majority of such cases.
- Usually, the lesions clear once the drug(s) are withdrawn.

Table 20.2 Drugs causing pemphigus

- D-penicillamine
- Captopril
- Rifampicin
- Phenylbutazone
- Piroxicam

Diagnosis of Pemphigus

Clinical

Positive **Nikolsky's sign**, i.e., peeling of the normal-looking skin on application of pressure during the active phase of the disease.

Histology

Demonstration of acantholytic cells in Tzanck smear (Table 20.3).

Immunopathology

Detection of IgG antibodies deposited at the intercellular area of lesion (in a **fishnet pattern**) in skin, by direct immunofluorescence test.

Serology

IgG antibodies in the serum are demonstrated by indirect immunofluorescence test. Titres of the circulating IgG antibodies usually correlate with the activity of disease.

Antibodies to desmoglein in serum DsgI and DsgIII.

Table 20.3 Diagnostic features of Tzanck smear in skin

Microscopic finding	Diagnosis
Acantholytic cells (large cells with enlarged nuclei and perinuclear halo).	Pemphigus.
Multinucleated giant cells (large cells with multiple nuclei).	Herpes simplex and herpes zoster.

Treatment

- The treatment for pemphigus is presented in Table 20.4. Once all the lesions have healed completely, one can start reducing the dosage of corticosteroids which can be withdrawn completely, while immunosuppressives may be continued in small doses (this has been found to prolong the remission).

Table 20.4 Treatment of pemphigus: At a glance

General treatment
- Cleaning of lesions with soap and water or compresses.
- Topical antibiotic, with or without corticosteroids.
- High protein diet.
- Chillies should be avoided in food.

Systemic Therapy

Systemic corticosteroids in adequate dose (started with 1–1.5 mg/kg of prednisolone) with or without immunosuppressive drugs like methotrexate, cyclophosphamide or azathioprine in adequate dose.
- **Dexamethasone–cyclophosphamide pulse** (DCP) therapy.
- Intramuscular gold sodium thiomalate 25–50 mg, once a week till the condition improves.
- IVIG.
- Biologic response modifiers like rituximab.

- In case there is relapse, corticosteroids may be started again in adequate dose.
- **Dexamethasone–cyclophosphamide pulse** (DCP) therapy: This consists of giving dexamethasone—100 mg in 500 ml 5% glucose transfused over 1–1½ hours on three consecutive days, along with cyclophosphamide—500 mg on second day. This regime is repeated at an interval of twenty-eight days. In between the two pulses, the patients take oral cyclophosphamide—50 mg, daily. This method of treatment has been found to be curative in pemphigus with very few side effects.
- Other medicines found to be useful in pemphigus include:
  i) Intramuscular gold sodium thiomalate 25–50 mg, once a week, till the patient shows improvement.
  ii) Plasma exchange.

Bullous Pemphigoid

Age

Usually develop in older people (Fig. 20.14).

Etiology

The blister occurs due to the separation of epidermis from the underlying dermis.

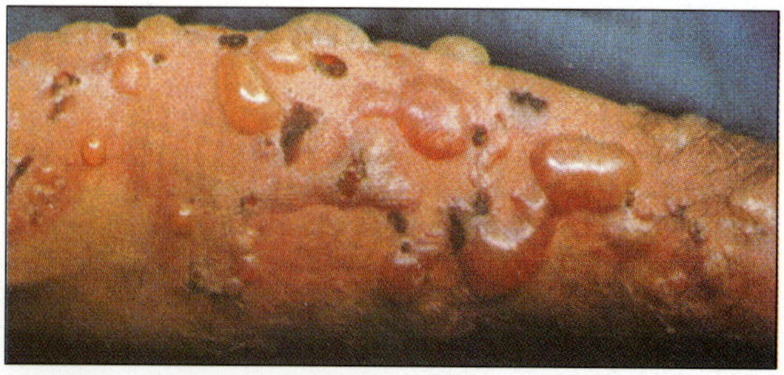

Fig. 20.14 Bullous pemphigoid

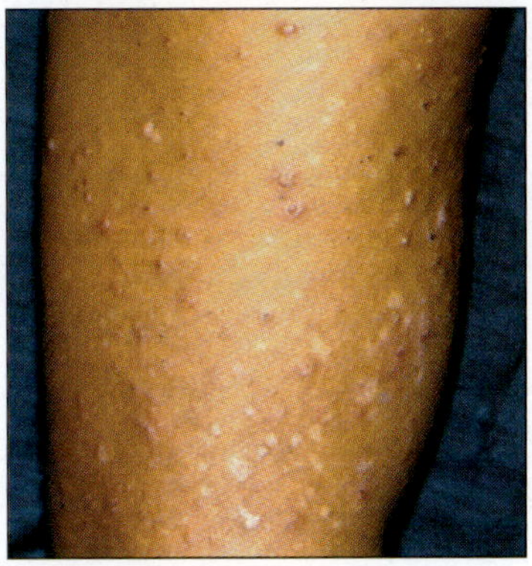

Fig. 20.15 Dermatitis herpetiformis

Clinical Features

- Generally, bullae are asymptomatic, large, tense and filled with clear fluid.
- They are usually surrounded by erythema.
- Bullae may be haemorrhagic.
- Lesions heal faster than the lesions of pemphigus.

Sites

- Predominantly present on flexor aspects of limbs and central part of the abdomen.
- May be seen scattered diffusely all over the body.
- Mucous membranes, by and large, are spared.

Course

Spontaneous remissions and relapses are quite frequent.

Diagnosis

- Biopsy.
- Demonstration of IgG antibodies and C3 (in a linear pattern) at the basement membrane zone by direct immunofluorescence test.
- IgG antibodies in the blood are diagnosed by indirect immunofluorescence test. The **titer does not correlate** with disease activity.

Treatment

- More protein in the diet.
- Lesions should be cleaned properly with soap and water.
- This condition should be treated on the line of pemphigus.

Dermatitis Herpetiformis

Age

Common in young adults and middle-aged people.

Clinical Features

- Severely itchy, urticarial, papular, papulo-vesicular or bullous lesions on an erythematous base (Fig. 20.15).
- Tendency for grouping is seen because of the presence of rapid excoriations.

Sites

- Extensors and buttocks are more frequently involved.
- Mucous membranes and face are usually not involved.
- Lesions tend to be symmetrical.

Course

- There is a tendency for remissions and relapses at variable intervals.
- A majority of cases have gluten-sensitive enteropathy. This results in atrophic villi in the small intestine.

Diagnosis

- Biopsy of early lesions reveals split at the dermo–epidermal junction and accumulation of polymorphs at the tips of the dermal papillae.
- Direct immunofluorescence shows granular deposits of IgA antibodies at the tips of dermal papillae.
- Indirect immunofluoroscence shows immune complex deposits.

Treatment

- Iodide in any form should be avoided as iodide has been seen to aggravate the disease.
- Use of gluten free diet.
- Local treatments are the same as that of pemphigus.
- Dapsone in a dose of 100 mg, twice daily in adults, and 25–50 mg twice daily in children, produces remission in a week's time.

For Non-responders to Dapsone

- Sulphapyridine: 3–4 gm daily in divided doses.
- Systemic corticosteroids as in pemphigus.

Benign Bullous Dermatosis of Childhood

It is a self-limiting blistering disease.

Age

Exclusively in children of 4–5 years of age.

Clinical Features

- The initial attacks are usually more severe than the subsequent recurrences.
- Vesicles and blisters are seen all over the body
- Eyes may be involved with redness, soreness, gritty sensation or conjunctivitis, which may occasionally lead to conjunctival scarring.
- The skin lesions are tense, usually situated on the normal skin, and they may be itchy.
- The lesions heal rapidly with hyperpigmentation and without scars.

Sites

- The lesions are more pronounced on the genitals, buttocks, inner part of the thighs and perioral areas.
- Occasionally, scalp and mouth may also be involved.

Diagnosis

- Skin biopsy shows subepidermal splits.
- Demonstration of linear IgA deposits in the basement membrane zone by direct immunofluorescence test.

Treatment

Dapsone 25–100 mg daily, till the clearance of lesions

For Non-responders to Dapsone

- Sulphapyridine: 3–4 gm, daily.
- Systemic corticosteroids, used as an alternative to sulphapyridine, lead to the clearance of the lesions.
- Local treatment remains the same as that of pemphigus.

Lupus Erythematosus

There are two types of lupus erythematosus:

i) **Discoid lupus erythematosus** (DLE), which is limited only to the skin.
ii) **Systemic lupus erythematosus** (SLE), which also involves other organs of the body.

Discoid Lupus Erythematosus

Age and Sex

- It occurs in all ages and both sexes.
- The occurrence is more in women between 25–45 years of age.

Clinical Features

- Seen as asymptomatic, well-defined, irregular or circular plaques of erythema: scaling, depigmentation, telangiectasia and atrophy of epidermis (Figs. 20.16 and 20.17).
- Scales are thick, large, rough and cannot be removed easily (**stuck-on crust**, Fig. 20.18).
- Follicular openings are dilated and filled with keratotic plugs after removing the scales (**carpet tag sign**).
- Borders of the lesions are usually hyperpigmented.
- Lesions on the scalp produce cicatricial alopecia (Fig. 20.19).
- In the oral mucosa, the lesions are whitish, but lack the lacy pattern of lichen planus.
- Some lesions regress spontaneously and heal after variable periods.

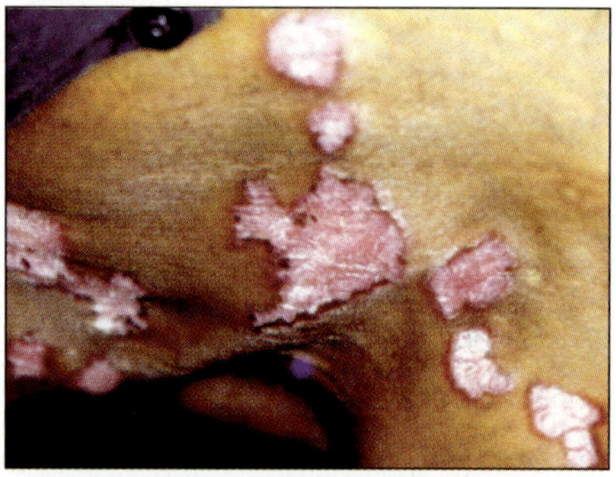

Fig. 20.16 Discoid lupus erythematosus

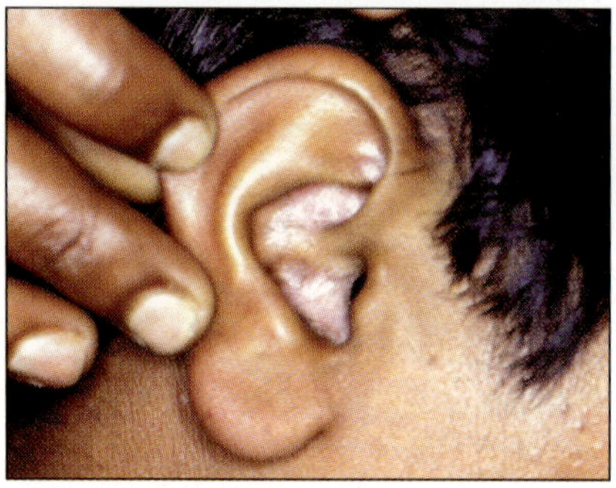

Fig. 20.17 Discoid lupus erythematosus: ear

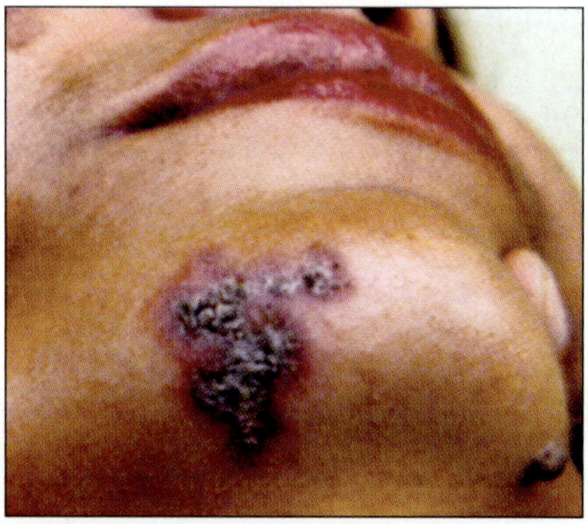

Fig. 20.18 Discoid lupus erythematosus: chin

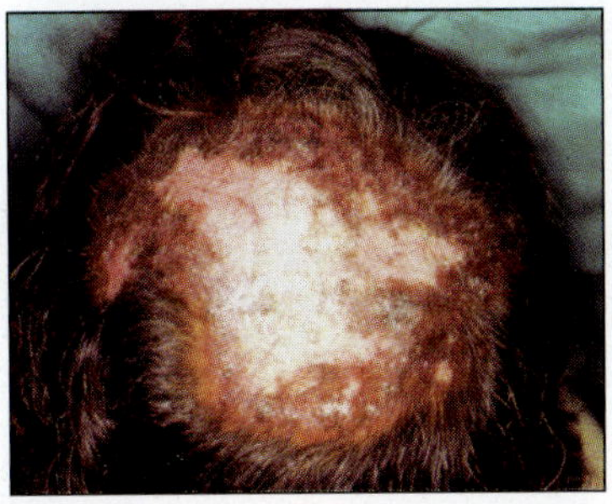

Fig. 20.19 Discoid lupus erythematosus: scalp (cicatricial alopecia)

Sites

Areas exposed to the sun, including the bridge of nose and surrounding areas (**butterfly region**).

Diagnosis

Skin biopsy from the lesions.

Differential Diagnosis

Lichen planus (Table 20.5).

Table 20.5 Difference between discoid lupus erythematosus and lichen planus

Discoid lupus erythematosus	Lichen planus
Lesions with central scarring surrounded by erythema.	Violaceous papules.
Scales adherent and prominent.	Scales minimal or no scales.
Follicular plugs present.	Wickham's striae present.
Photosensitivity present.	Intensely itchy.
Face and ears are common sites.	Wrists and shins are common sites.

Treatment

The overall management of DLE is presented in Table 20.6.

Table 20.6 Management of DLE: At a glance

- Protect from sunlight by clothes, umbrella and sunscreens.
- Topical corticosteroids, massaged twice daily.

For non-responsive or widespread lesions:

- 3–4 courses of chloroquine sulphate, 200 mg twice daily for 2–3 weeks.

For lesions still non-responsive:

- Oral corticosteroids: 20–30 mg prednisolone, daily.

Other forms of treatment

- Oral thalidomide.
- Cyclophosphamide.
- Azathioprine.

Systemic Lupus Erythematosus

Sex

Females.

Clinical Features

General Symptoms

- Fever, weakness, fatigue, weight loss and loss of appetite.
- Arthralgia or arthritis of small joints of hands and feet.
- Diffuse alopecia due to general toxaemia of the disease (Fig. 20.25).
- Cicatricial alopecia on the scalp.
- Superficial ulcerations in the oral, nasal and genital mucosae.
- Raynaud's phenomenon.
- Generalised lymphadenopathy.
- Hepatosplenomegaly are quite frequent.
- Amenorrhoea and menorrhagia.
- Pleuritis and pneumonitis.
- Cardiac involvement (Table 20.7).
- Epilepsy.
- Peripheral neuropathy.
- Mental disturbances.
- Glomerulonephritis.

Table 20.7 Cardiac involvement in SLE

- Pericarditis
- Myocarditis
- Pericardial rub
- Effusion
- Coronary vasculitis
- Occasionally, endocarditis

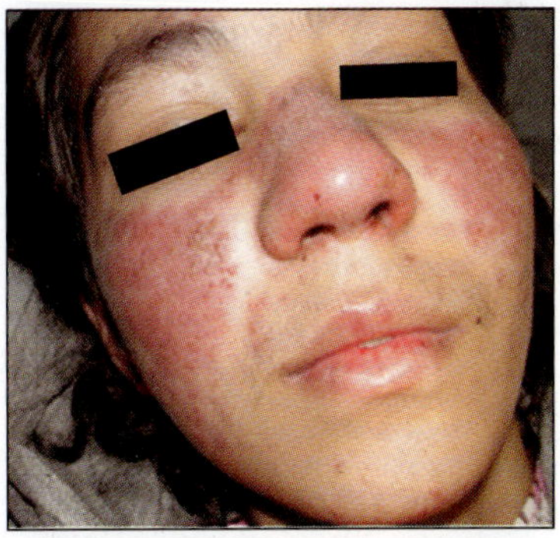

Fig. 20.20 Systemic lupus erythematosus: face

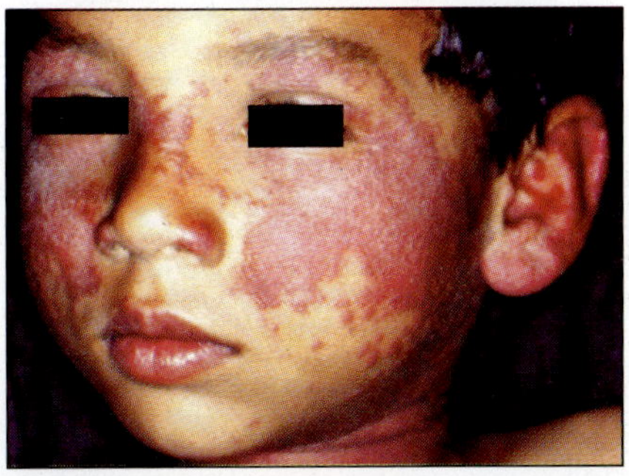

Fig. 20.21 Systemic lupus erythematosus: macules on face

Skin lesions

- Ill-defined erythematous macules.
- Dusky-red discolouration (Figs 20.20 and 20.21) on the cheeks, bridge of the nose, forehead, chin (Fig. 20.22), external ear, V area of the chest, dorsum of hands (Fig. 20.23), forearms and (less commonly) other areas (Fig. 20.24).
- Occasionally, urticaria, maculo-papules, purpura, bullae, urticarial vasculitis or livido-reticularis are present.
- Telangiectasia may be seen on posterior nail-fold.
- Small infarcts on the finger-tips may be present.
- Superficial gangrene of the fingers and toes may occur.

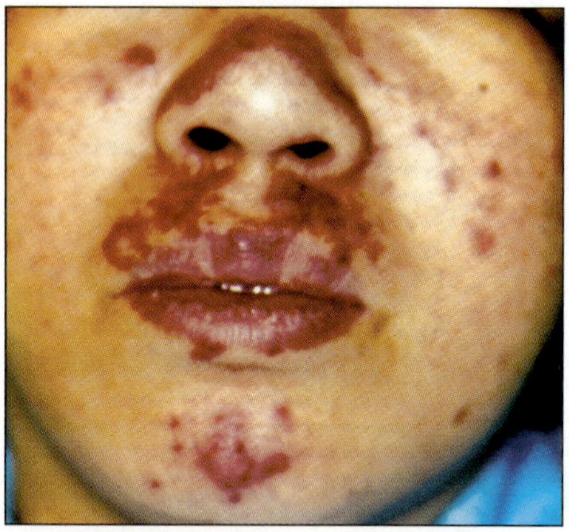

Fig. 20.22 SLE: bridge of nose and chin

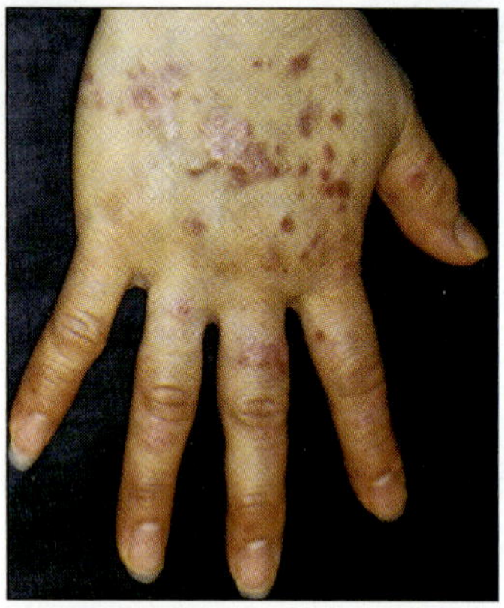

Fig. 20.23 SLE: dorsum of hand

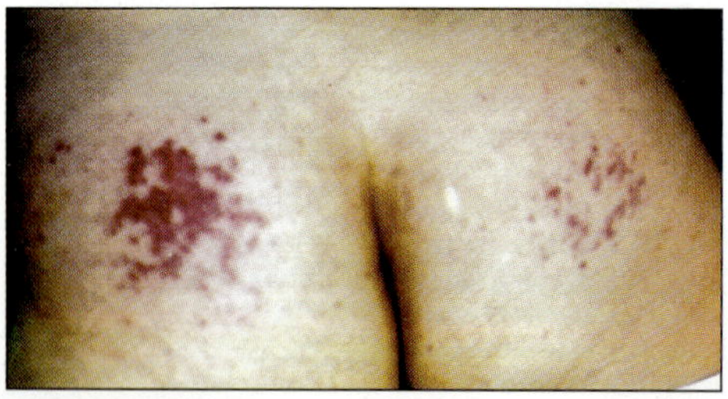

Fig. 20.24 SLE: buttocks

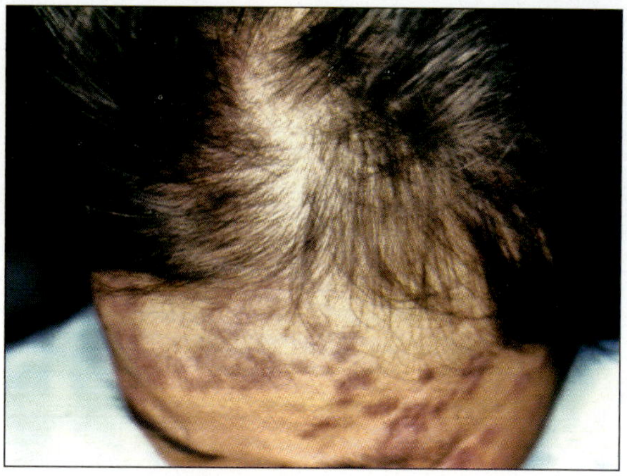

Fig. 20.25 Diffuse alopecia: SLE

Diagnosis

Skin biopsy for histopathology and direct immuno-ophthalmic involvement (Table 20.8).

Table 20.8 Immuno-opthalmic involvement in SLE

Conjunctivitis.
Uveitis.
Periorbital oedema.
Haemorrhage.
Optic nerve atrophy.

- Fluorescence staining from the lesion and from normal skin show deposition of IgG antibodies at the basement membrane zone.
- Serum for **auto-antibodies** such as:
  i) **Antinuclear antibodies**(ANF) present in 90% of cases.
  ii) Anti-DNA antibodies in almost all active cases.
  iii) Anti-Sm antibodies in 15–25%, but their presence seems to be specific.
- Raised ESR.
- Anaemia.
- Leucopenia.
- Thrombocytopenia.
- Reversal of albumin/globulin ratio.
- Biological false-positive VDRL test.
- Hypergamma-globulinaemia.

Treatment

- Prognosis is not very poor.
- Systemic corticosteroids and various immunosuppressive agents, in a dose and manner as used for the treatment of pemphigus, have been found to be useful in SLE.
- Dexamethasone cyclophosphamide pulse (DCP) therapy, as used in pemphigus, has also been found curative in SLE.

Scleroderma

Scleroderma occurs in two forms:
i) A localised form called morphoea.
ii) Systemic form called systemic sclerosis.

Morphoea

Sex

Most commonly in females.

Clinical Features

- Asymptomatic, mildly hyperpigmented, indurated, circumscribed area with atrophy of the epidermis which results in shiny and wrinkled appearance (Figs 20.26 and 20.27).
- Initially, the lesions are pale and they increase in size.
- But after several months or years, the lesions start regressing spontaneously, become depressed and atrophic with loss of hair.
- Usually 1–2 patches are present.
- Lesion on hairy areas produces cicatricial alopecia.

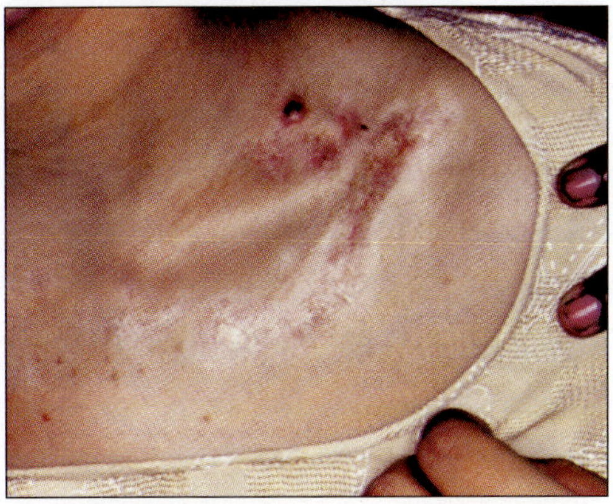

Fig. 20.26 Morphoea: localised

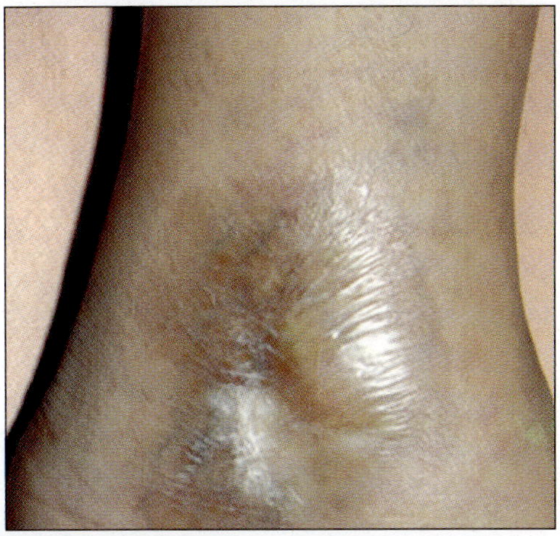

Fig. 20.27 Morphoea: ankle

Sites

- The lesions are usually seen on the extremities.
- They may be seen on any part of the body.

Generalised Morphoea

- Occasionally, multiple, large plaques are seen all-over the trunk and extremities (Fig. 20.28).
- Intervening skin between the two patches is usually normal.

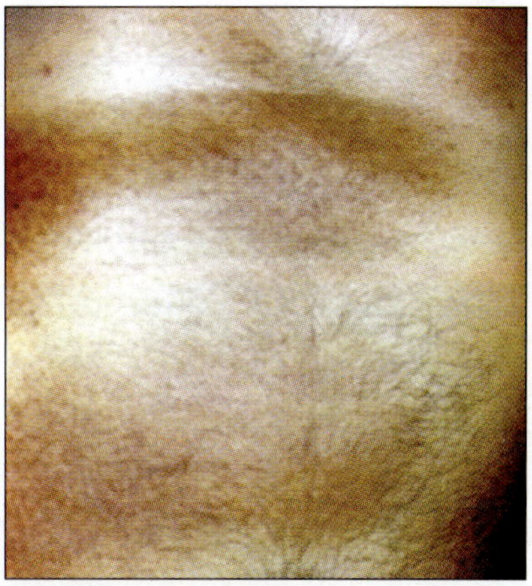

Fig. 20.28 Morphoea: generalised

Linear Morphoea

- Linear elongated plaques, usually located on the extremities or on the forehead (Fig. 20.29).
- Often associated with atrophy of the underlying subcutaneous tissues, muscles, and even bones.

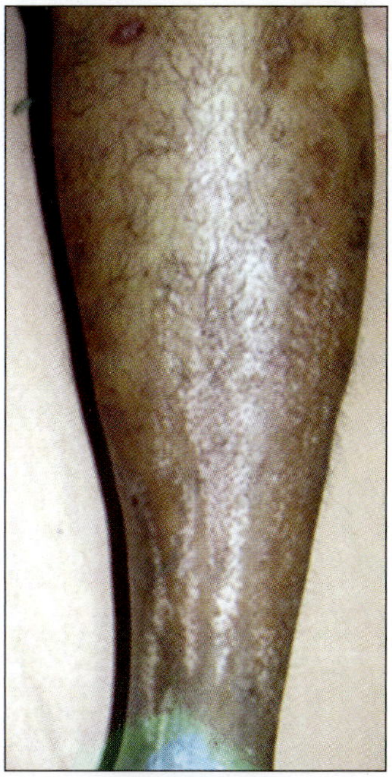

Fig. 20.29 Linear morphoea: leg

En Coup De Sabre

When the linear lesion is situated on the forehead and scalp, it is called en coup de sabre.

Guttate Morphea

Occasionally, multiple small ivory white spots of 2–3 mm size are present on the chest, neck, shoulders and legs. They are believed to be lesions of lichen sclerosus et atrophicus (Table 20.9).

Table 20.9 Lichen sclerosis et atrophicus (LSA) and morphoea

LSA	Morphoea
Begins as discrete small lesions which become confluent.	Indurated plaques.
Ivory colour.	Brown, though initially may be ivory-white.
Follicular plugs prominent.	Follicular plugs absent.

Diagnosis

Skin biopsy.

Treatment

- Majority of the lesions regress spontaneously in 3–5 years.
- The regression can be accelerated by:
  i) Systemic corticosteroids: 15–20 mg prednisolone, daily for 3–6 months.
  ii) Topical corticosteroids are usually not effective.

Systemic Sclerosis

Sex

Usually in women.

Clinical Features

- Raynaud's phenomenon (Fig. 20.30) in majority of the patients where fingers and toes become cold and blue on exposure to cold, especially seen in winter months.

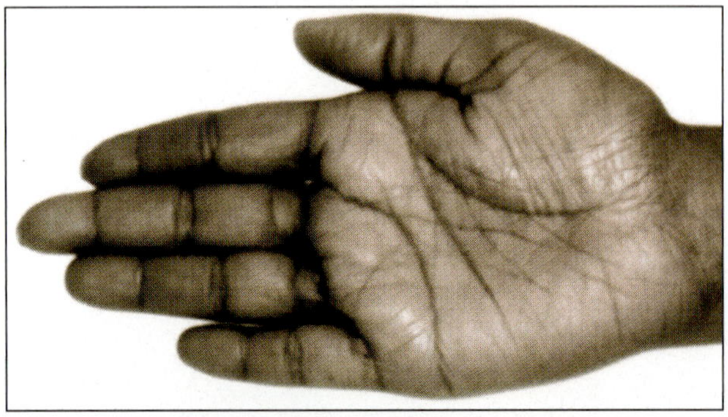

Fig. 20.30 Systemic sclerosis: Raynaud's phenomenon

- Pain and stiffness in the fingers.
- Skin changes occur in about 90% of cases, e.g., generalised thickening and darkening of the skin which is bound down on the underlying structures and cannot be lifted up into a fold.
- Skin looks shiny due to, atrophy of epidermis.
- Lesions are more prominent, initially at the peripheral parts of the body like hands, feet and face but ultimately spread proximally and involve the whole body.
- Due to disappearance of the naso-labial folds and furrows on the forehead, the face looks expressionless (Fig. 20.31) with pinched nose (**beaking nose**) and thin lips (**purse string lips**, Fig. 20.32).

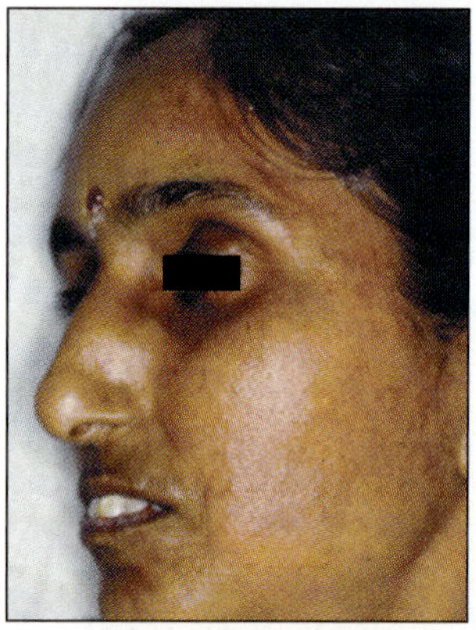

Fig. 20.31 Systemic sclerosis: expresionless face

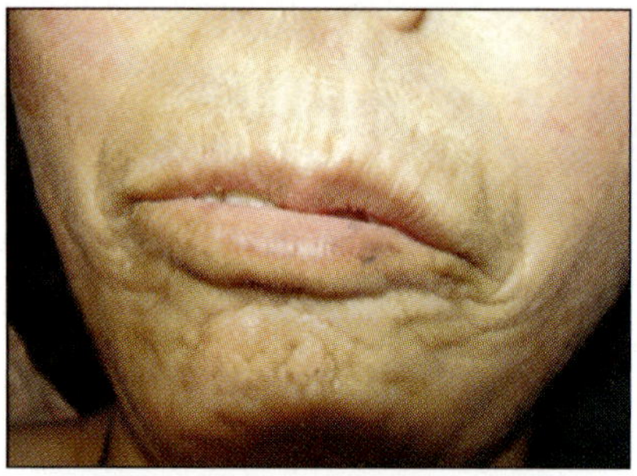

Fig. 20.32 Systemic sclerosis: mouth

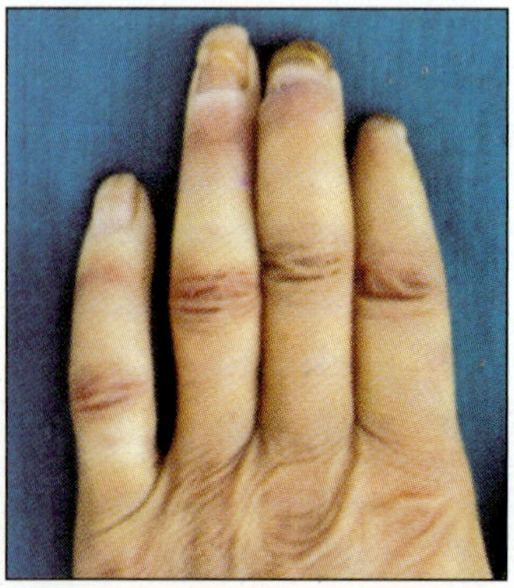

Fig. 20.33 Systemic sclerosis: thin and tapered fingers

- The fingers become thin and tapered (Fig. 20.33).
- In long-standing cases, absorption of the terminal phalanges is seen with shortening of the corresponding nails (Figs 20.34–20.37).
- Skin may show punctate spots of depigmentation on the face, neck, arms and upper trunk (Fig. 20.38).

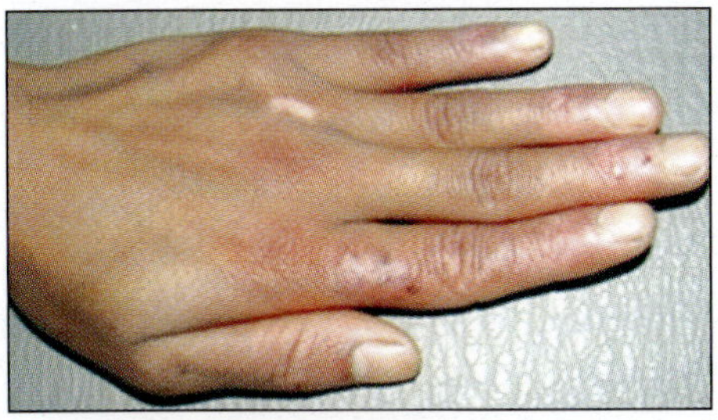

Fig. 20.34 Systemic sclerosis: hand

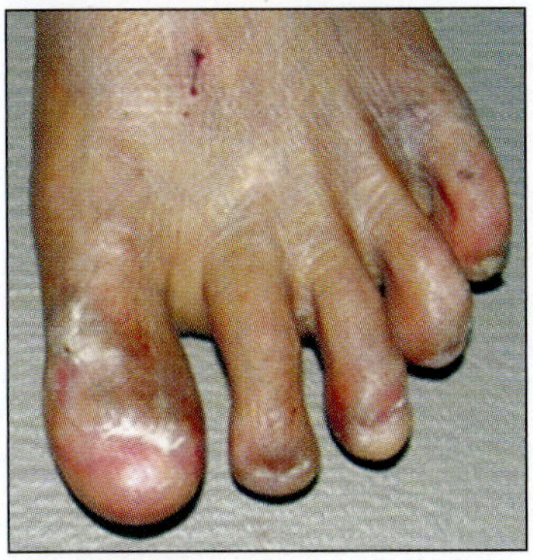

Fig. 20.35 Systemic sclerosis: toes

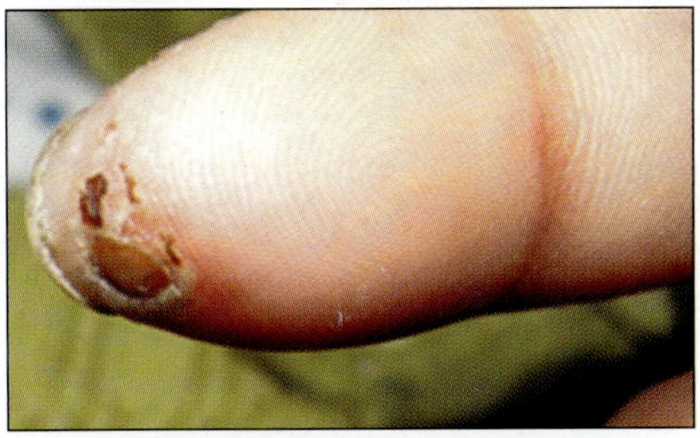

Fig. 20.36 Systemic sclerosis: ulcer tip finger

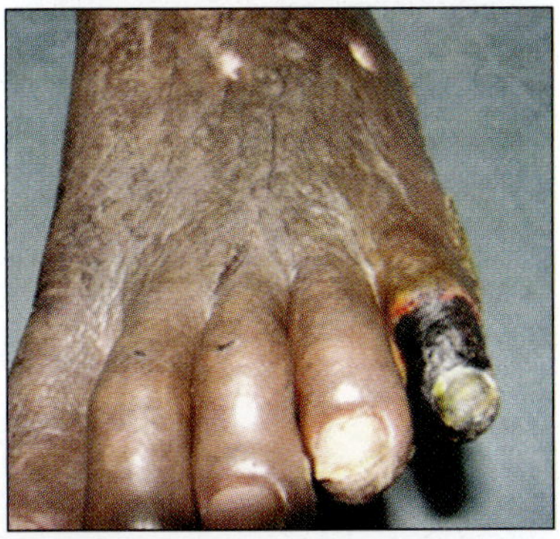

Fig. 20.37 Systemic sclerosis: gangrene

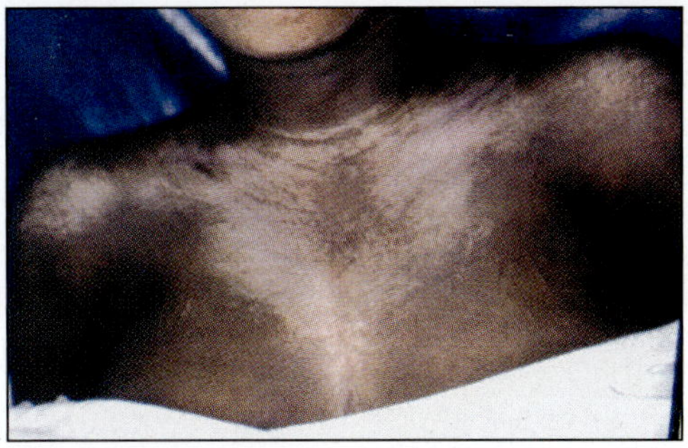

Fig. 20.38 Systemic sclerosis: depigmentation on chest

Internal Organs' Involvement

Gastrointestinal

Gastrointestinal involvement presents as:
- Difficulty in swallowing.
- Esophagitis.
- Symptoms of peptic ulcer.
- Recurrent diarrhoea and constipation.

Respiratory

Respiratory involvement present as dyspnoea due to the thickening of interstitial membrane.

Renal

Renal involvement may manifest as:
- Uraemia.
- Renal hypertension.
- Renal failure, which is the chief cause of fatalities.

Other Complications

Some patients complain of:
- Arthralgia or arthritis.
- Fever.
- Amenorrhea.
- Calcinosis.

Diagnosis

- Skin biopsy from the lesions.
- Antinuclear antibodies with nucleolar or speckled pattern in the serum are present in most of the active patients.
- Scl-70 is very specific, but not present in all the cases.
- X-ray of the chest shows increased bronchopulmonary markings or changes of emphysema or interstitial lung disease.
- X-ray of the hand shows osteoporosis, thinning and absorption of the phalangeal bones or calcium deposits in the skin.
- Barium meal studies may show lack of peristalsis and dilatation of the oesophagus.
- Similar changes are noticed in the small intestines.

- Pulmonary function tests to assess the extent of respiratory impairment.
- Renal function tests for the presence of albumin in the urine and raised blood urea.
- Electrocardiographs for detecting the cardiac involvement.

Treatment

The drugs used for the treatment of systemic sclerosis are presented in Table 20.10. Other precautions to prevent the complications are as follows:

- Protect from cold during winter.
- Vasodilators like nefedipine, 10–20 mg, daily.
- Avoidance of smoking.

Table 20.10 Drugs used in the treatment of systemic sclerosis

- Systemic corticosteroids.
- D-penicillamine: 250–1500 mg/day.
- Colchicine.
- Cyclophosphamide.
- Azathioprine.
- Cyclosporin.
- Plasmapheresis.

With variable result

Recently, dexamethasone cyclophosphamide pulse therapy (DCP) using dexamethasone 100 mg in 500 ml, 5% glucose intravenously for three consecutive days and cyclophosphamide 500 mg on day 2 and 50 mg daily, orally in between pulse, repeated at monthly intervals for 2–3 years, has been found to arrest and reverse the pathological changes to a variable extent in majority of the patients.

Dermatomyositis

It is an autoimmune disorder involving the skin, muscle and blood vessels.

Age

Two varieties of this condition are seen. They are as follows:

- Childhood variety seen mostly in children under the age of 10 years.
- Adulthood variety seen between 40–60 years of age.

Sex

The frequency of occurrence in women is twice as much as in men.

Clinical Features

There may be difficulty in speech and swallowing.

Muscles

- Aching, painful, tender muscles with weakness, and later on atrophy.
- Difficulty in going upstairs or rising from a chair.
- In women, difficulty in raising the arm high enough to comb the hair.
- Recurrent bursitis of shoulders and hips may precede the myositis and effusion of joints.
- The most frequently involved muscles are that of limbs, girdles, proximal part of limbs, pharynx and tongue. However, muscles involvement is not uniform.

Skin Rash

- Purplish-red, heliotropic erythema involving eyelids, upper cheeks, forehead and temples. This rash confirms the diagnosis (Fig. 20.39).
- **Gottron's papules**: Voilaceus, atrophic papules are seen over the knuckles and pressure points.

Calcinosis Cutis

- Presence of hard calcium in the skin.
- More than 90% patients with calcinosis are women.
- Majority of children with dermatomyositis have calcinosis.
- Calcinosis is a good sign for survival, but the functional recovery is less.
- Contracture develops in 5–10% of patients.
- Occasionally, patients may have cardiomyopathy, Raynaud's phenomenon and arthralgia or arthritis.

Nail Fold

Telangiectasia and haemorrhage.

Carcinoma

- About 30–40% of adult dermatomyositis are associated with underlying internal malignancy.
- Common tumours include tumour of lung, breast, female genital tract, stomach, rectum, kidney or testis.

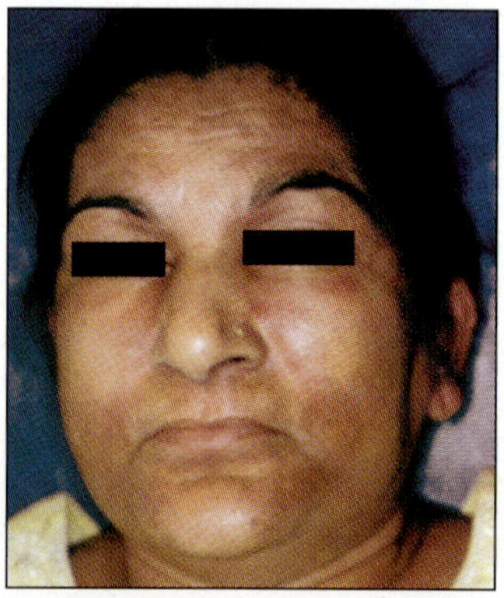

Fig. 20.39 Dermatomyositis

- Dermatomyositis usually gets worst with the progress of neoplasm, but may improve when the neoplasm is treated.

Diagnosis

- Skin biopsy from muscles.
- Elevated muscle enzyme, such as follows:
  - i) Creatine phosphokinase (CPK) (specific and sensitive).
  - ii) Serum aldolase.
  - iii) SGOT, SGPT, LDH.
  - iv) Electromyography.
  - v) ANA usually negative.

Course

- Majority of the deaths are due to underlying carcinoma.
- Precipitating factors include the following:
  - i) Acute pulmonary infiltrations.
  - ii) Dysphasia.
  - iii) Increasing age.
  - iv) Children have better prognosis.

Treatment

- Rest in acute phase.
- Exclude an underlying carcinoma in adults.

Systemic Corticosteroids

Initial dose of 60 to 120 mg of prednisolone, daily. The dose should be gradually reduced as the patient improves.

Immunosuppressive (As steroid sparing agents)

- Methotrexate 10–15 mg/daily.
- Azathioprine 1–2 mg/daily.
- Cyclophosphamide 100 mg/daily.
- These therapies are required for some years till the disease is burnt out totally.
- Recently dexamethasone cyclophosphamide pulse therapy (DCP) as given in pemphigus and SLE has been found to be curative.

CHAPTER 21

Skin Disorders in Systemic Diseases

SYSTEMIC DISEASES WITH SKIN MANIFESTATIONS

Systemic diseases that may have skin manifestations are endocrine diseases, renal diseases, internal malignancies, metabolic diseases and malnutrition.

Ëndocrine Diseases

Ëndocrine diseases which have skin lesions associated with them are:

- Diabetes mellitus.
- Thyroid disorders.
- Adrenal gland disorders like Addison's disease and Cushing's syndrome.

Diabetes Mellitus

Skin Manifestations

The skin manifestations of diabetes are presented in Table 21.1.

Table 21.1 Cutaneous manifestations of diabetes

Infections:	Other dermatoses:
• Pyogenic	• Xanthomas
• Candidiasis	• Neuropathic foot ulcers
• Diabetic dermopathy	• Sclerodactyly
• Acanthisis nigricans	
• Necrobiosis lipoidica	

Infection

Sometimes infections, especially pyogenic and candida, are the first manifestations of diabetes.

Pyogenic Infection

- Recurrent furuncles and carbuncles frequently caused by *Staphylococcus aureus* may be the presenting features.
- Infection is usually extensive and requires aggressive treatment.

Candida Infection

Recurrent balanoposthitis or candidal vulvovaginitis may be the first manifestation of undiagnosed diabetes.

Diabetic Dermopathy

- It occurs due to microangiopathy and very commonly affects the shins in cases of long standing diabetes.
- Presents as small, dull-red papules (Fig. 21.1)with scales. Papules slowly subside leaving small, brown depressed scars (Fig. 21.2).

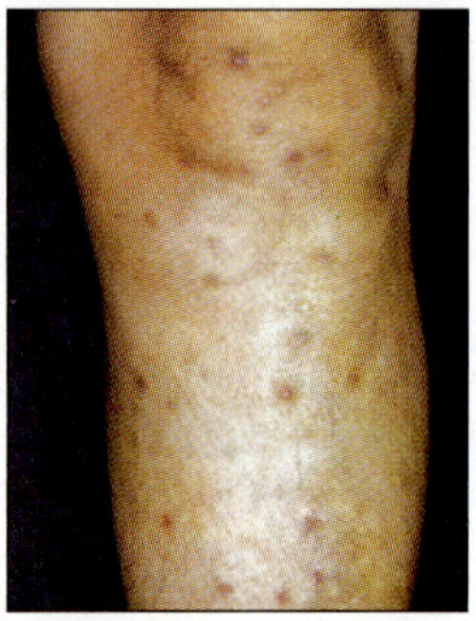

Fig. 21.1 Diabetic dermopathy: active

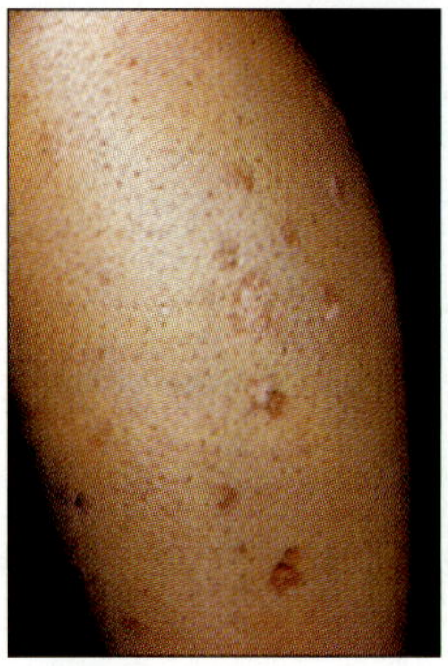

Fig. 21.2 Diabetic dermopathy: scars

Acanthosis Nigricans

- It usually occurs in insulin resistant diabetics.
- Presents as hyperpigmented thick areas on neck, axillae, inguinal and inframammary folds.

Necrobiosis Lipoidica

- Majority of patients with necrobiosis have diabetes and impaired glucose tolerance. However, less than 2% diabetics develop necrobiosis lipoidica.
- More frequently occurs on shins as single or multiple, asymptomatic, indurated, annular, yellowish-brown plaques that may ulcerate.

Granuloma Annulare

- Extensive and atypical lesions that often have glucose intolerance.
- Skin-coloured erythematous papules arranged in an annular pattern (Fig. 21.3).

- Commonly seen on the knuckles and dorsal aspect of hands.

Pruritus

- Skin in majority of diabetics becomes dry, more so in winter.
- Generalised itching is present all over body.

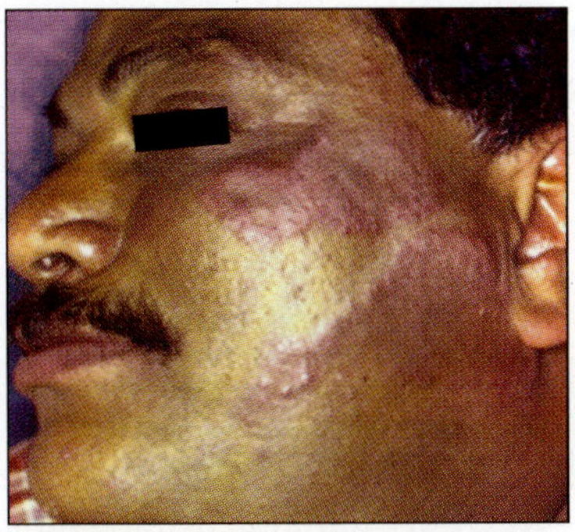

Fig. 21.3 Granuloma annulare: face

Diabetic Neuropathy

- It is more commonly seen in elderly due to the impairment of autonomic vasomotor response.
- Presents initially as pain, hyperesthesia and paraesthesia on the feet.
- Later on, blisters (Fig. 21.4) appear on the tip of the toes.

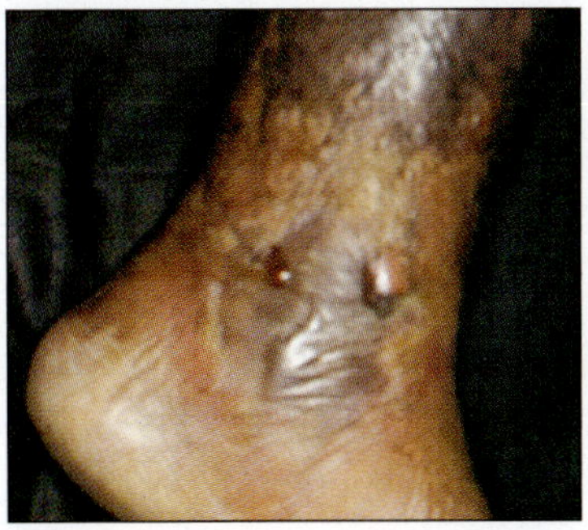

Fig. 21.4 Diabetic bullae

Thyroid Disorders

Hypothyroidism

Skin Manifestations

Skin appears dry, pale and cold.

Face

- Face has a broad nose, thick lips and long thick tongue.
- Face may appear expressionless.

Myxedema

Generalised, non-pitting edema.

Hair

Hair is dry, coarse and brittle. There is loss of hair which may be patchy or diffuse. Supraciliary madarosis of lateral third of eye-brow is seen.

Hyperthyroidism

- Palmoplanter hyperhidrosis.
- Flushing of face with palmar erythema.
- Hyperpigmentation of face as well as vitiligo are commonly associated.
- Pretibial myxedema.

Adrenal Gland Disorders

Addison's Disease

Etiology

The cutaneous pigmentation seen in this disease is due to an increased secretion of melanotropic hormones.

Clinical features

- Pigmentation is diffuse, but more intense in the areas exposed to sunlight, flexors, sites of pressure, traction and creases of palms and soles.
- Pigmented areas like nipples and genitals become more dark.
- Pigmentation in buccal mucosa is almost always present.

Treatment

Pigmentation gets cleared by the oral administration of corticosteroids.

Cushing's Syndrome

Etiology

In Cushing's syndrome, there is an over-production of glucocorticoids by the suprarenal glands.

Clinical Features

- Due to redistribution of subcutaneous fat presenting as moon facies (Fig. 21.5), buffalo hump, pot-belly and slender limbs.

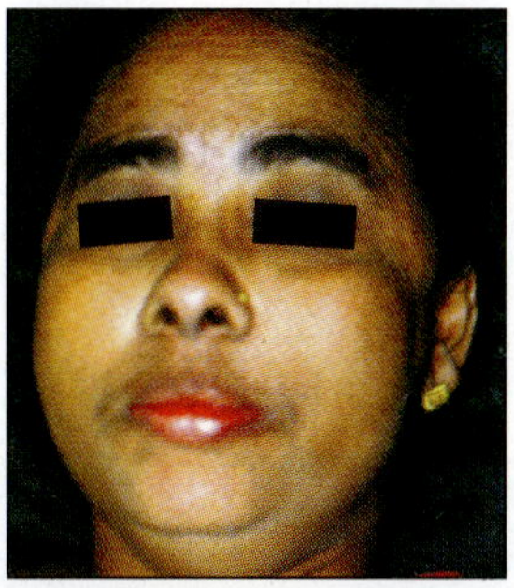

Fig. 21.5 Cushing's syndrome: moon facies

- Purplish **striaeatrophicans** are commonly seen **on trunk** and limb.
- Hirsutism is present.
- Acneiform eruptions.
- Addisonian pigmentation.
- Infections by both candida and atypical dermatophyte.

Skin Manifestations in Renal Disorder

Skin changes observed in renal disorder are as follows:

- Dry skin with fine scaling and itching.
- Pallor due to anaemia.
- Muddy-brown discolouration of skin.
- Increased nail pigmentation, usually on distal half.
- Purpura.
- Calcinosis cutis, presenting as tender, woody, infiltrated, nodular plaques around the axillae, thighs, large joints and perineum.

Skin Manifestations in Liver Disorders

Skin lesions in hepatic disorders, especially in hepatic failure, are as follows:

- Jaundice.
- Spider naevi and palmar erythema.
- Telangiectasia.
- Purpura.
- White nail bed due to hypo-albuminaemia.
- Diffuse pigmentation.
- Loss of axillary and pubic hair.
- Pruritus due to increased bile salt.

Skin Manifestations in Internal Malignancies

Cutaneous lesions due to internal malignancy can be divided broadly into four groups:

- Cutaneous metastasis.
- Genodermatoses.
- Cutaneous markers of exposure to a carcinogen.
- Paraneoplastic syndromes.

Cutaneous Metastases

Cutaneous metastases may be due to the following causes:

- Direct spread of tumour to skin as in Paget's disease of breast.
- Spread through the blood from distant sites like adenocarcinoma of stomach, large bowel, ovaries, kidneys or lung.

Genodermatoses

Genodermatoses with an increased predisposition to internal neoplasm include the following conditions:

- **Peutz–Jeghers Syndrome**: Pigmentation of lips, oral mucosa and perioral area with frequent association of polyposis of small intestine and occasionally carcinomatous change.
- **Palmoplantar keratoderma**, especially tylosis and esophageal carcinoma.
- **Neurofibromatosis**: Sarcomatous changes in deep lesion is occasionally seen.
- Mucosal neuromata, medullary thyroid carcinoma and phaeochromocytoma (**Sipple's syndrome**) with neuromata. Risk of medullary thyroid carcinoma is very high in the presence of neuromata.
- Association of multiple sebaceous adenomata, especially of trunk, with gastrointestinal carcinoma.

Cutaneous Markers of Exposure to Carcinogens

Cutaneous markers of exposure to a carcinogen may be categorised as follows:

Exposure to Arsenic

Exposure to arsenic produces pigmentation, keratosis, superficial basal cell carcinoma and internal carcinoma, especially of bronchus.

Bowen Disease

Bowen disease on covered skin is discovered with a high degree of internal malignancy within 5–10 years of diagnosis of skin manifestation.

Nicotinic Staining

Nicotinic staining of the fingers indicates the predisposition of bronchus towards tobacco-linked neoplasia.

Radiation

Radiation induced dermatitis (Fig. 21.6) increases the risk of carcinoma of the underlying tissue, especially thyroid carcinoma.

Paraneoplastic Syndrome

Acanthosis Nigricans

When the thickening and pigmentation of the skin of flexors (Fig. 21.7) develops for the first time in an adult with the absence of obesity and negative family history, it may be associated with gastric carcinoma. It is generally itchy.

Dermatomyositis

When this occurs in adults, it may be associated with carcinoma.

Digital Ischaemia

Atypical Raynaud's phenomenon of late onset with persistent pain may be a reliable marker of internal malignancy.

Annular Erythemas

Annular erythemas (Fig. 21.8), especially erythema gyratum repens, are frequently associated with internal malignancy.

Necrolytic Migratory Erythema

It is usually associated with islet cell carcinoma of pancreas.

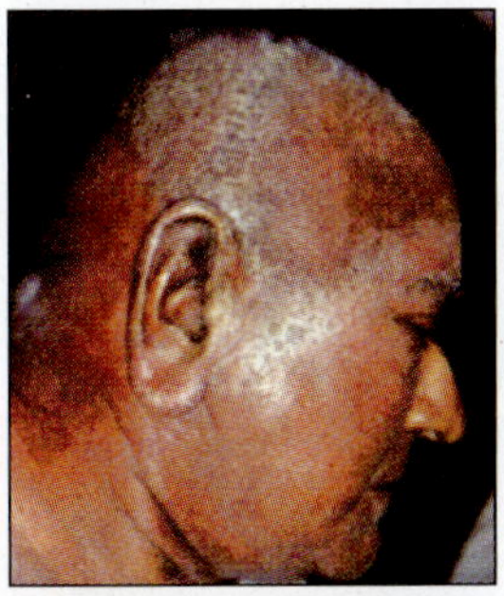

Fig. 21.6 Radiodermatitis

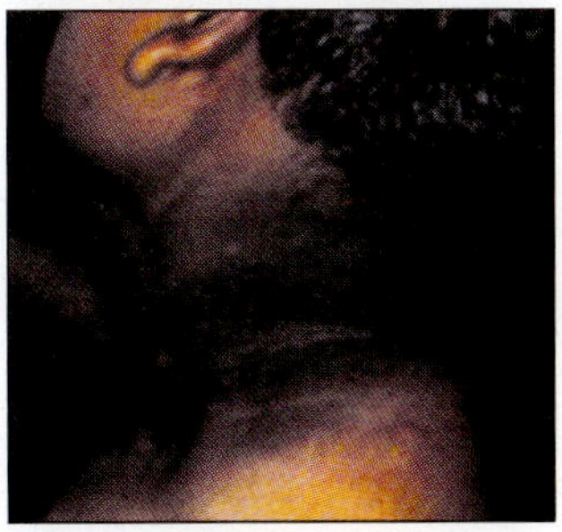

Fig. 21.7 Acanthosis nigricans

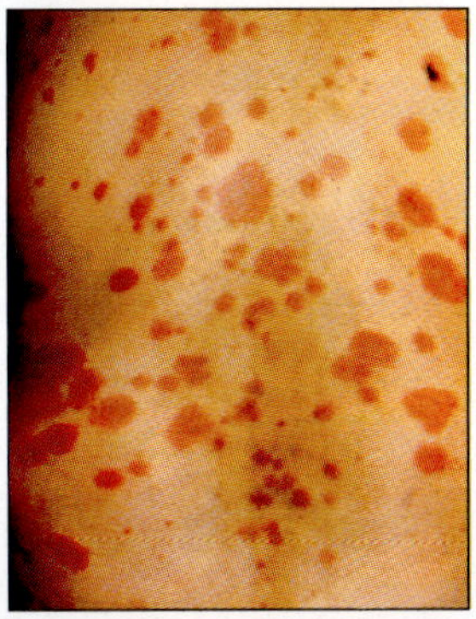

Fig. 21.8 Annular erythema

Paraneoplastic Pemphigus

- Skin lesions of pemphigus along with painful mucosal, especially oral lesions.
- Associated with thymoma and lymphoma.

Migratory Thrombophlebitis

- Multiple, superficial and deep venous thrombosis.
- Many cases show underlying malignancy, especially carcinoma of pancreas.

Acquired ichthyosis

- Late onset of ichthyosis like lesions (Fig. 21.9).
- May occasionally be associated with Hodgkin's disease and other neoplasms.

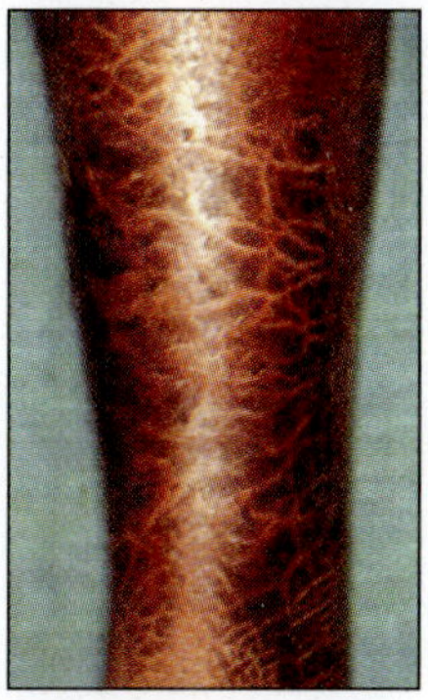

Fig. 21.9 Acquired ichthyosis

Pruritus

- The presence of severe intractable pruritus, especially of nostrils, is a well-recognised symptom of brain tumours.
- Generalised severe pruritus is seen in Hodgkin's tumour.

Pyoderma Gangrenosum

This condition is sometimes associated with leukemia (Fig. 21.10).

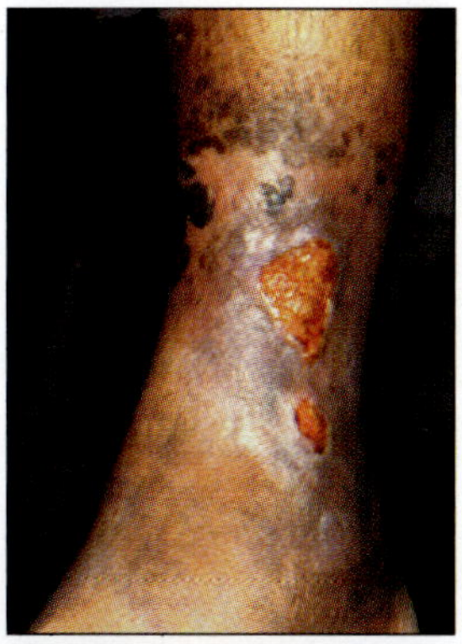

Fig. 21.10 Pyoderma gangrenosum

Erythroderma

Erythroderma may be the presentation of mycosis fungoides. It may be associated with the underlying lymphoma or leukemia.

Leser–Trelat Sign

- Sudden development of large numbers of seborrhoeic keratosis with pruritus.
- Alhough its occurrence is rare, it is a reliable marker of internal malignancy.

Eruptive Keratoacanthoma

This may be associated with the carcinoma of fallopion tubes and stem cell leukaemia.

Unilateral lymphoedema

Sudden onset of unilateral lymphoedema over the age of 40–45 suggests the obstruction of abdominal lymphatics from malignant deposits or a pelvic neoplasm.

Herpes Zoster

Herpes zoster (Fig. 21.11) occurring with great severity and frequent dissemination may be associated with reticulosis—a lympho proliferative disorder.

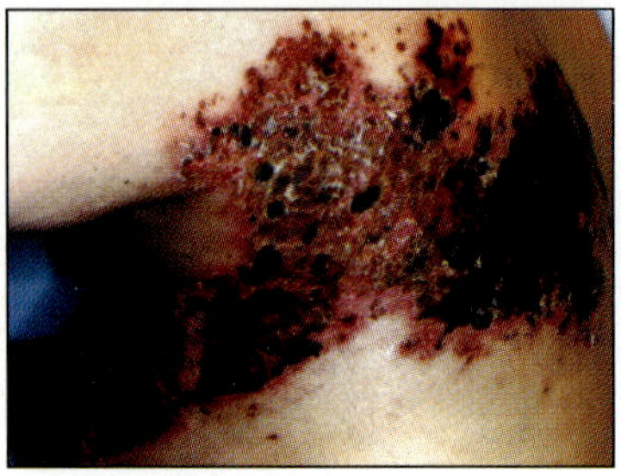

Fig. 21.11 Herpes zoster in reticulosis

Acquired Hypertrichosis Lanuginosa

This is a rare condition associated with carcinoma in most of the cases.

Graft versus Host Reaction

Reactions involve predominantly the following organs:

- Intestinal tract: Diarrhoea.
- Liver: Liver dysfunction.
- Skin: Skin lesions.

Acute Reaction

- Occurs 7–10 days after transplantation.
- Macular eruptions appear on the trunk followed by face and hands.
- Within the first six weeks, more florid eruptions develop like diffuse erythema and scaling. Lichenoid lesion or bullae appear and they may look like toxic epidermal necrosis.

Chronic stage

- Occurs after 3–12 months.
- Macular or maculopapular lesions turn to lichenoid.
- Lesions of skin and buccal mucosae look like lichen planus (Fig. 21.12).
- Later on, develop atrophy, dermal sclerosis and reticulate pigmentation.

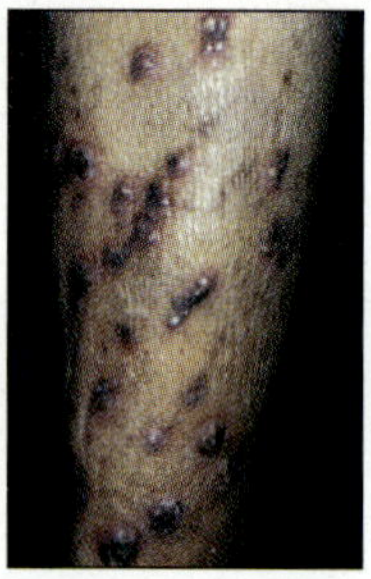

Fig. 21.12 Lichenoid eruption: graft versus host reaction

Treatment

- Antibiotics to reduce the infection from gut.
- Immunosuppressive drugs may also diminish the severity of condition.

CHAPTER 22

Tumours of the Skin

A tumour is are an abnormal growth of tissue due to some stimulus. They usually develop late in life and are not seen at birth. Depending upon their tendency to metastasize, they may be benign or malignant (Table 22.1).

Table 22.1 Benign tumours of the skin

Seborrhoeic keratosis	Tricho-epithelioma
Dermatosis papulosa nigra (DPN)	Milia
Skin tag	Syringoma

Seborrhoeic Keratosis

- The lesions may be pedunculated when present on the eyelids or on the flexors.
- Sudden appearance of a large number of seborrhoeic keratoses may be associated with internal malignancy. This is called **Leser–Trelat sign.**

Size

The size of lesions may vary from 1 mm to several centimeters.

Etiology

Occurs due to the accumulation of immature keratinocytes between the basal cells and stratum corneum.

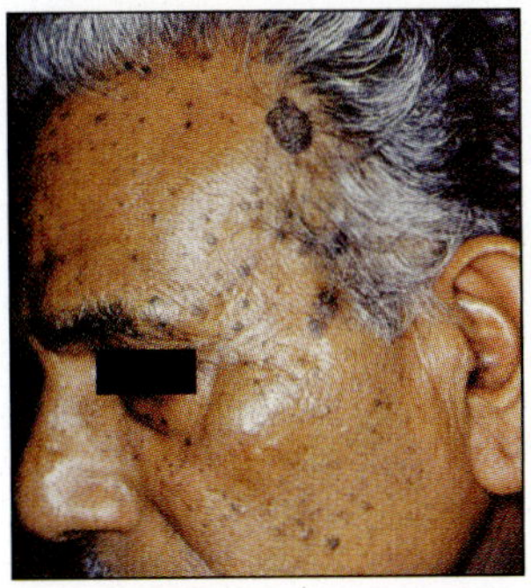

Fig. 22.1 Seborrhoeic keratosis

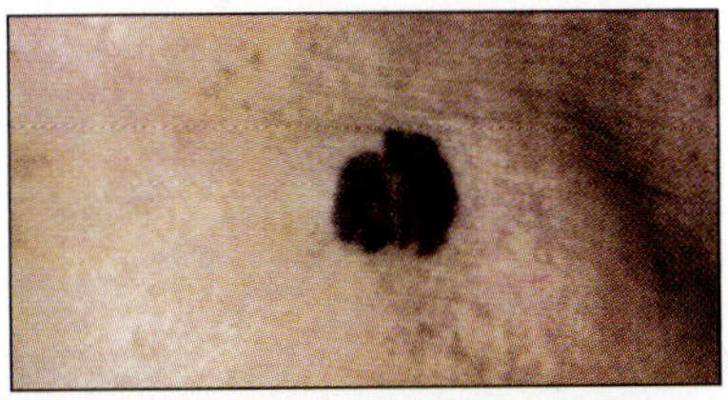

Fig. 22.2 Seborrhoeic keratosis: single lesion

Clinical Features

- Hyperpigmented papules with lustureless granular surface are seen.
- Sometimes a dirty-yellow, loosely adherent, greasy keratin is present on the surface of the papules.

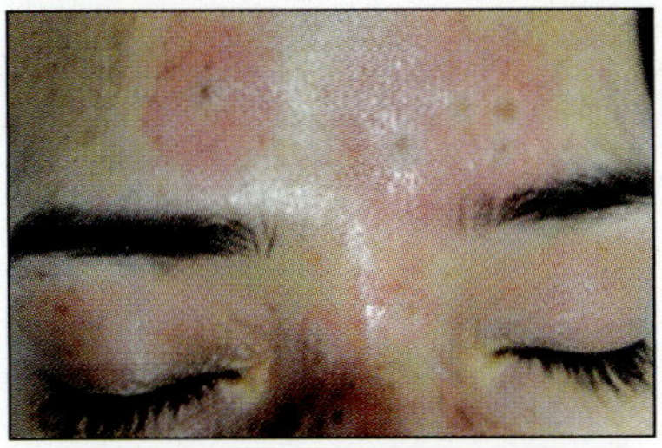

Fig. 22.3 Seborrhoeic keratosis: during cryotherapy

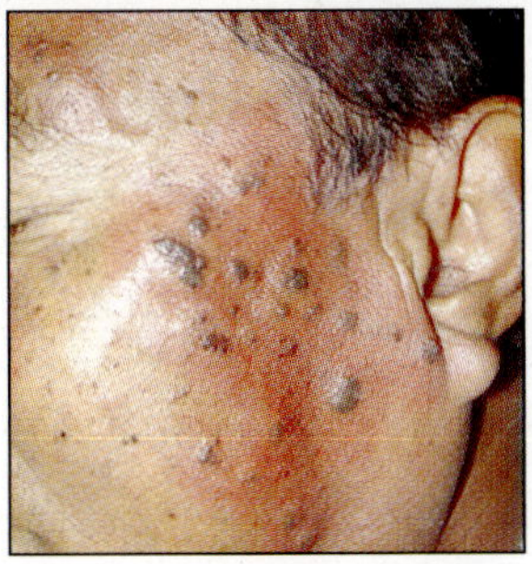

Fig. 22.4 Seborrhoeic keratosis: immediately after cryotherapy

Sites

Areas rich in pilosebaceous follicles, especially on the face (Fig. 22.1) and upper trunk.

Table 22.2 Difference between verruca vulgaris (VV) and seborrhoeic keratosis (SK)

VV	SK
Appears at any age.	Usually appears after 50 years of age
Trauma prone sites.	Face, upper trunk, upper extremities.
Verrucous, firm papules with dry surface.	Hyperpigmented, greasy papules, 'stuck on'appearance.

Dermatosis Papulosa Nigra (DPN)

Clinical Features

- Seen early in life in dark-skinned patients.

- Morphologically, it is similar to seborrhoeic keratosis (Fig. 22.5).

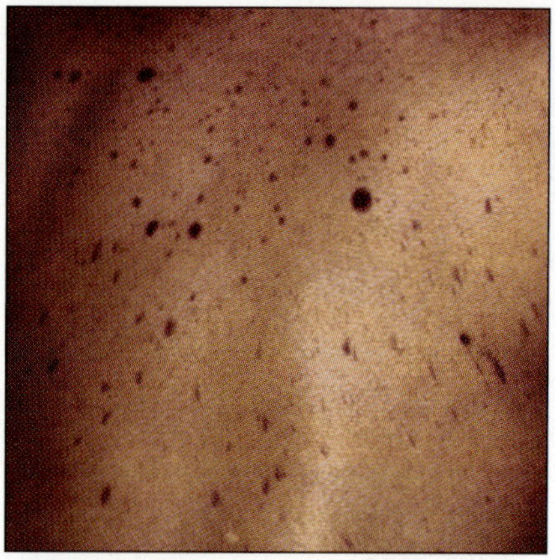

Fig. 22.5 Dermatosis papulosa nigra (DPN): back

Size

1–5 mm in diameter.

Sites

- Present on the forehead and malar region of the face.
- Occasionally seen on the neck, chest and back.

Treatment

Both seborrhoeic keratosis and dermatosis papulosa nigra may be removed with electrocautery, cryosurgery and lasers with good cosmetic result (Figs 22.2–22.4).

Skin Tag

Synonym

Acrochordon.

Age

Middle-aged and elderly.

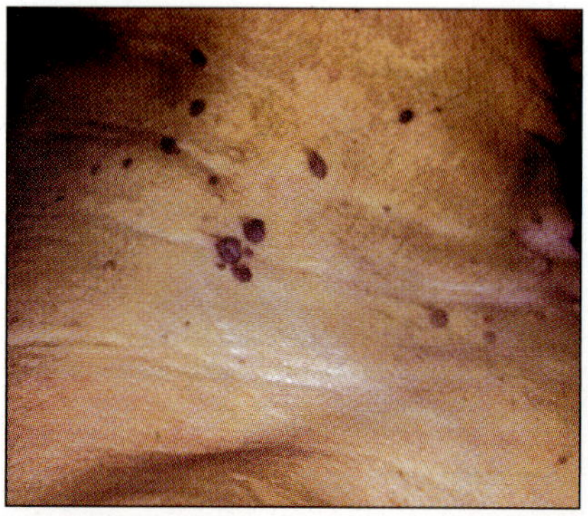

Fig. 22.6 Skin tags: neck

Clinical Features

- Soft, pedunculated and often pigmented protrusions (Figs 22.6 and 22.7) of few millimeters size are seen.
- The lesions are usually rounded and elastic.
- Majority of the lesions are composed of loose fibrous tissues.

Sites

Neck and flexors like axillae and groin.

Treatment

- Destructionofthelesionsbyelectrocautery,cryosurgery and lasers even without local anaesthesia.
- New lesions are likely to reappear, thus periodical destruction by electrocautery, cryosurgery or lasers may be required.

Trichoepithelioma

Tumour of hair follicle.

Etiology

It is a hereditary disorder, inherited through autosomal dominant genes.

Age

Usually appears at puberty.

Clinical Features

- Seen as bilaterally symmetrical, multiple, small, rounded papules.
- Commonly seen on the cheeks, eyelids and nasolabial folds.
- May be seen on other parts of the face, upper trunk and even on the arms.

Treatment

Destruction by electrocoagulation or lasers.

Milia

Pathology

Small subepidermal keratin cysts.

Etiology

It may occur after the following:
- Second degree burns.
- Epidermolysis bullosa.
- Dermabrasion.

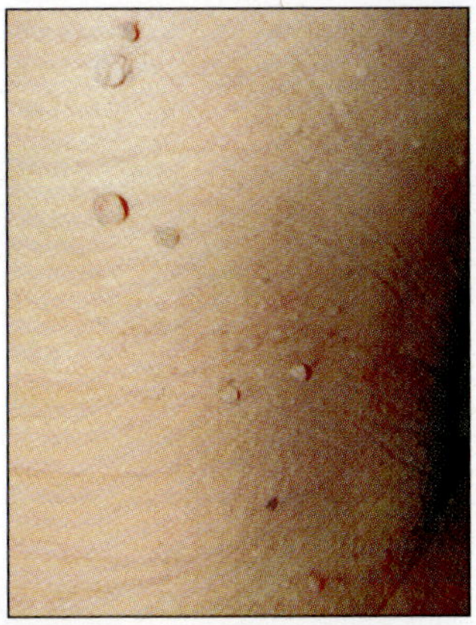

Fig. 22.7 Skin tags

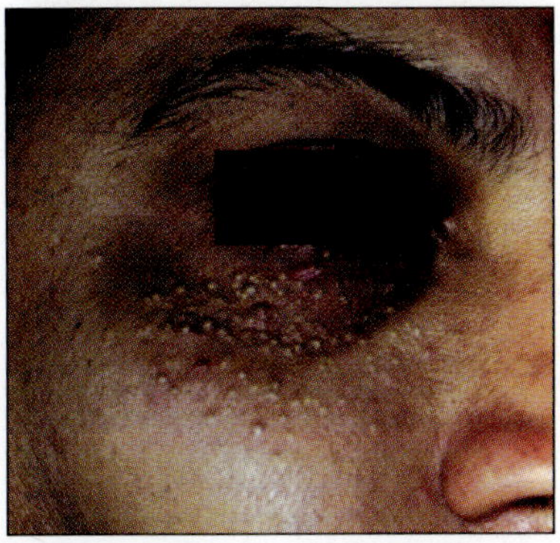

Fig. 22.8 Milia: around eye

Clinical Features

- Whitish or yellowish tiny papules (Figs 22.8 and 22.9).
- 1–2 mm in size.
- Usually seen on the cheeks and around eyelids.

Treatment

Puncturing and expressing the individual lesions by simple needle or electrocautery needle.

Syringoma

Etiology

Due to the malformation of sweat ducts.

Sex

Commonly seen in women.

Age

Usually occurs at adolescence.

Clinical Features

- Yellowish or skin-coloured papules which look cystic and translucent in some patients
- Surface of the papules are round or flat with characteristic acuminate margins (Fig. 22.10).

Sites

- On the eyelids and upper cheeks.
- Occasionally on the chest, and even on neck.

Size

1–3 mm in size.

Treatment

Destruction by electrocautery, lasers or cryotherapy (Fig. 22.11).

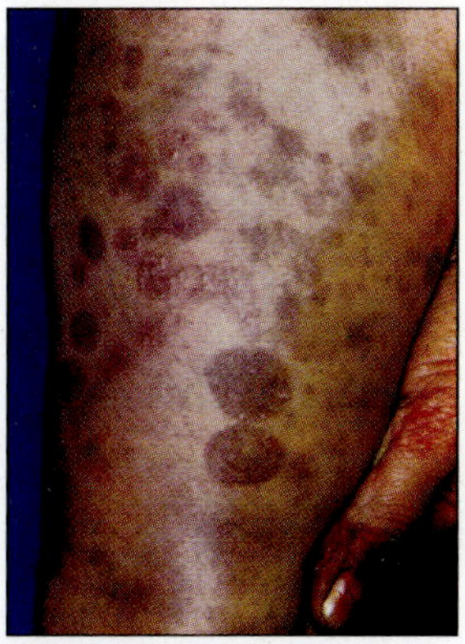

Fig. 22.9 Milia: on healing lichen planus

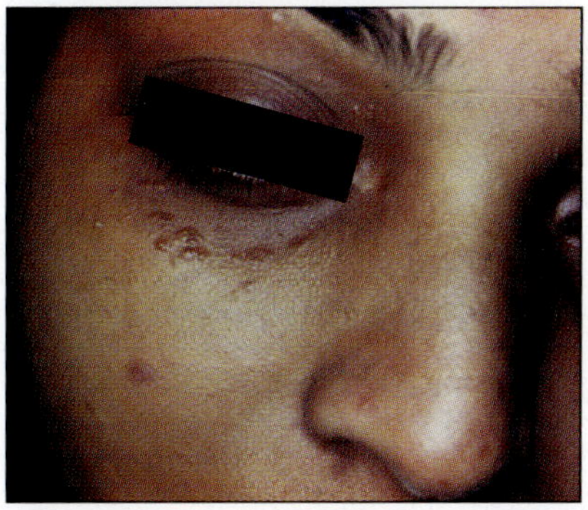

Fig. 22.10 Syringoma

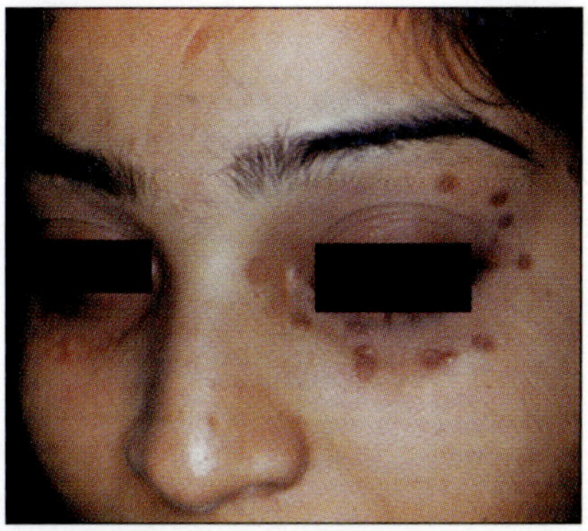

Fig. 22.11 Syringoma after cryotherapy

Lipoma

It is a benign tumour composed of mature fat cells found in the subcutaneous tissue.

Clinical Features

- Subcutaneous, often lobulated nodules (Fig. 22.12), seen with soft putty-like consistency.
- The overlying skin is normal and moves freely over the lipoma.
- Sometimes a lipoma is painful due to the pressure on the surrounding nerve.
- Fat necrosis may cause enlargement, pain and tenderness.

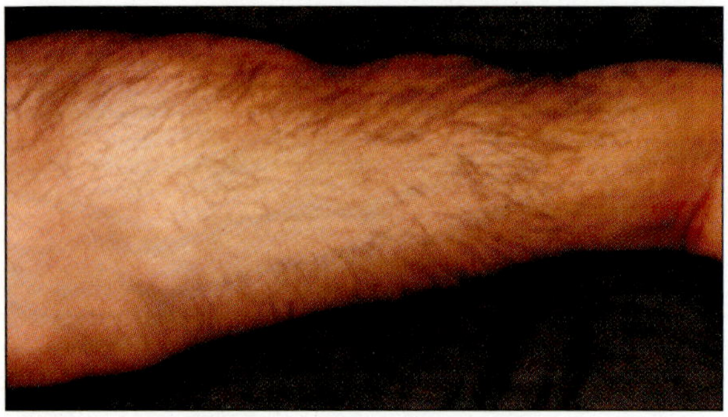

Fig. 22.12 Lipoma: arm

Sites

Neck, shoulders, upper arms, back and thigh.

Differential Diagnosis

Sebaceous Cyst

The presence of central punctum in a sebaceous cyst distinguishes it from a lipoma.

Treatment

- Small lesions may be ignored.
- Complete removal by surgery.

Sebaceous Cyst

Commonly single, may be multiple in the scrotum (Fig. 22.13).

Sex

Males are more frequently affected.

Clinical Features

- Firm, pale-yellow, spherical, dermal cysts attached to the epidermis (Fig. 22.13).
- Central punctum may be present (Fig. 22.14).
- It may be asymptomatic, or may get painful when inflamed.

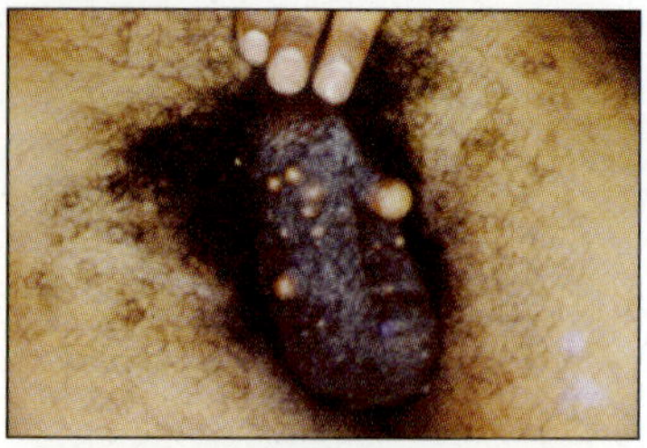

Fig. 22.13 Sebaceus cyst: scrotum

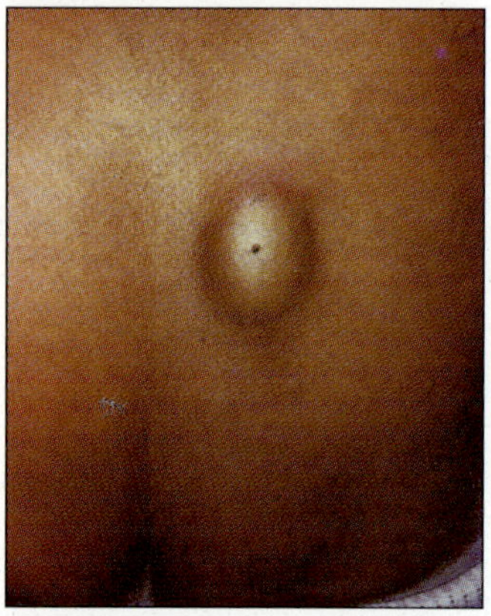

Fig. 22.14 Sebaceus cyst: back

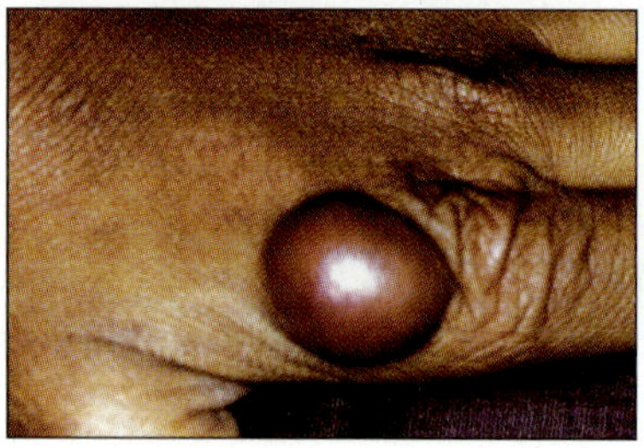

Fig. 22.15 Dermoid cyst

Sites

Face, trunk and scrotum are very frequently involved.

Differential Diagnosis

Dermoid cyst (Fig. 22.15); dermatoid cyst does not have a punctum in the centre.

Treatment

Enucleation is done, recurrence is common if a small portion is left.

Dermoid Cyst

- Uncommon occurrence.
- It is an embryonic epithelium-lined cavity which is filled with semisolid material.

Clinical Features

- Oval, firm, smooth swelling.
- Deep seated in the skin.
- Less mobile than other cysts.

Sites

Face, especially around the eye.

Treatment

Excision and curettage.

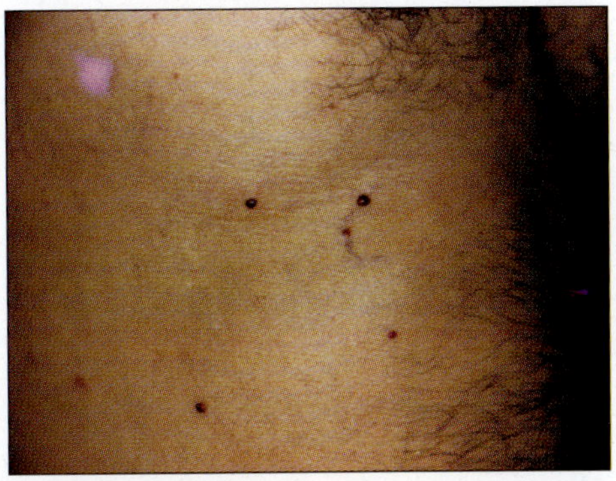

Fig. 22.16 De morgan angioma

De Morgan Angioma

This condition is similar to a capillary angioma.

Synonyms

- Cherry angioma.
- Campbell de Morgan spot.
- Senile angioma.

Etiology

Occurs with ageing.

Pathology

Similar to capillary angioma.

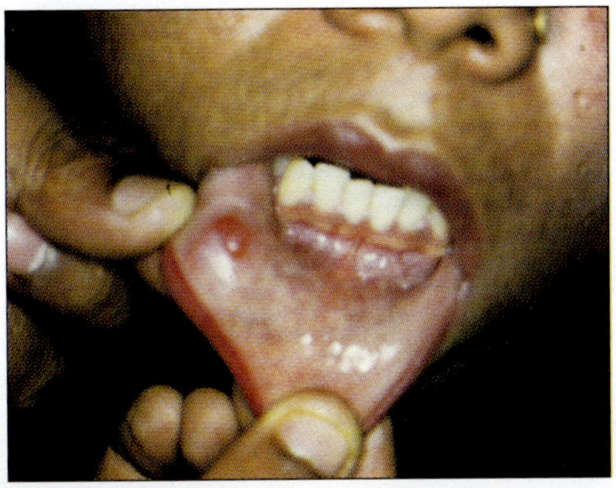

Fig. 22.17 Mucous cyst

Clinical Features

- Dome shaped, purplish or cherry-red, smooth surfaced lesion (Fig. 22.16).
- Many lesions may appear over a period of a few months.

Treatment

Destruction of lesions by cryotherapy or electrocoagulation.

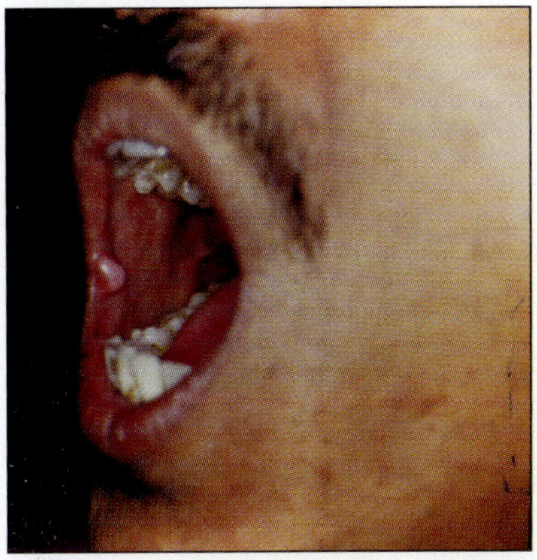

Fig. 22.18 Mucous cyst: after cryotherapy

Mucous Cyst

Mucous cyst, also known as mucocele, is a fluid-filled swelling that occurs on the lip or mouth (Figs. 22.17 and 22.18). The cyst develops when a salivary duct is plugged with mucus. The cyst is usually temporary and painless. However, a chronic cyst may require surgical removal.

Dermal Cyst

Dermal cyst looks like a sebaceous cyst, but it does not have a punctum.

Basal Cell Carcinoma

- It is a locally malignant tumour that rarely shows metastasis.
- The tumour arises from the basal cell layer of the epidermis.

Site

Commonly seen on the face.

Types

Papulonodules

It is the most common variety. The lesions are usually small, pearly, raised and rounded .

Pigmented Basal Cell Carcinoma

Occasionally, the pigment is seen on the surface. This condition is called pigmented basal cell carcinoma (Figs 22.19–22.21).

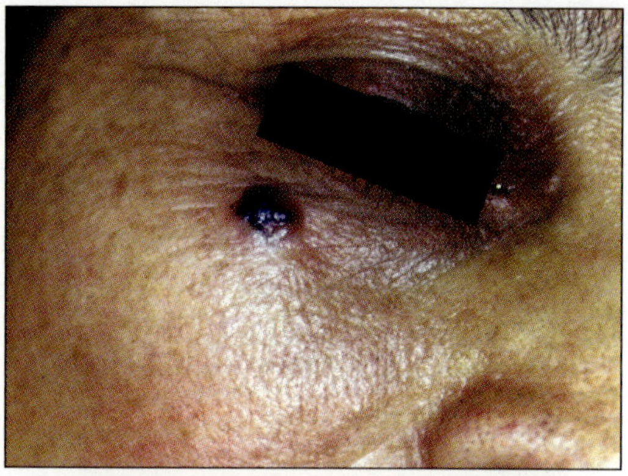

Fig. 22.19 Basal cell carcinoma

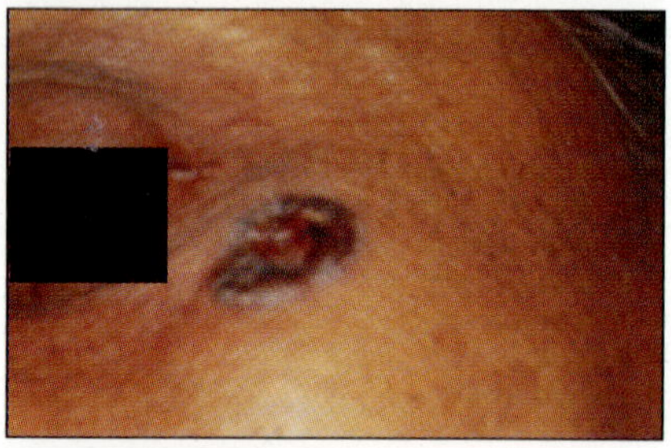

Fig. 22.20 Basal cell carcinoma

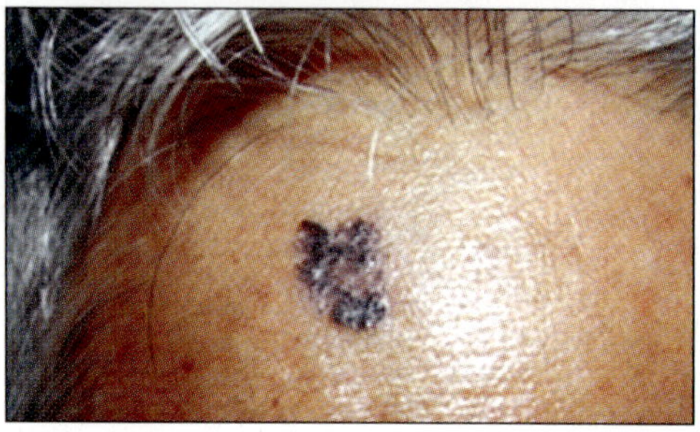

Fig. 22.21 Basal cell carcinoma

Clinical Features

- The lesions grow slowly with well-defined margins.
- Nodules increase in size and show ulceration during the later stage.
- In some patients, the centre becomes atrophic and scaly.

Rodent Ulcer

- In some patients, the tumour ulcerates, resulting in an indurated raised edge. The floor of the ulcer is depressed below the skin surface and appears fleshy.
- If left, the ulcers may spread deeply in periphery and cause great destruction of the surrounding tissues including eyes, nose, ears, bones of face and skull (Fig. 22.22).
- In other types, the lesion produces intense fibrosis of the skin leading to a thickened plaque.

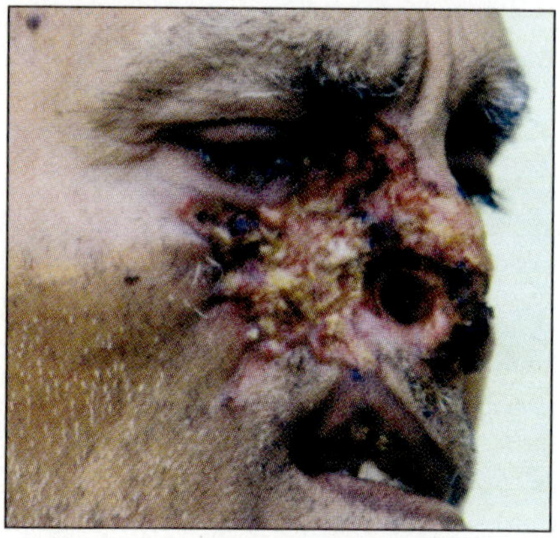

Fig. 22.22 Basal cell carcinoma: rodent ulcer

Diagnosis

Confirmed by biopsy and histopathological examination of the lesion.

Treatment

The treatment for rodent ulcer involves one of the following course:

- Excision (generally with a 0.5 cm thick skin margin) with primary closure.
- Excision with sliding full-thickness skin graft.
- Cryosurgery or curettage of lesion.

Squamous Cell Carcinoma

- It is a malignant tumour that arises from the keratinocytes in epidermis or its appendages.
- It has a tendency to spread locally to the surrounding tissues.
- Usually metastasizes to distant organs through the lymphatics.

Types

There are two types of squamous cell carcinomas:

Squamous Cell Carcinoma de Novo

When the tumour arises from the normal skin.

Squamous Cell Carcinoma

When the tumour arises from one of the following pre-existing skin lesions:

- Chronic ulcers.
- Lupus vulgaris.
- Discoid lupus erythematosus.
- Burn scar, etc.

Clinical Features

- Indurated verrucous nodule(s), or plaques which increases in size and ulcerate.
- The lesions have irregular, elevated, everted margins and look like cauliflower (Fig. 22.23).
- Bleed easily on touch.
- On the lips and genitals, the lesions present as fissures, erosions or ulcers which fail to heal and bleed repeatedly (Fig. 22.24).
- In the early stages in a few patients, the tumour is well-differentiated and presents as elongations covered with keratotic crust which shed later on leaving an ulcer (Fig. 22.25) or eroded tumour with irregular indurated margins.

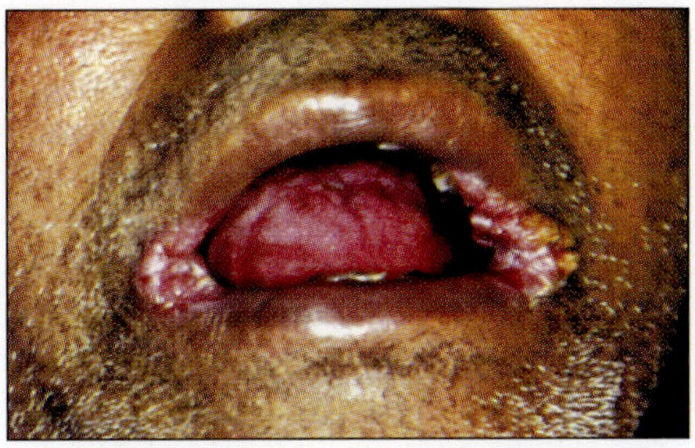

Fig. 22.23 Squamous cell carcinoma: cauliflower lesion

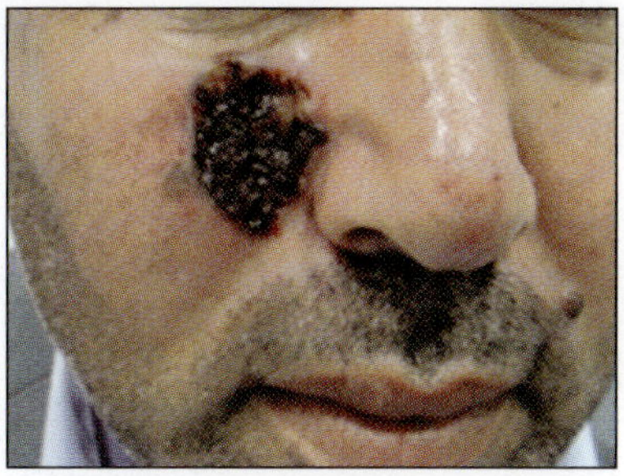

Fig. 22.24 Squamous cell carcinoma

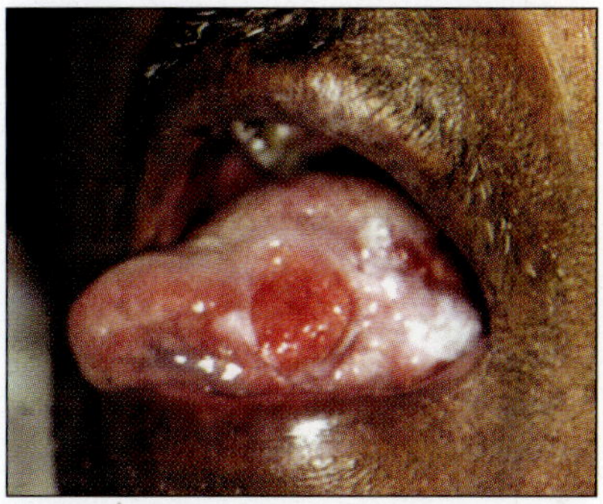

Fig. 22.25 Squamous cell carcinoma: ulcer

Diagnosis

Biopsy samples are taken for histopathological examination.

Management

Excision with a 0.5 cm or larger skin margin, and/or radiotherapy.

CHAPTER 23

Sexually Transmitted Diseases

INTRODUCTION

The diseases that occur through sexual intercourse, or its related activities, are called **sexually transmitted diseases** (STD). They are presented in Table 23.1. Sometimes these diseases may also occur through nonsexual route.

Table 23.1 Common sexually transmitted diseases and their causes

Traditional	Causative Organism
Syphilis	*Treponema pallidum*
Gonorrhoea	*Neisseria gonorrhoea*
Chancroid	*Haemophilus ducreyi*
Lympho-granuloma venereum	*Chlamydia trachomatis*
Donovanosis	*Donovania granulomatis*
Recent Inclusion	
Non-specific urethritis (NSU)	*Chlamydia trachomatis*
Herpes progenitalis	*Herpes hominis*
Venereal warts	*Human papilloma virus (H.P.V.)*
Molluscum contagiosum	Pox group of virus
Pediculosis occurring on genital area	*Phthiriasis pubis*
Scabies	*Sarcoptus scabiei*

Syphilis

Etiology

Syphilis is caused by a spirochaete called *Treponema pallidum*.

Mode of Transmission

Usually transmitted through sexual intercourse. Sometimes, it may get transmitted through the following non-sexual routes:

- Blood transfusions.
- Handling of infected materials.
- Congenital syphilis is transmitted to the offspring through the placenta during pregnancy.

Course

The course of the disease, if untreated, is presented in Table 23.2.

Table 23.2 Phases of acquired syphilis

Primary syphilis
↓
Secondary syphilis
↓
Latent syphilis
↓
Tertiary syphilis
↓
Gumma | Cardiac syphilis | Neuro syphilis

Primary Syphilis

- Incubation period varies from 9–90 days.
- Lesions usually appear 2–4 weeks after the contact.

Clinical Features

- Painless, indurated, well-defined ulcer called **Hunterian chancre** (Figs 23.1–23.3) is seen on the genitals.
- Regional lymph nodes get enlarged within 7–10 days after the appearance of the chancre.
- The enlarged lymph nodes are non-tender, discrete, multiple and firm (**lead shots**).
- **In males**, the ulcer is usually located at one of the following locations:
  i) Coronal sulcus.
  ii) Glans penis.
  iii) Mucosal surface of prepuce.
  iv) Shaft of penis.

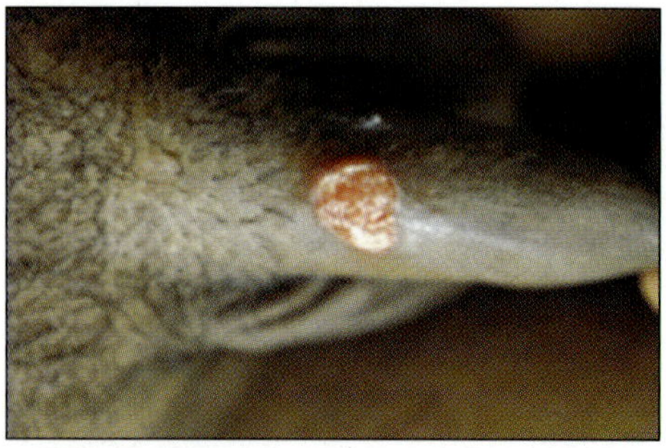

Fig. 23.1 Primary chancre

- **In females**, the common sites are as follows:
  i) Labia majora.
  ii) Labia minora or clitoris.

iii) When it is present on the vaginal wall or cervix uteri, it may not be visible.

- These ulcers heal spontaneously in 3–8 weeks time, leaving behind a thin, atrophic scar.

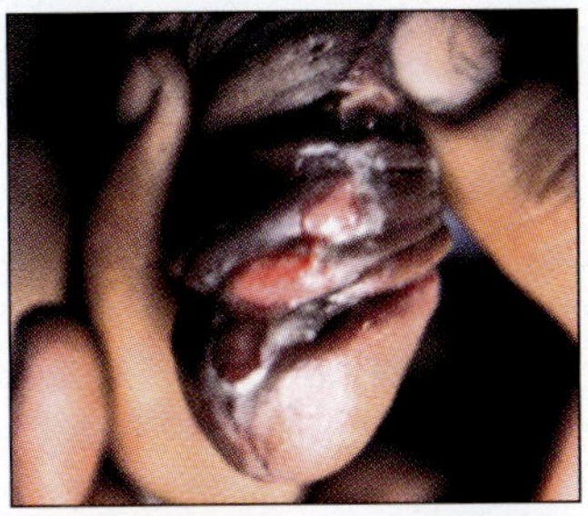

Fig. 23.2 Primary chancre: glans

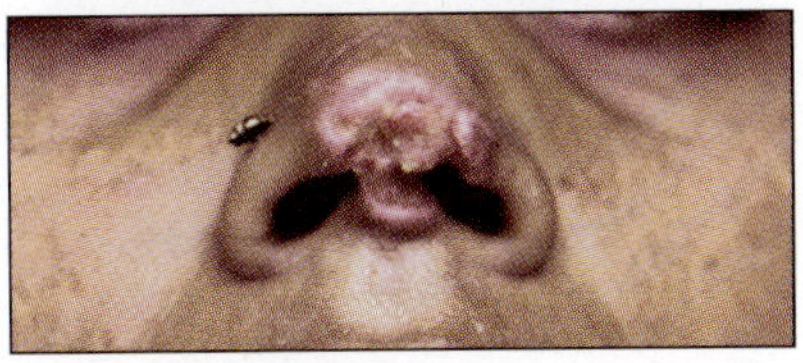

Fig. 23.3 Primary chancre: nose

Diagnosis

- Confirmed by demonstration of brightly illuminated spiral *Treponema pallidum* against a dark background in the serous exudate obtained from the ulcer in dark-ground microscopic examination.
- Direct fluorescence antibody test will show apple green fluorescence.
- Serological test for syphilis, especially VDRL test, becomes positive 1–2 weeks after the appearance of ulcer. Serological tests are of two types:
  i) **Non-Treponemal Tests**: These tests include VDRL and RPR. Non-treponemal tests are good screening tests. These tests become negative on treatment and thus are used for follow-ups also.
  ii) **Treponemal Tests**: These testes include TPHA, FTA, TPI and others. Treponemal tests are more specific and they do not become negative on treatment.

Secondary Syphilis

Incubation Period

6–8 weeks after the appearance of primary chancre.

Clinical Features

Constitutional Symptoms

- Headache.
- Malaise.
- Anorexia.
- Loss of weight.
- Low grade fever.
- Pain in muscles, bones and joints, worst in night.

Cutaneous Lesions

- They are asymptomatic, generalised, bilateral and symmetrical.
- They consist of erythematous macules called **roseolar syphilide**.
- Papules called **papular syphilide** are the most commonly seen cutaneous lesions (Fig. 23.4). These papules may later on coalesce to form annular lesions. There is deep dermal tenderness on pressing the lesions (**Buschke–Ollendroff sign**).
- Papulosquamous lesions are also seen in secondary syphilis (Figs 23.5 and 23.6).
- **Condyloma lata** (Fig. 23.8), a condition in which the papular lesions present in warm and moist areas erode superficially such as:
  i) Between the buttocks.
  ii) Lateral surface of scrotum.
  iii) Vulva.
  iv) Groin.
  v) Around the anus.
  vi) Other skin folds.

They usually become large and fleshy with broad base and flat top. These are very infectious.

Vesicles or bullae have never been reported in secondary syphilis.

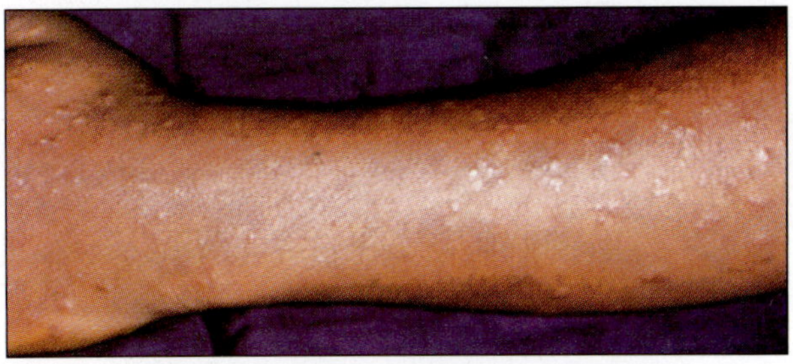

Fig. 23.4 Secondary syphilis: papules on arm

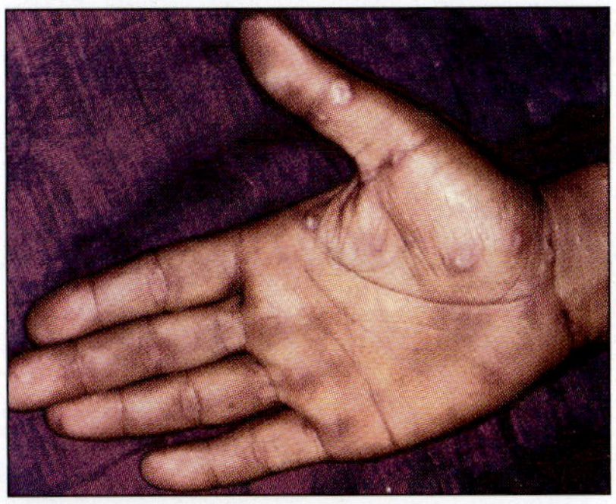

Fig. 23.5 Secondary syphilis: palm

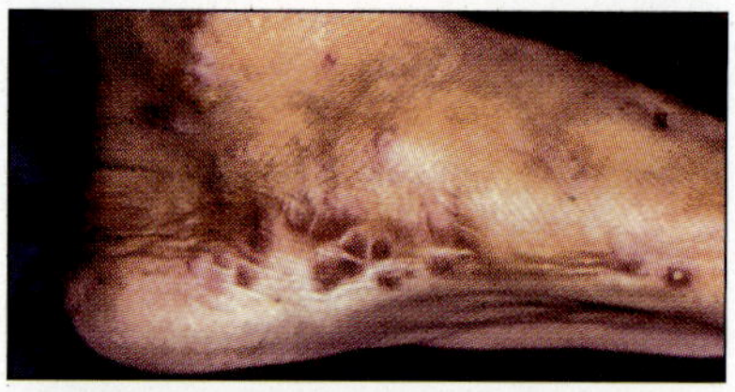

Fig. 23.6 Secondary syphilis: sole

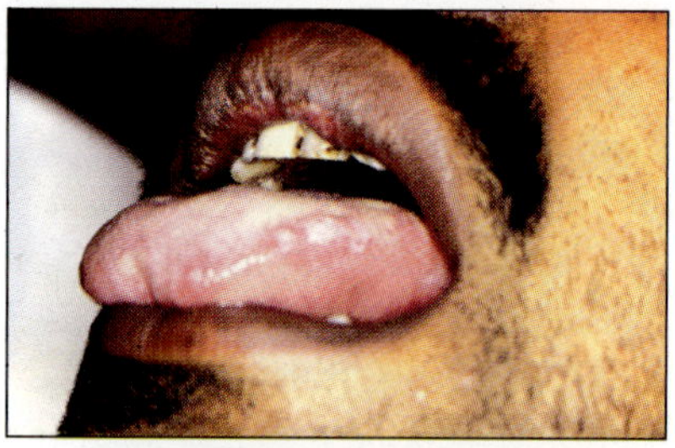

Fig. 23.7 Secondary syphilis: mucosal lesion tongue

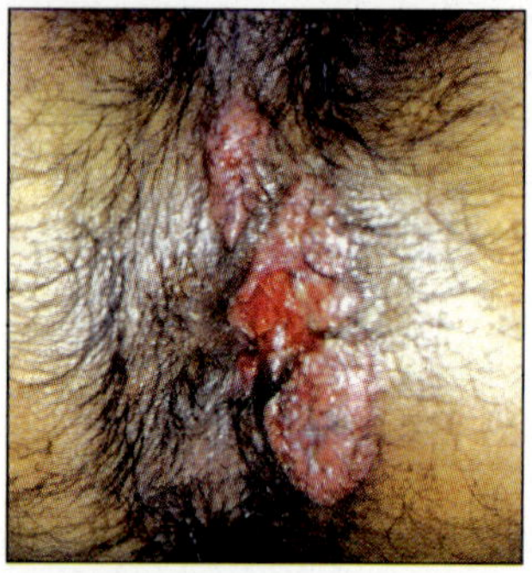

Fig. 23.8 Condyloma lata: anus

Other Manifestations

- **Generalised Lymphadenopathy**: The nodes are non-tender, discrete and rubbery in consistency.
- Erythematous, pigmented and scaly lesions on palms (Fig. 23.5) and soles (Fig. 23.6).
- **Syphilitic Alopecia**: Patchy loss of hair from the scalp.
- **Snail Track Ulcers**: Superficial, linear or zig-zag ulcers on the mucous membranes of the mouth (Fig. 23.7).
- Occasionally, some patients may develop uveitis, hepatitis, arthritis, meningitis or cranial nerve palsies.

Diagnosis

- Demonstration of *Treponema pallidum* in the exudate from the skin and mucosal lesions, especially of condyloma lata.
- Both, VDRL and TPHA, tests are positive in almost all the patients.
- **Prezone Phenomenon**: Sometimes, very high titre of VDRL test may become false negative.
- VDRL test becomes positive on serial dilution of the serum in prezone phenomenon.
- Lesions of secondary syphilis also heal spontaneously even without treatment.
- Recurrences are common and may continue for as long as up to two years.

Latent Syphilis

- This is the period after the secondary syphilis, when there are no signs and symptoms of syphilis in any organ, but the VDRL and TPHA tests are positive in the blood while negative in the cerebrospinal fluid.
- This is usually a non-contagious phase.
- A woman may deliver a newborn with congenital syphilis during this phase.

Incubation Period

Varies from a few years to even rest of the patient's life.

Tertiary Syphilis

The earliest lesion of tertiary syphilis is called **Gumma**.

Incubation Period

3–10 years after the primary infection.

Clinical Features

Gumma may show the following characteristics:

- Nodular gumma is round, dull-red in colour and involves the whole thickness of the skin.
- Psoriasiform or subcutaneous gumma is a round, painless, subcutaneous nodule with dull-red discolouration.
- Gumma leaves punched-out ulcer when it breaks down.
- Gumma commonly involves the skin, mucous membranes, subcutaneous and submucosal tissues, bones, joints, muscles, heart, kidneys, brain, lymph nodes and in fact, any tissue of the body.
- Gumma produces the symptoms of space-occupying lesions in the internal organs; or fracture if present in the bone.
- Gumma of the skin heals with tissue-paper scar.
- Infectivity of the disease is almost nil in the tertiary stage. The other presentations of tertiary syphilis include:
  i) Cardiovascular syphilis.
  ii) Neurosyphilis.

Due to adequate treatment of early syphilis, secondary and tertiary syphilis are rarely seen these days.

Diagnosis

- Biopsy of gummatous lesion shows a characteristic granulomatous histopathology.
- Serological tests for syphilis (VDRL and TPHA) are usually positive, but occasionally may become negative.

Treatment

- Counselling and education about sexual abstinence (till the lesions heal).
- Use of barrier methods and presumptive treatment of partners is an important component of treatment.
- Treatment for syphilis is summarised in Tables 23.3 and 23.4.

Table 23.3 Treatment of syphilis

Penicillin is the drug of choice.
For primary and secondary stage:
Benzathine penicillin 2.4 million units, as a single intramuscular injection.
Procaine penicillin 6 lac units, intramuscular injection daily for 10 days.
For latent and tertiary syphilis:
Benzathine penicillin 3 million units, weekly for three weeks.
Procaine penicillin 6 lac units, intramuscularly daily for 20 days.

Table 23.4 Treatment to patients allergic to penicillin

Tetracycline.
Erythromycin.
Chloramphenicol.
Cephalexin.
Each in a dose of 2 gm per day.
For primary and secondary syphilis, for 10–15 days.
For latent and tertiary syphilis, for 20 days.

Gonorrhoea

Etiology

Caused by a gram negative intracellular diplococcus called *Neisseria gonorrhea.*

Mode of Transmission

Usually through sexual contact.

Incubation period

2–10 days.

Clinical Features

- **Urethritis**: Males develop burning micturition and frequent urination followed by pus discharge from the urethra (Fig. 23.9).
- **In females**, the infection usually occurs in cervix uteri and has the following symptoms:
  i) Purulent cervical discharge.
  ii) Vagina is not involved, except in the prepubertal girls (due to the presence of stratified epithelium in adults).
- Infection of urethra usually presents as dysuria.
- Urethral discharge is usually not seen in females.
- Asymptomatic gonococcal infection is very common in females. It is occasionally in males, as a result of contact with a female patient.
- If treatment is neglected, or if the disease is refractory to treatment, it may have the following consequences:
  i) Infection may spread to prostate, seminal vesicles or epididymis in males. This may produce prostatitis, seminal vesiculitis and epididymitis.
  ii) It may even lead to fibrous stricture of the urethra.
  iii) Occasionally, it may produce arthritis, hepatitis, septicaemia, generalised skin rashes, carditis and even meningitis.

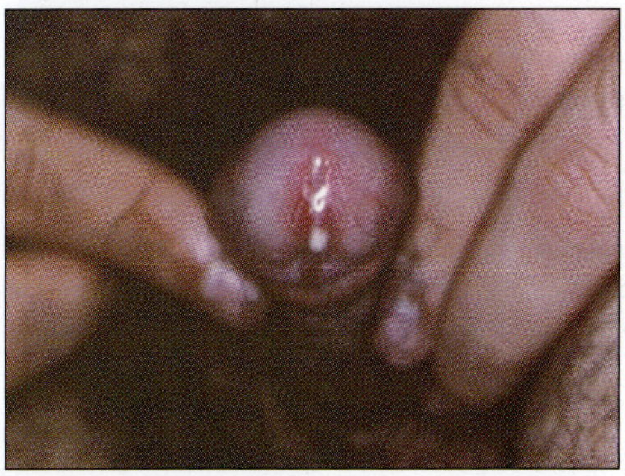

Fig. 23.9 Gonococcal urethritis

Diagnosis

- Demonstrating gram negative intracellular kidney shaped diplococci in the smear prepared from pus discharge or secretion stained with Gram's stain. The material is obtained from the anterior urethra in males: and cervix, urethra or rectum from the females. If there is no discharge, the penile shaft can be squeezed from behind (milking the urethra).
- Culturing the organism on enriched media or selective media (modified Thayer–Martin medium and Chacko–Nair medium) and identifying the organism by one of the following methods:
  i) Sugar fermentation test.
  ii) Serological tests.
  iii) Oxidase test.

Treatment

- Treatment for gonococcal infection is presented in Table 23.5.
- Counselling and education about sexual abstinence (till the lesions heal).
- Use of barrier methods and presumptive treatment of partners is an important component of the treatment.

Table 23.5 Treatment of gonococcal infection

- Procain penicillin: A single dose of 24 lac units intra-muscularly with 1 gm of probenecid orally.
- Norfloxacin: Oral administration of a single dose of 800 mg.
- Ofloxacin: 200 mg.
- Ampicillin: 2 gm.
- Ciprofloxacin: 2 gm in two divided doses, given at an interval of 12 hours.
- Tetracycline/erythromycin: 500 mg every 6 hourly for 2 days.
- Doxycycline: 100 mg, twice daily for 2 days.

Chancroid

Synonym

Soft chancre or ulcus molle.

Etiology

Caused by *Haemophilus ducreyi*—a short, slender, gram negative, rod shaped organism with rounded ends.

Incubation period

1–5 days.

Clinical Features

- Ulcers are superficial, well-defined, soft, tender with reddish granulation tissue on the floor (Figs 23.10 and 23.11). They bleed on touch.

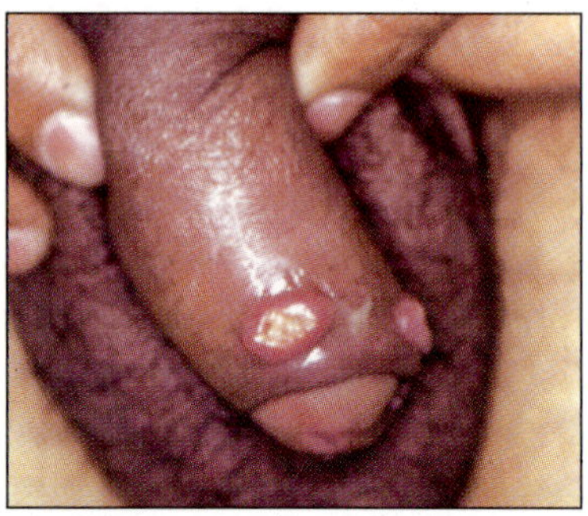

Fig. 23.10 Chancroid

- Usually multiple, the lesions spread in continuity.
- Within a few days, the inguinal lymph nodes (bubo) become enlarged, tender and get matted together with the formation of unilocular abscess (Figs 23.12 and 23.13) which ruptures through a single sinus (Fig. 23.14).
- Lymphadenopathy is usually unilateral.
- Lesions tend to heal spontaneously even without any treatment.

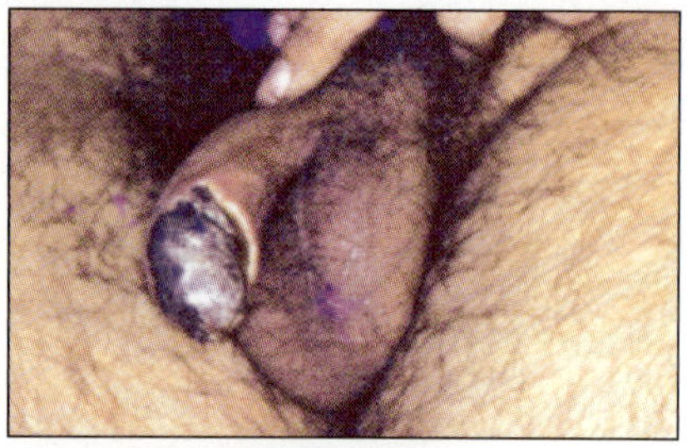

Fig. 23.11 Chancroid: phagedenic ulcer

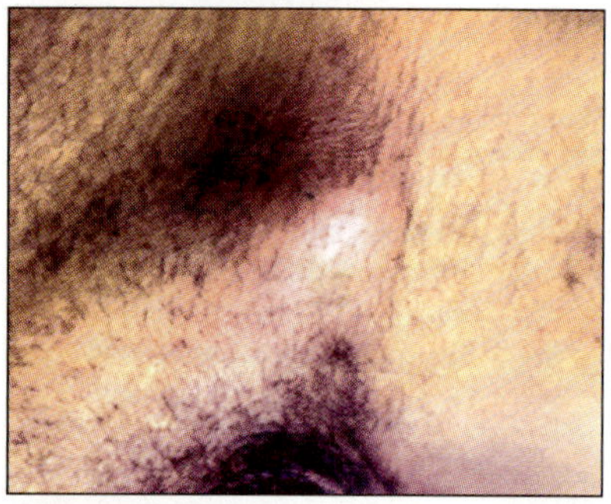

Fig. 23.12 Chancroidal bubo

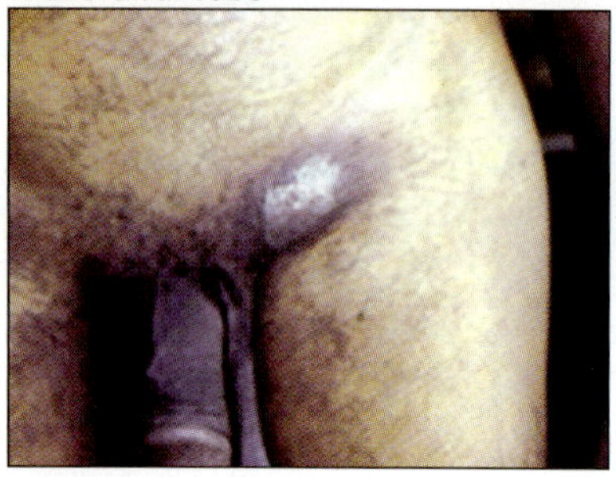

Fig. 23.13 Chancroidal bubo

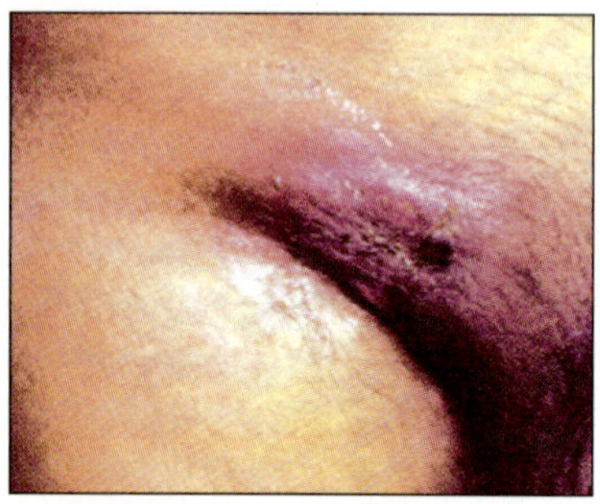

Fig. 23.14 Ruptured buboes chancroid

Diagnosis

- Usually made clinically by exclusion of other causes for genital ulcers (Table 23.6).

Table 23.6 Difference between chancroid and chancre

Chancroid	Chancre
Multiple ulcers.	Single ulcer.
Painful.	Painless.
Irregular, ragged margins.	Well-defined margins.
Not indurated.	Button-like induration.
Bleeds on pressure.	Serum exudes on pressure.
Inflammatory lymphadenopathy (bubo).	Shotty lymphadenopathy.

- In about 30% of cases, it is possible to demonstrate the haemophilus ducreyi in the smear made directly from the ulcers or pus aspirated from an unruptured lymph node (bubo) and stained with Gram's stain.
- Haemophilus ducreyi is seen as groups of gram negative bacilli often lying in chains giving the appearance of a **school of fish formation**.
- Antigen detection is done by immunofluoroscence technique.

Organism is fastidious.

Culture may be tried on media containing whole human blood or defibrinated rabbit blood.

Treatment

- Co-trimoxazole (trimethoprim 160 mg and sulfamethoxazole 800 mg): 1 tablet, twice daily for 10 days.
- Oral tetracycline or erythromycin: 500 mg, six hourly for 10 days.
- Doxycycline, ciprofloxacin, streptomycin, cephalexin, chloramphenicol or ceftriaxone, in usual doses for 10–12 days are also effective.
- An important component of treatment is counselling and education about sexual abstinence (till the lesions heal).
- Use of barrier methods and presumptive treatment of partners.

Lymphogranuloma Venereum

Etiology

Caused by a virus like organism called *Chlamydia trachomatis*.

Transmission

Through sex.

Incubation Period

Usually less than a week.

Clinical Features

Skin Lesions

- Transient, very small vesicles or ulcers present on the genitals, usually missed by the patient.
- Thus, the initial lesions that are noticed are the tender, matted and often suppurated, inguinal lymph nodes.
- These suppurated lymph nodes, on rupture, form multiple sinuses that discharge purulent material.
- Enlargement of lymph nodes above and below inguinal ligament produces the groove in the bubo called **groove sign**.

Constitutional Symptoms

Headache, anorexia, nausea, arthralgia, loss of weight, fever and chills may be present in a few patients.

Late Manifestation

Late manifestations common in females (if untreated) are as follows:

- **Esthiomene** or genital elephantiasis.
- Anal stricture, perineal sinuses and rectovagina fistulae (**watering can perineum**).

Investigation

- Demonstration of causative agent can be done through smear, culture or direct immunofluoroscence test.
- Hypergammaglobulinaemia with increased total serum protein.
- **Complement Fixation Test**: Detection of antibodies reaction, in increasing dilution, is highly suggestive of lymphogranuloma venereum.

Treatment

- Sulphonamides are still the drugs of choice, especially sulphadiazine—5 gm daily in divided doses.
- Co-trimoxazole (trimethaprim 160 mg and sulfamethoxazole 800 mg) twice daily, for 7–10 days.
- Tetracycline 500 mg, four time daily for 7–10 days.
- Counselling and education about sexual abstinence (till the lesions heal).
- Use of barrier methods and presumptive treatment of partners is an important component of treatment.

Donovanosis

Synonym

Granuloma inguinale.

Etiology

It is caused by an organism called *Donovania granulomatis*.

Incubation period

3 days to 6 months, or even few years.

Clinical Features

- Round, elevated, velvety and granulomatous ulcers (Fig. 23.15).
- Ulcers are painless, friable and they bleed on touch.
- Sometimes a subcutaneous lesion in the inguinal area (called **pseudobubos**) may be mistaken for enlarged lymph gland.
- Lesions spread slowly by **continuity** (Table 23.7).

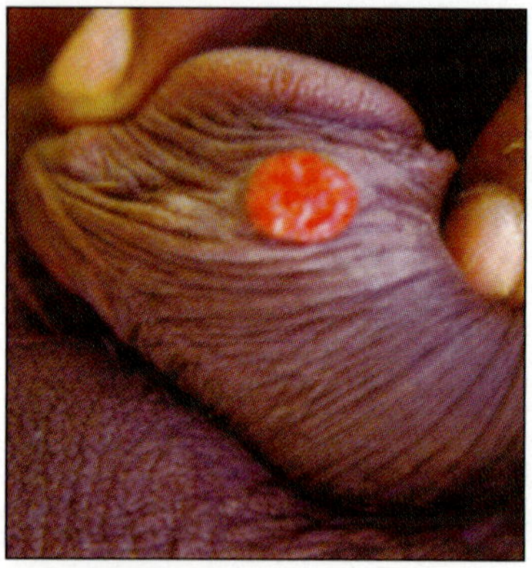

Fig. 23.15 Donovanosis

Diagnosis

Demonstrating safety pin like organisms inside the macrophages in a smear prepared from the granulation tissue and stained with **Giemsa's stain**.

Treatment

- Streptomycin: 1 gm intramuscularly, twice daily for 10–20 days.
- Alternatively, oral tetracycline or erythromycin 500 mg, 6 hourly for 10–20 days.
- Counselling and education about sexual abstinence (till the lesions heal).
- Use of barrier methods and presumptive treatment of partners is an important component of treatment.

Table 23.7 Difference between donovanosis and chancroid

Chancroid	Donovanosis
Painful.	Asymptomatic.
Multiple lesions.	Single/few lesions.
Soft ulcers.	Firm.
Dirty-looking floor which bleeds on touch.	Beefy-red floor which bleeds on touch.
Unilateral, inflammatory lymphadenopathy.	No lymphadenopathy.

SYNDROMIC MANAGEMENT OF STDS

Syndromic management is a practical optimised approach to control the STDs at the peripheral rural areas considering the availability of limited resources. The syndrome is diagnosed based upon the presence of a group of symptoms such as urethral or vaginal discharge or genital ulcer. Standardised therapeutic regimens are given to cover the majority of microbes causing the syndrome in that geographical zone (Table 23.8).

Table 23.8 Syndromic management of STD

Kit number	Colour	Syndrome	Contents
1	Grey	Urethral discharge/ painful micturition/ cervical discharge/ painful scrotal swelling	Tab Azithromycin 1 gm (OD STAT) +Tab Cefixime 400 mg OD STAT
2	Green	Vaginal discharge	Tab Secnidazole 2 gm (OD STAT) + Cap Fluconazole 150 mg (OD STAT)
3	White	Non-herpetic genital ulcer	Inj Benzathine Penicillin 2.4 MU+ Tab Azithromycin 1 gm (single dose)
4	Blue	Non herpetic genital ulcer	If allergic to penicillin, Doxycycline 100 mg (BD for 15 days) + Azithromycin 1 gm (single dose)
5	Red	Herpetic genital ulcer	Tab Acyclovir 400 mg TDS for 7 days
6	Yellow	Lower abdominal pain	Tab Cefixime 400 mg OD stat+Tab Metronidazole 400 mg BD x 14 days + Doxycycline100 mg BD x 14 days
7	Black	Inguinal bubo	Tab Azithromycin 1 gm (single dose) +Tab Doxycycline100 mg BD x 21 days

Important Considerations for Syndromic Management

- Educate and counsel the client and sexual partner(s) regarding STI/RTI, safer sex practices and the importance of taking complete treatment.
- Treat partner(s).
- Advise sexual abstinence or use of condom during the course of treatment.
- Provide condoms, educate about correct and consistent use.
- If symptoms persist, assess whether it is due to re-infection and advise prompt referral.

Reference Link

http://naco.gov.in/sites/default/files/Syndromic% 20Poster_REDUCED.pdf

CHAPTER 24

Acquired Immunodeficiency Syndrome (AIDS)

INTRODUCTION

It is a disease indicative of a defect in the **cell-mediated immunity** (CMI) in a person with no known cause for immunodeficiency. It is caused by a lymphotropic retrovirus called **human immunodeficiency virus** (HIV).

The HIV virus is of two types–HIV-1 and HIV-2:

- HIV-1 is responsible for almost all the infections in USA and Europe.
- HIV-2 is responsible for the infections in West Africa.
- In India, the majority of infections are due to HIV-1 and a few due to both or only by HIV-2.

HIV is present in the following body-fluids:

- Blood.
- Genital secretions.
- Breast milk.

Epidemiology

Table 24.1 Occurrence of AIDS

	Global
Number of people living with HIV (2012)	35,300,000
New cases detected (adults and children) (2012)	2,300,000

In India, adult (15–49 years) HIV prevalence was estimated at 0.26% (0.22%–0.32%) in 2015.

In 2015, adult HIV prevalence was estimated at 0.30% among males and at 0.22% among females

Transmission of HIV

- Through homosexual or heterosexual contact with the infected person.
- Exposure to the infected body fluids, especially blood and blood products.
- Prenatal exposure to the infected mother during pregnancy.

Pathogenesis

- Once HIV is in the human body; it enters into CD4 lymphocyte in the blood, where it uses an enzyme called **reverse transcriptase** and converts its RNA into DNA.
- HIV not only infects CD4 cells but also certain sanctuary sites like the central nervous system.
- During the early stage of infection, a viral reservoir is established in resting memory CD4 cell lymphocytes.
- Since these cells have a very long half-life, possibility of a cure with the presently available anti-retroviral therapy is not possible.
- HIV DNA then enters the nucleus of CD4 cell and inserts itself to cell DNA.
- HIV DNA then instructs the cell to make many copies of the original virus.
- With the help of the protease enzyme, the new viral particles are assembled.
- These newly formed viruses then leave the cell and are ready to infect the other CD4 cells (Fig. 24.1).
- Thus, there is a continuous and rapid replication of HIV with simultaneous destruction of CD4 cells throughout the course of HIV infection.

Clinical spectrum of HIV

Table 24.2 Clinical varieties of AIDS

Four groups:
• Primary HIV Infection.
• Asymptomatic HIV infection.
• Symptomatic HIV disease.
• Advanced HIV disease.

(I) Primary HIV Infection

Usually asymptomatic, except in 10–20% of patients.

Incubation period

3–6 weeks.

Clinical Features

- Influenza.
- Infectious mononucleosis.
- Aseptic meningitis.
- Malaise, sore throat.
- Fever, rigor.
- Headache.
- Lethargy, anorexia.
- Nausea.

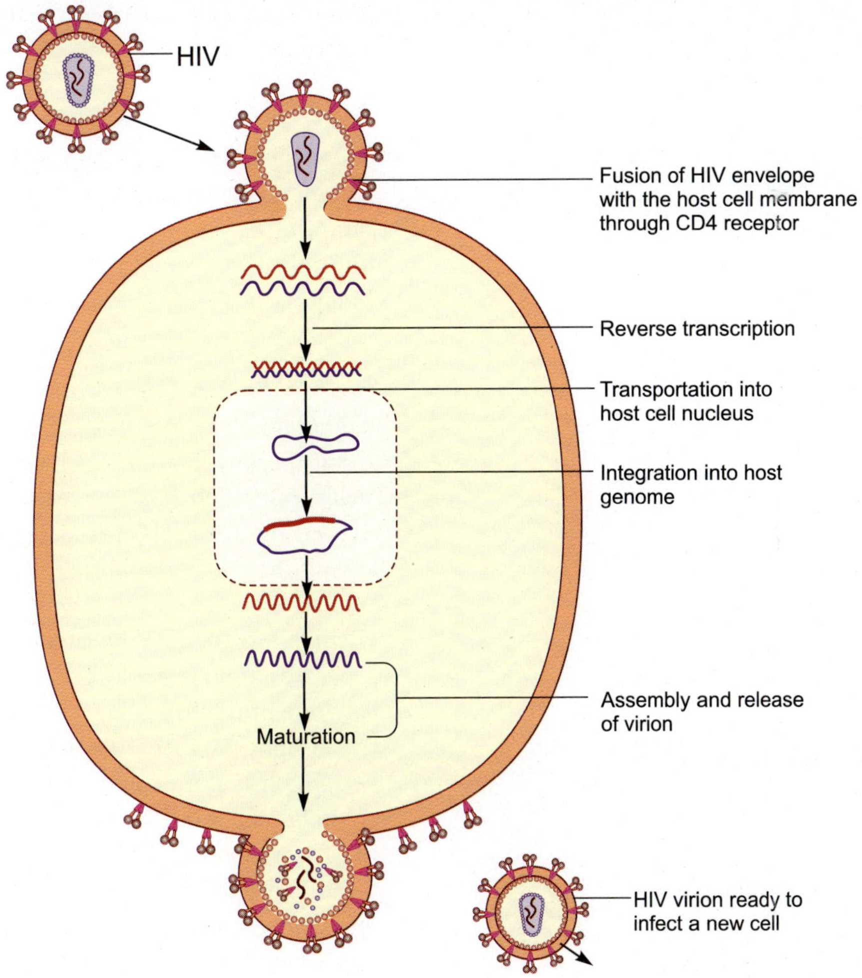

Fig. 24.1 Pathogenesis of HIV

- Myalgia, arthralgia, stiff neck.
- Abdominal pain, diarrhoea.
- Cramps.
- Photophobia.

Skin lesion

- Acute urticaria.
- Erythematous maculopapular rash.
- May have generalised lymphadenopathy.
- Oral erosions, glossitis.
- Genital ulcers.
- Palatal and esophageal ulcers.
- Oropharyngeal candidiasis.
- Opportunistic infections.

Diagnosis

- Positive seroconversion by ensyme linked immunosorbent assay.
- Confirmed by **Western blot** test.

Other Findings

- Leucopenia.
- Increased ESR.
- CSF lymphocytosis.
- Pleocytosis.
- P24 antigenemia.
- Culture from blood and CSF.

(II) Asymptomatic HIV Infection

- Lasts for several years (the mean duration is about 10 years).
- Peripheral blood CD4 cell-count is usually more than 500 cells/mm3.

(III) Symptomatic HIV Disease

Divided into two phases:

- Early phase.
- Late phase.

Early Phase

CD4 cell count continues to decrease further.

Constitutional symptoms

- Fever.
- Unexplained weight loss.
- Recurrent diarrhoea.
- Fatigue and headache.

Skin Lesions

- Seborrhoeic dermatitis.
- Folliculitis.
- Recurrent herpes simplex.
- Oral hairy leukoplakia.

Late Phase

- Risk of developing opportunistic infections or malignancies increases.
- CD4 cell count less than 200 cells/mm^2.
- May have generalised lymphadenopathy.
- Oral erosions, glossitis.
- Genital ulcers.
- Palatal and esophageal ulcers.
- Oropharyngeal candidiasis.
- Opportunistic infections.

Common opportunistic infections in India

- Tuberculosis (pulmonary and extra pulmonary).
- Atypical *Mycobacterium avium* infection.
- Oropharyngeal candidiasis.
- Herpes zoster.
- Herpes simplex.
- Toxoplasmosis.
- Cryptococcal meningitis.
- *Pneumocystis carinii* pneumonia (PCP).
- Cytomegalovirus retinitis.
- Cryptosporidial diarrhoea.

Neoplasms Associated with HIV

Kaposi's sarcoma.
Non-Hodgkin's lymphoma.
Fast growing squamous cell carcinoma.
Basal cell carcinoma.

Kaposi's Sarcoma in HIV

- Multifocal, widespread lesions.
- Lesions involve the skin, oral mucosa, lymph nodes and visceral organs like the GI tract, lungs, liver and spleen.
- Single or several red to purple macules, rapidly progressing to papules, nodules and plaques are present mostly on head, neck, trunk, arms or mucosae.

Advanced HIV Disease

- CD4 cell count is less than 50 cells/mm^2.
- Patient usually has the following AIDS related symptoms:
- Multiple opportunistic infections.
- Malignancies.

Incubation period of AIDS

The incubation period of AIDS is usually 10–12 years. Without therapy, the CD4 cell count declines by 40 to 80 cells/mm^2 each year.

According to WHO, a person should fulfill the following two criteria before he is declared having AIDS:

- Positive test for HIV by two tests preferably on two separate samples of blood
- Any one of the following:
  i) Weight loss of 10% body weight or cachexia which is not explainable by any other non HIV related condition
  ii) Chronic, constant or intermittent, diarrhoea of one month duration.
  iii) Disseminated, miliary or extra-pulmonary tuberculosis,
  iv) Candidiasis of the esophagus presenting as dysphagia, and oral candidiasis.
  v) Neurological impairment restricting the daily activities not related to trauma etc.
  vi) Kaposi's sarcoma.

Diagnosis

Detection of antibodies against HIV is done by the following tests:

- **Enzyme linked immuno-sorbent assays** (ELISA) that become positive only 3–4 weeks after the infection.
- Western blot (WB) test.
- HIV specific antibodies become positive about 22–27 days after the acute infection.

Western Blot Test

- Done to confirm the Elisa positive serum.
- Detects antibodies against specific HIV protein.
- May also not be positive during the initial 3–4 weeks of infection.

False Positives in HIV Diagnosis

Table 24.3 lists the conditions which may present false positive results for HIV.

Table 24.3 False positive test for HIV

- Multiparous women.
- Recent recipient of influenza or hepatitis B vaccine.
- Multiple blood transfusions.
- Haematological malignancies.
- Auto-immune disorders.
- Multiple myeloma.
- Primary biliary cirrhosis.
- Alcoholic hepatitis.

Other Tests

Some other tests for AIDS are as follows:

- CD4 cell counts measure the level of the following:
  i) Immune suppression.
  ii) Viral load.
- Viral culture: Not very sensitive.
- Detection of antigen p24.
- **Polymerase chain reaction** (PCR) that detects the virus antigen, is very sensitive.

Treatment

With the triple drug regimen (Tables 24.4 and 24.5), referred to as **highly active anti-retroviral therapy** (HAART), the HIV infection is now considered a chronic disease manageable over the course of many years.

HIV develops a very fast resistance to any drug, when used alone. The use of a minimum of three antiviral drugs at a time, has proven to inhibit the viral replication below the limit of detection.

Asymptomatic Patient

- ART therapy should be initiated when the CD4 cell count goes below 350 cells/mm^2.
- When the viral load (HIV RNA) is above 30–55,000 copies/ml.

Symptomatic Patient

All the symptomatic patients (wasting, thrush or unexplained fever for more than two weeks) should be treated with ART therapy irrespective of CD4 cell counts or plasma viral load.

Progress

The progress of the disease is monitored periodically by viral load and CD4 cell counts.

Table 24.4 Aims of HAART

a) To inhibit the viral replication and keep it as low as possible. Maintain it to a lower level as long as possible.
b) To increase the CD4 cell counts. Restore the immune response.

These drugs act on two enzymes:
Protease
Reverse transcriptase.
Two groups of drug are available for the treatment of HIV:
I. Protease inhibitors (PI's).
II. Reverse transcriptase inhibitors.
- Nucleoside reverse transcriptase inhibitors (NRTIs).
- Non-nucleoside reverse transcriptase inhibitors (NNRTIs).

Table 24.5 Antiretroviral drugs with their usual doses

Nucleoside Reverse Transcriptase Inhibitors	Non-Nucleoside Reverse Transcriptase Inhibitors (NRTIs)	Protease Inhibitors (PIs)
Zidovudine 300 mg BID	Nevirapine 200 mg BID	Indinavir 800 mg OD
Stavudine 30–40 mg BID	Efavirenz 600 mg HS	Nelfinavir 1250 mg OD
Lamivudine 150 mg BID	Delavirdine 400 mg TDS	Ritonavir 600 mg BID
Didanosine 125–200 mg BID		Saquinavir 1200 mg TDS
Zalcitabine 0.75 mg TDS		Amprenavir 1200 mg BID
Abacavir		Lopinavir/Ritonavir caps BID

Miscellaneous Disorders

The diseases whose etiology is still not clear, have been grouped in this chapter.

Pityriasis Alba

Synonym

Pityriasis simplex.

Etiology

Believed to occur due to saprophytic *Staphylococcus*.

Age

Occurs mainly in children.

Clinical Features

- Presents as asymptomatic, hypopigmented, mildly scaly, ill-defined macules (Fig. 25.1).
- The lesions need to be differentiated from leprosy (Table 25.1).

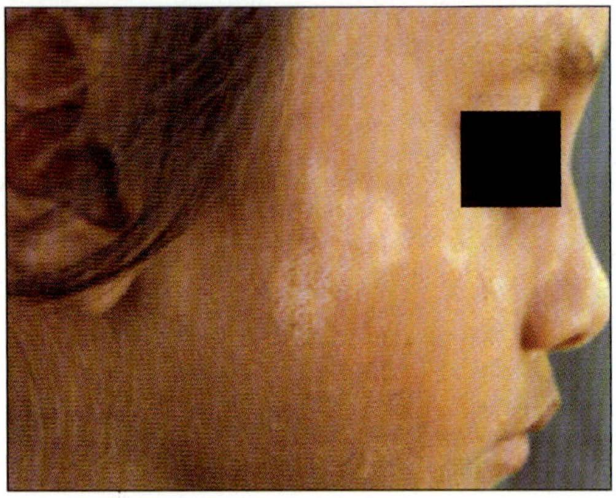

Fig. 25.1 Pityriasis alba

Sites

- Usually on cheeks and other parts of the face.
- Occasionally, it may be seen on other parts of the body.

Course

- The lesions usually disappear spontaneously after persisting for a long period.
- Recurrences are frequent.
- This condition is extremely rare after puberty.

Treatment

- Many patients may not require any treatment except the explanation and assurance that it is a self-limiting disease.
- Topical antibiotic and corticosteroid creams clear the lesions.

Table 25.1 Differences between Pityraisis alba and indeterminate leprosy

Pityriasis Alba	Indeterminate Leprosy
Scaly, hypopigmented macules.	Hypopigmented macule with atrophy.
Sensation normal.	Hypoaesthesia or normal sensation.
Nerves not thickened.	Nerve may be thickened.
Mostly children are affected.	Age no bar.
Face commonly involved.	Any part of the body may be affected.

Pityriasis Rosea

Etiology

Not known.

Clinical Features

- There is a sudden eruption of asymptomatic or itchy, oval or circular, erythematous and scaly lesions.
- Fine bran-like scales, free at the centre and attached at the periphery of the lesions are seen (Fig. 25.2).

Sites

- The lesions are present on the trunk and upper arm and are parallel to the ribs (**fir-tree appearance**).
- Occasionally the lesions are found only on the extremities and rarely on the face.
- One can see a single lesion appearing 2–3 days prior to the main eruptions, called **herald patch** (Fig. 25.3). Sometimes it is confused with tinea corporis (Table 25.2).

Course

Lesions continue to appear during the next 2–3 weeks and then start subsiding spontaneously and disappear completely within 6–8 weeks without leaving any marks (Table 25.3).

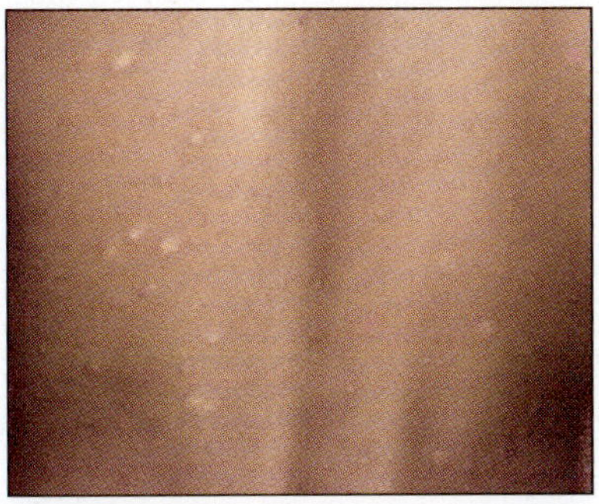

Fig. 25.2 Pityriasis rosea

Table 25.2 Differences between herald patch and tinea corporis

Tinea Corporis	Herald Patch
Itching is prominent.	Asymptomatic or mildly itchy.
Annular lesion with papulo-vesicles and scales at the periphery.	Annular lesion with scales attached to periphery.
Fungal hyphae seen in KOH preparation.	Fungal hyphae not seen.

Table 25.3 Evolution of pityriasis rosea

Herald Patch

↓ Phase of evolution (7–20 days)

Many smaller lesions which enlarge slowly and increase in number

↓ Phase of resolution (6–8 weeks)

Mild pigmentary changes which fade away slowly

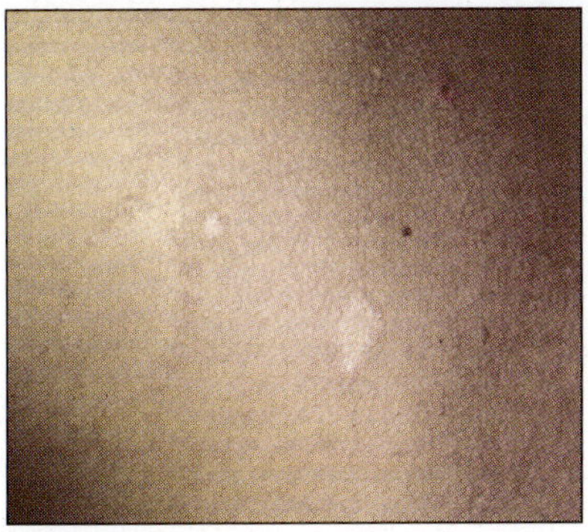

Fig. 25.3 Pityriasis rosea: herald patch

Investigations

As the lesions of secondary stage of syphilis may sometimes be similar (Table 25.4) VDRL test should be done whenever there is any doubt. The lesions should be differentiated from those of pityriasis lichenoides chronica (Table 25.5).

Table 25.4 Pityriasis rosea and secondary syphilis

Pityriasis Rosea	Secondary Syphilis
Annular lesions with scales attached to periphery.	Maculopapular and papulo-squamous lesion.
Oral lesions usually absent.	Mouth, genitals, perianal areas, palms and soles may have lesions.
Lymphadenopathy usually absent.	Lymphadenopathy frequently present.
Negative serology.	Serology for syphilis and dark ground microscopy positive.

Table 25.5 Pityriasis lichenoides chronica (PLC) and pityriasis rosea (PR)

PLC	PR
Longer course of remissions and relapses.	Self limiting course.
Erythematous papules.	Erythematous annular lesions.
Mica-like scale.	Herald patch seen with scales in periphery.
Heals with hypopigmentation.	Heals with hyperpigmentation.

Treatment

- Since the disease has a self-limiting course, it is better not to give any treatment, except assurance.
- Occasionally, symptomatic treatment may be prescribed, e.g., oral antihistamine or soothing agent like calamine lotion for itching.
- Corticosteroids—topical or oral—should be avoided.
- An attack usually produces a lifelong immunity in the majority of cases.

Psoriasis

Psoriasis is a papulosquamous disorder characterised by the presence of papules and plaques that are covered by scales.

Etiology

- The exact cause is not known.
- Inherited as an autosomal dominant character with irregular penetrance.
- In 10–30% of the cases, more than one member in the family is found to have psoriasis.
- Exposure to certain drugs is a predisposing factor (Table 25.6).

Table 25.6 Drugs that precipitate or aggravate psoriasis

- Chloroquine.
- Lithium.
- Indomethacin.

Immune Mechanism

Helper T cells get stimulated leading to the production of cytokines that stimulate keratinocytes leading to their faster proliferation.

The time taken for transfer of epidermal cells from basal cell layer to outer surface of skin is drastically reduced from the normal one month to 3–5 days. This results in the formation of immature epidermal cells which are shed as scales.

Age and Sex

Seen in both the sexes and it may occur at any age.

Clinical Features

Different types of psoriasis are presented in Table 25.7.

Table 25.7 Types of psoriasis

• Plaque-type psoriasis. • Guttate psoriasis. • Pustular psoriasis. • Erythrodermic psoriasis.
*Rupioid psoriasis is a variant where the lesions appear conical because of the heaped up scaling (Fig. 25.18).

Plaque Type Psoriasis

- Commonly manifests as well-defined erythematous scaly plaques (Figs 25.4–25.6) which become silvery on attempt to scrape.

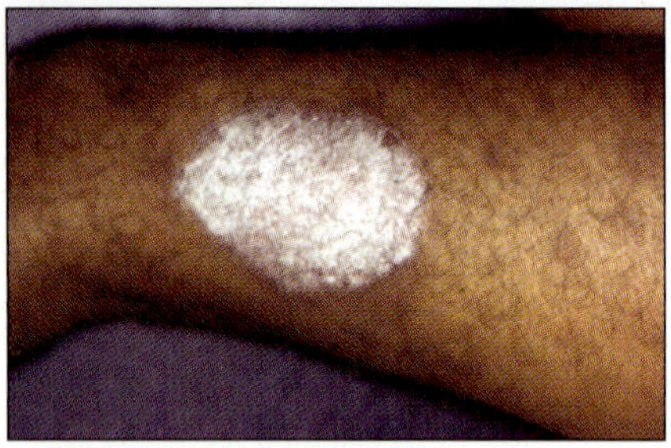

Fig. 25.4 Psoriasis: plaque on arm

- The lesions vary in shape and size (Fig 25.8–25.16).

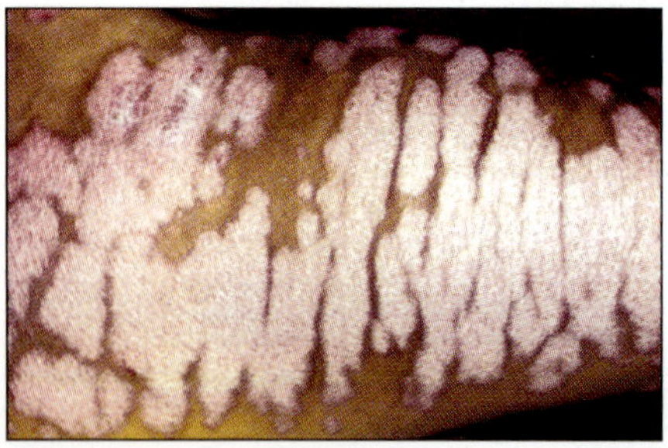

Fig. 25.5 Psoriasis: shoulder back

- Sometimes some of them coalesce to form large gyrate or geographical patterns (Fig. 25.7).
- May be completely asymptomatic or some patients may have severe itching

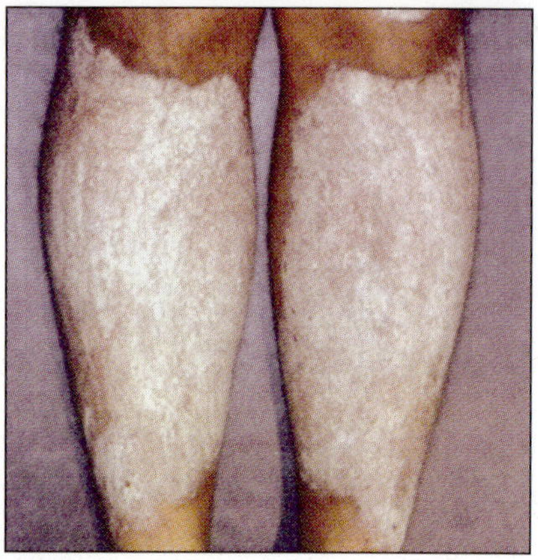

Fig. 25.6 Psoriasis: plaque on whole legs

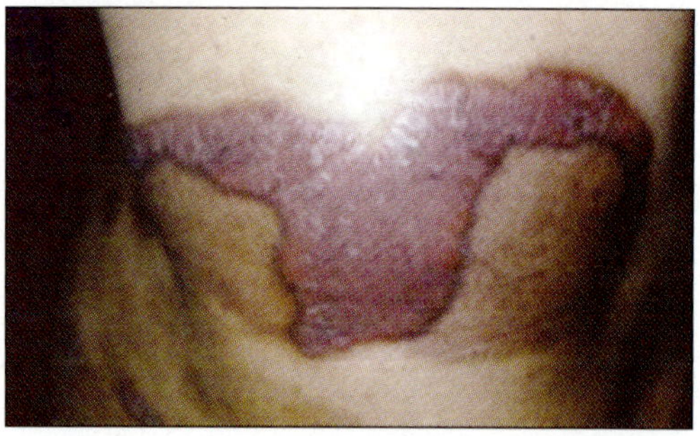

Fig. 25.7 Psoriasis: geographical pattern

- The lesions worsen during winter and improve, or even clear during the summer months.
- Spontaneous remissions and relapses at variable intervals are quite frequent.
- Joint involvement mimicks rheumatoid arthritis. In psoriasis, distal interphalyngeal joints are involved.
- The serum is negative for rheumatoid factor.

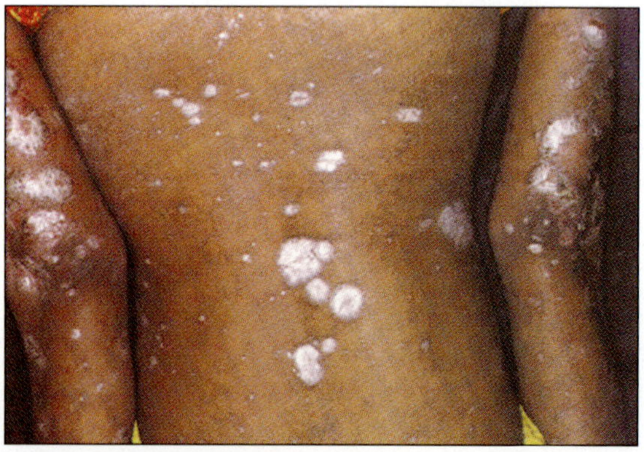

Fig. 25.8 Psoriasis: lesion on back

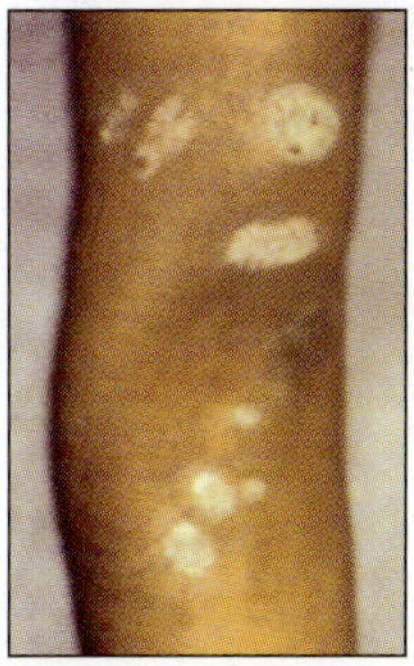

Fig. 25.9 Psoriasis: elbow

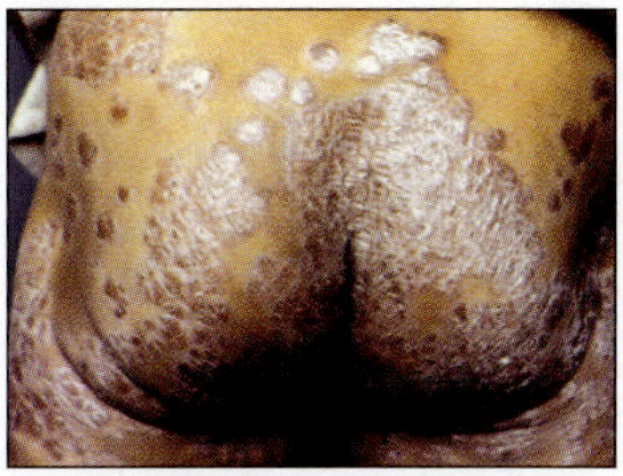

Fig. 25.10 Psoriasis: buttocks

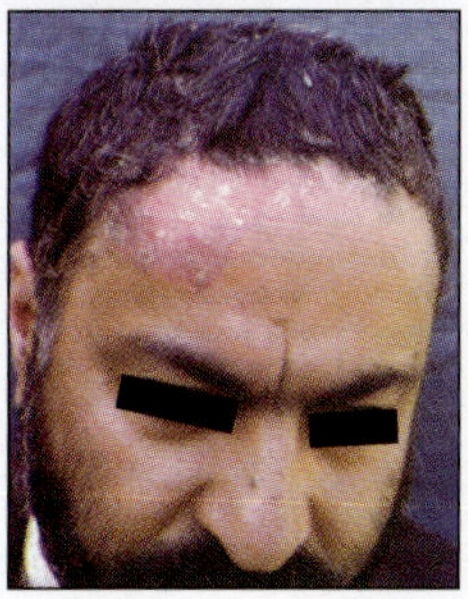

Fig. 25.11 Psoriasis: scalp

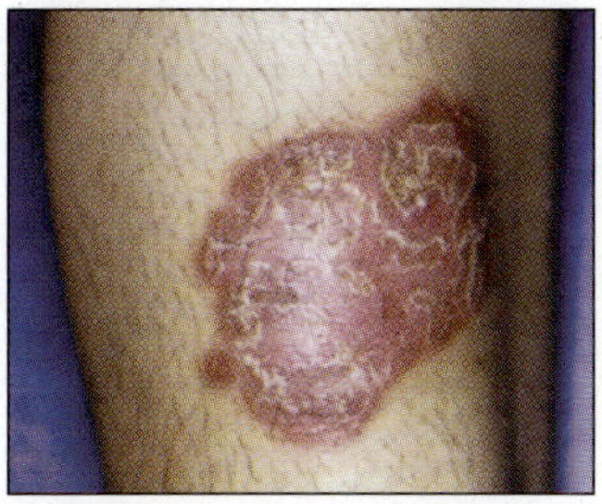

Fig. 25.12 Psoriasis: erythematous lesion

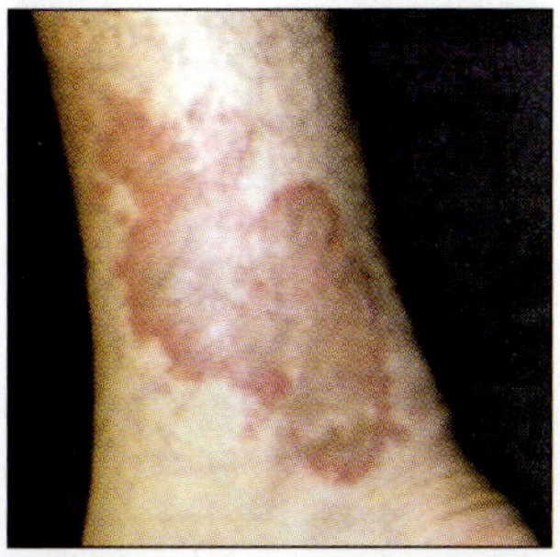

Fig. 25.13 Psoriasis: leg

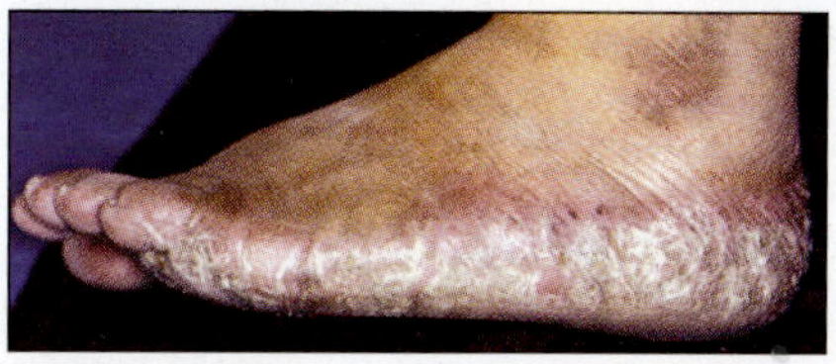

Fig. 25.14 Psoriasis: foot

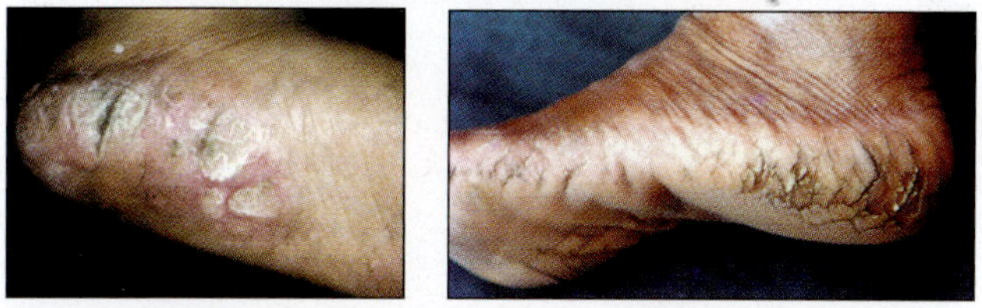

(a) (b)

Fig. 25.15 (a) Psoriasis: foot; (b) Fissure foot: no erythema or induration

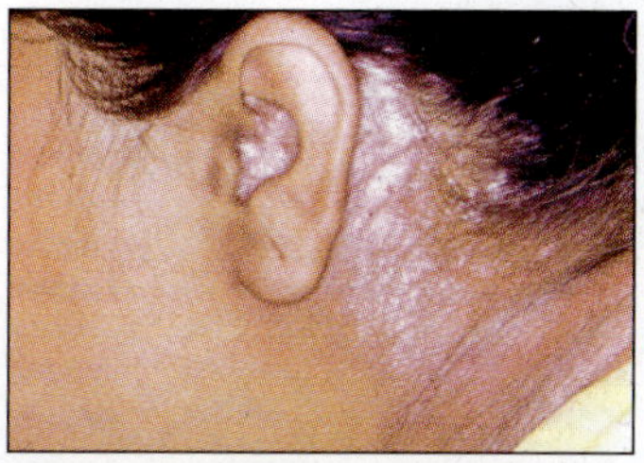

Fig. 25.16 Psoriasis: post auricular area

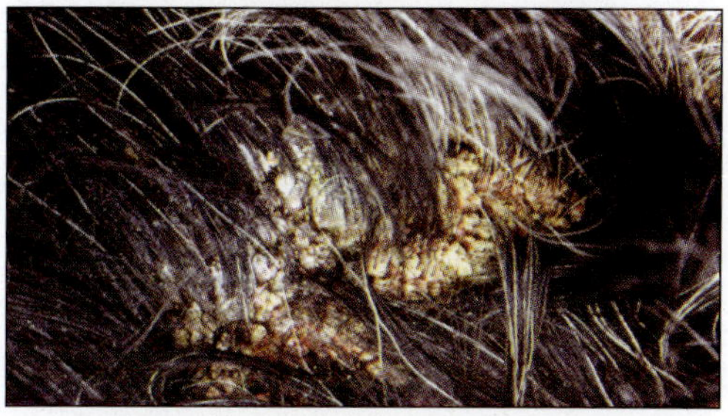

Fig. 25.17 Pityriasis amentacea: on scalp

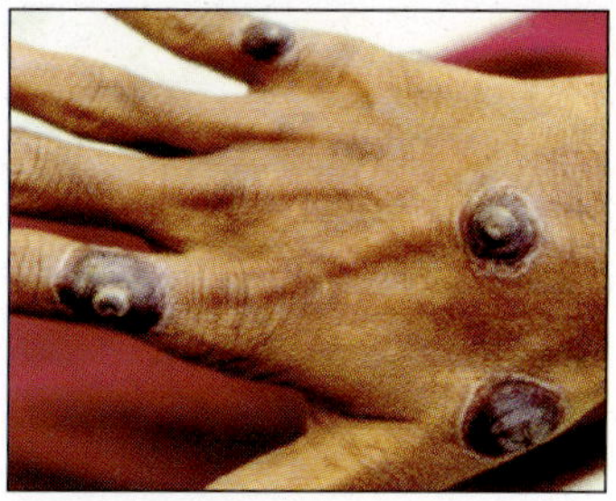

Fig. 25.18 Psoriasis: rupioid lesion

Nail Changes

Seen in a few patients only, these changes are as follows:

- Multiple, pin-point pits on the nail plates (Fig. 25.19).

- Separation of the nail plate from the nail-bed, called onycholysis (Fig. 25.20). This presents as an area of yellowish discolouration.
- Brownish discolouration, thickening and irregularity of the nail plate called onychodystrophy (Table 25.8).

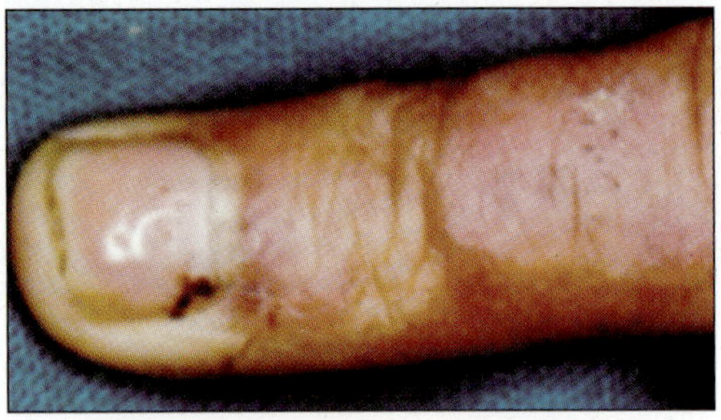

Fig. 25.19 Nail psoriasis: pitting

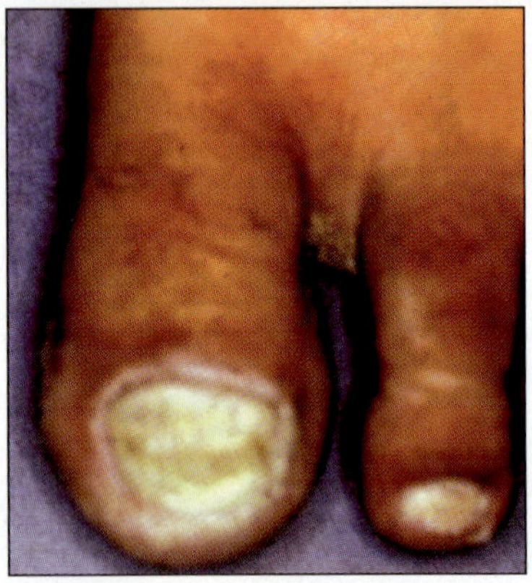

Fig. 25.20 Nail psoriasis: onycholysis

Table 25.8 Differences in condition of nails in psoriasis and tinea unguim

Psoriasis of nails	Tinea unguim
Symmetrical involvement of several nails.	Asymmetrical involvement of a few nails.
Begins proximally.	Usually begins distally.
Pitting of nails very frequent.	Pitting not seen.
Subungual debris does not crumble.	Subungual debris friable.

Guttate Psoriasis

- Occasionally some patients, usually children, suddenly develop numerous erythematous and scaly papules 0.5 to 1 cm in size resembling psoriasis (Fig. 25.21).
- The lesions may occur 2–4 weeks after an infection with group-A beta-haemolytic streptococci.
- These lesions usually clear spontaneously but may recur.
- Sometimes they persist and change into plaques producing plaque-type psoriasis.

Table 25.9 Difference between guttate psoriasis and pityriasis rosea

Guttate Psoriasis	Pityriasis Rosea
Plaques with silvery scales attachment. Appear in crops, sometimes after streptococcal sore throat.	Annular lesions with scales attached in periphery. Herald patch appears first, followed by secondary lesions which appear in crops.

Pustular Psoriasis

- It presents as superficial, tiny pustules (Fig. 25.22) over the existing psoriasis plaques, or even on the normal skin.
- Pustules are sterile and contain a large number of polymorphs.
- The lesions of pustular psoriasis may be limited to palms and soles without any systemic symptoms, or may appear all over the body with fever and toxaemia.

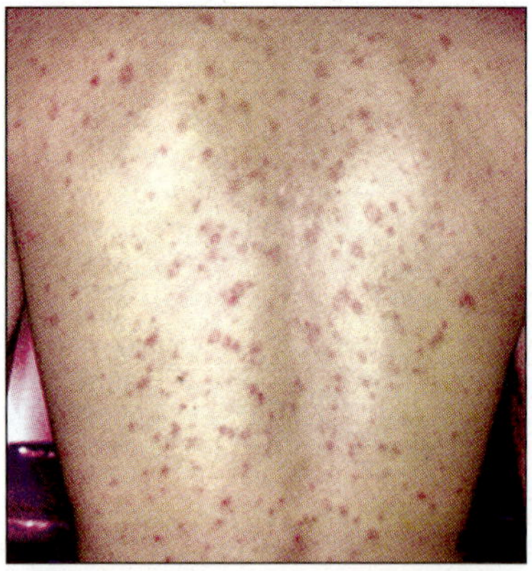

Fig. 25.21 Guttate psoriasis

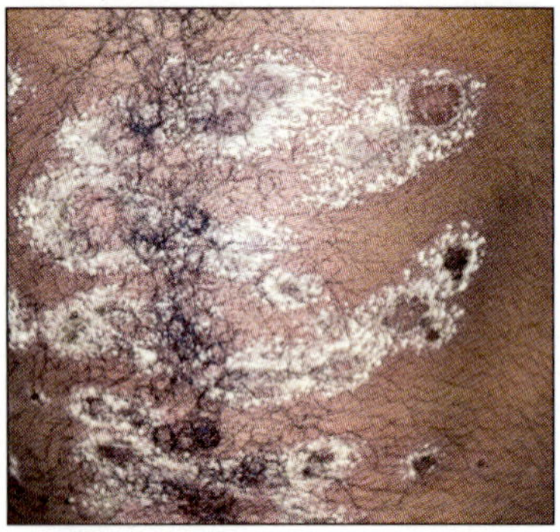

Fig. 25.22 Pustular psoriasis

Erythrodermic Psoriasis

- Erythrodermic psoriasis may occur, due to excessive treatment with topical irritants or may even appear spontaneously. The lesions become extremely itchy with erythema and scaling (Fig. 25.23).
- Chills and rigor may be associated.

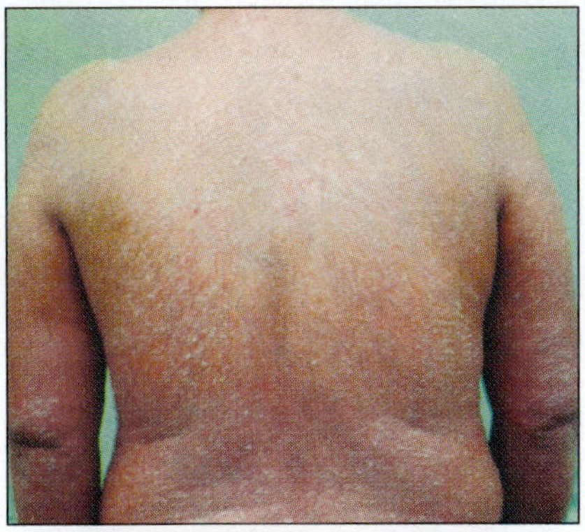

Fig. 25.23 Psoriasis: erythroderma

Koebner's Phenomena

- Sometimes new lesions of psoriasis develop in a linear fashion along the lines of scratches or trauma (Fig. 25.24).
- This is seen in the active phase of psoriasis.
- Trauma precipitates the formation of new psoriasis lesions. That is why psoriatic lesions are frequently seen on the extensor surfaces of elbows and knees.

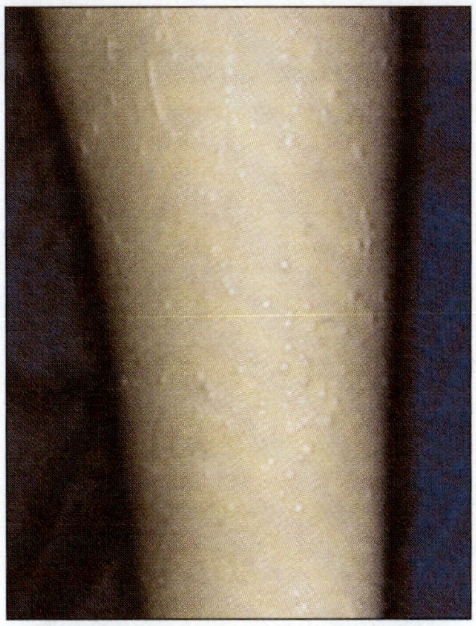

Fig. 25.24 Koebner's phenomenon: psoriasis

Sites

- Extensors of the extremities, especially elbows, (Fig 25.9), knees, sacral region of back (Fig. 25.10), scalp (Fig. 25.11) are the most favoured sites.
- When the lesions are localised to any of the flexural areas of the body, it is called flexural psoriasis.

Diagnosis

The disease is to be differentiated from the similar-looking lesions of seborrhoeic dermatitis (Table 25.10), discoid eczema, pityriasis rosea and secondary syphilis. Psoriasis is confirmed by the following tests:

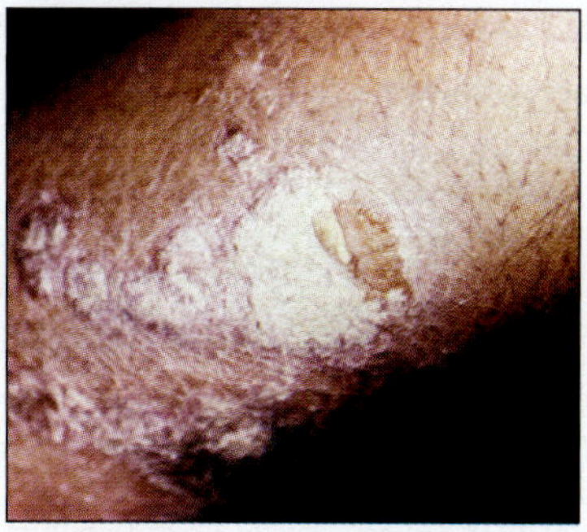

Fig. 25.25 Grattage test

- **Grattage Test**: When an attempt is made to scrape the psoriatic plaque, it becomes silvery. On further scrapping, a thin membrane of skin (Berkley's membrane) is visible, with further scrapping it results in multiple pin-point bleeding spots known as Auspitz sign and the whole process is called Grattage test (Fig. 25.25).
- Skin biopsy.

Table 25.10 Difference between psoriasis and seborrhoeic dermatitis

Psoriasis	Seborrhoeic dermatitis
Well-defined.	Less defined.
Indurated plaques.	Not indurated.
Erythema marked.	Erythema less.
Silvery scales.	Scaling greasy and yellow.
Scalp and forehead, elbows, knees and lower back. Facial lesions less common.	Scalp, nasolabial folds, retroauricular region, presternal and interscapular region, axilla and groins.

Treatment

The entire treatment is divided into four phases:

Phase1: Treatment with azathioprine pulse therapy continued till the clearance of all lesions. Along with this, other medicines like methotrexate, coal tar, cyclosporin etc. are also given for fast clearance of the lesions.

Phase 2: Patients remains without lesions but continues azathioprine pulse therapy for 9 months.

Phase 3: After phase II, IHD is stopped but CLD is continued for 9 months.

Phase 4: If there is no lesion, the patient is followed-up without any treatment for as long as possible.

Photochemotherapy

This is used along with tar in the treatment of psoriasis. If given in large enough doses (20–30

Table 25.11 Management of psoriasis: At a Glance

Few plaques of psoriasis:
- Topical tar preparation.
- Topical corticosteroids.
- Dithranol ointment.
- Regular use of the treatment will keep the skin free from the lesions.

Guttate psoriasis:

Systemic antibiotics in full dose.

Pustular psoriasis, erythrodermic psoriasis or extensive plaque psoriasis
- Methotrexate: 15–22.5 mg, weekly. Folic acid: 5 mg, weekly is added to prevent any side effects.
- Psoralens: 15–20 mg daily with exposure to artificial UVR (PUVA) or to sunlight (PUVASOL).
- Cyclosporine.
- Hydroxyurea.
- Retinoids: 25–50 mg, daily.
- Patient should be encouraged to get exposed maximally to sunlight and avoid trauma during the active phase. Patients with scalp lesions should preferably apply tar-lotion at night, followed by shampooing the next morning.
- **Recently azathioprine pulse therapy** (APT) has been found curative in psoriasis. This consists of giving intermittent high dose (IHD) azathioprine 500 mg orally on three consecutive days and is repeated on a monthly basis. In between IHD, the patients are given continued low dose (CLD) azathioprine 100 mg daily orally with minimum side-effects.
- Emollients are used as adjuncts to the systemic therapy.

Joules cm^2), it was found beneficial to psoriasis. The term PUVA means 'psoralens + ultra violet A'. Psoralens are materials that make the skin more sensitive to UV light. Various type of psoralens are—8-methoxypsorlen (8-MOP), methoxypsorlens and 4,5,8 trimethoxypsoralen (TMP). The combination results in the inhibition of epidermal DNA synthesis in humans. Sun is a potent source of the UVA light. Immediate side-effects of this therapy include nausea, headache, pruritus, dizziness, fatique or drowsiness and erythema. Long-term side-effects include carcinoma and fibrosarcoma.

Lichen Planus

Etiology

- Not known exactly.
- Histopathologically, the findings suggest an immunological response to an agent present in the basal cell layer of the epidermis.

Clinical Features

- Extremely itchy, violaceous, flat-topped papules (Figs 25.26 and 25.27).
- Large lesions may show whitish criss-cross streaks on their surface called **Wickham's striae.**

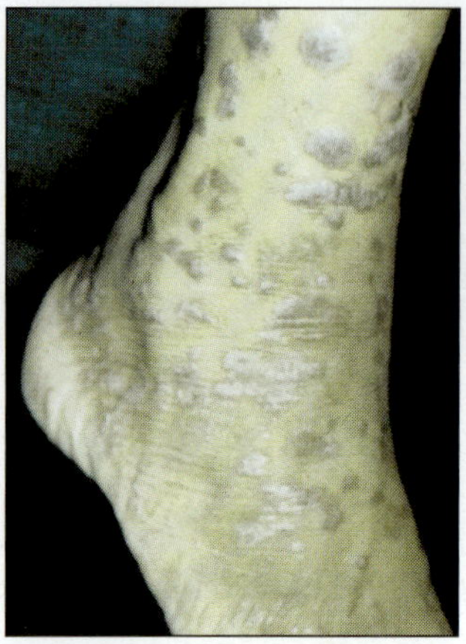

Fig. 25.26 Lichen planus foot: early lesion

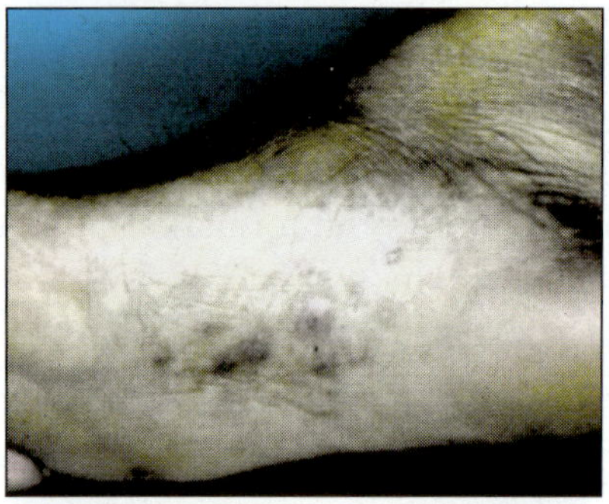

Fig. 25.27 Lichen planus: sole

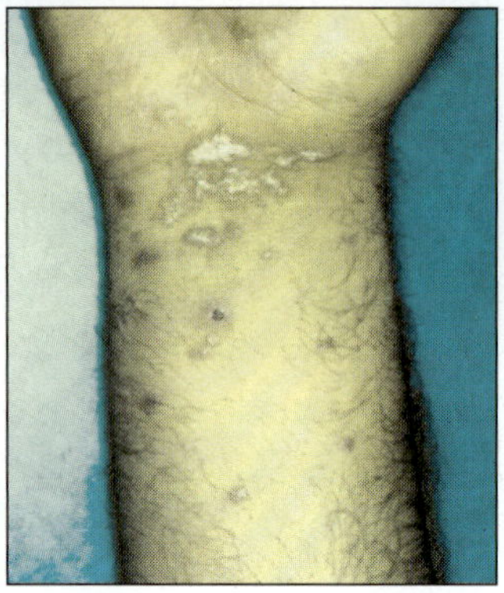

Fig. 25.28 Lichen planus: wrist

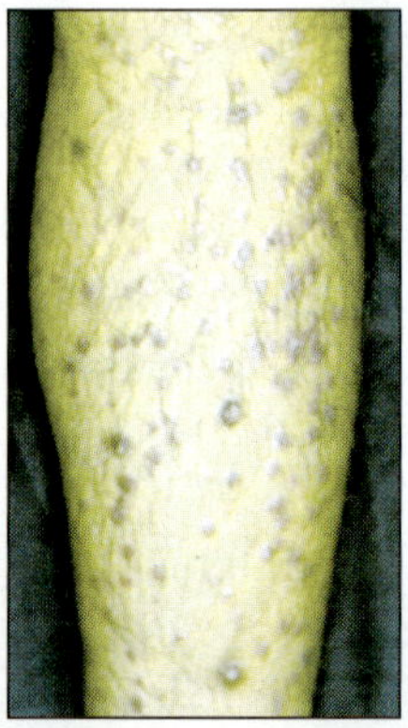

Fig. 25.29 Lichen planus: leg

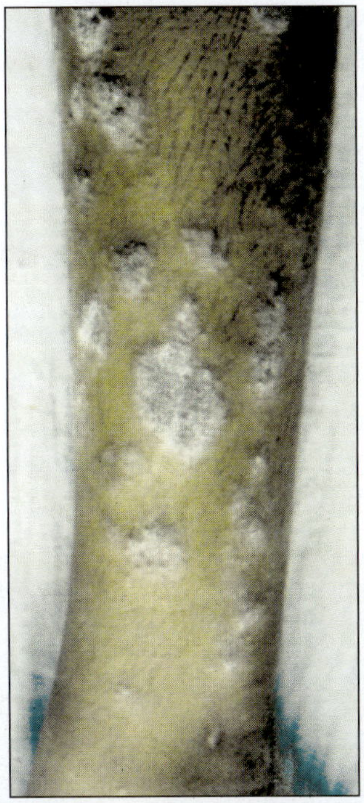

Fig. 25.30 Lichen planus: scaly lesion

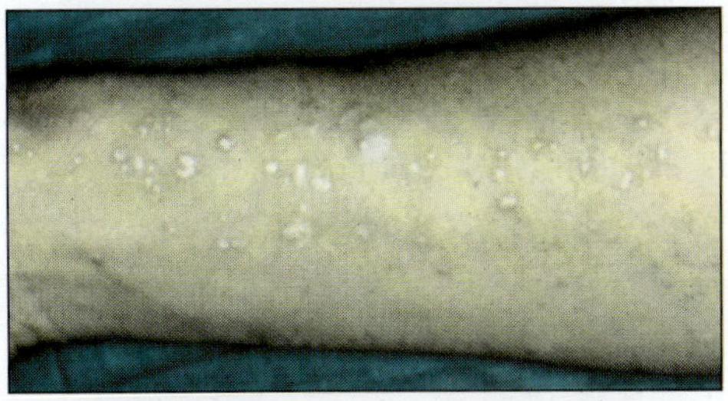

Fig. 25.31 Lichen planus: arm

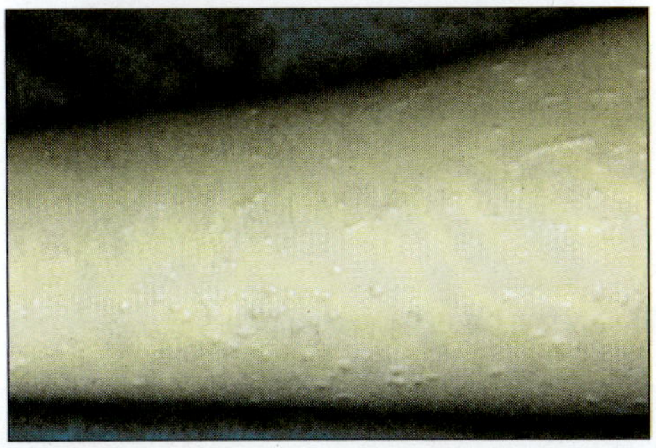

Fig. 25.32 Lichen planus: Koebner's phenomenon

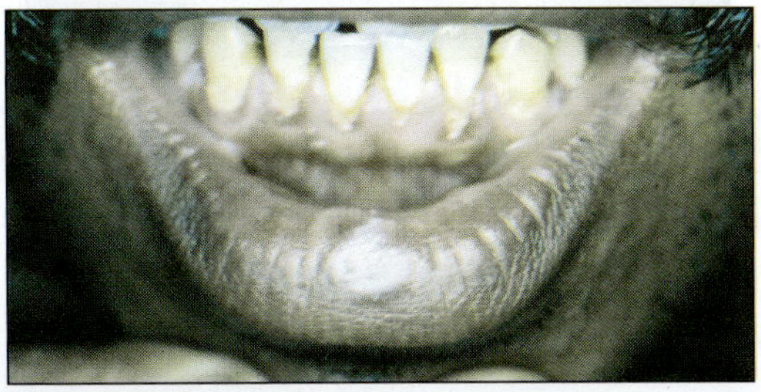

Fig. 25.33 Lichen planus: lower lip

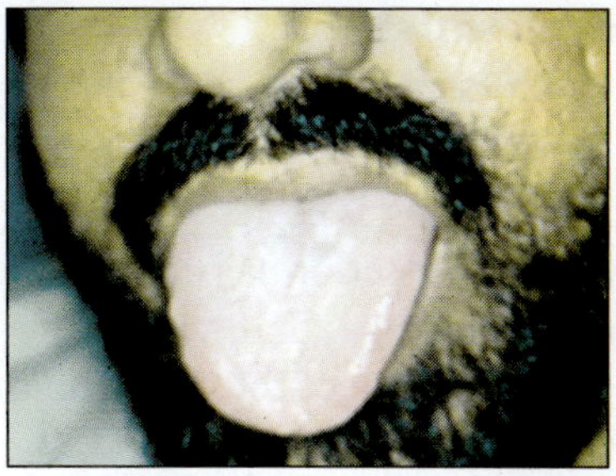

Fig. 25.34 Lichen planus: tongue

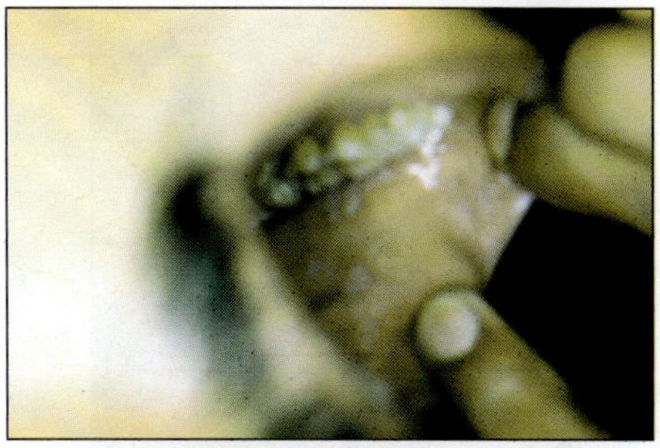

Fig. 25.35 Lichen planus: buccal mucosa

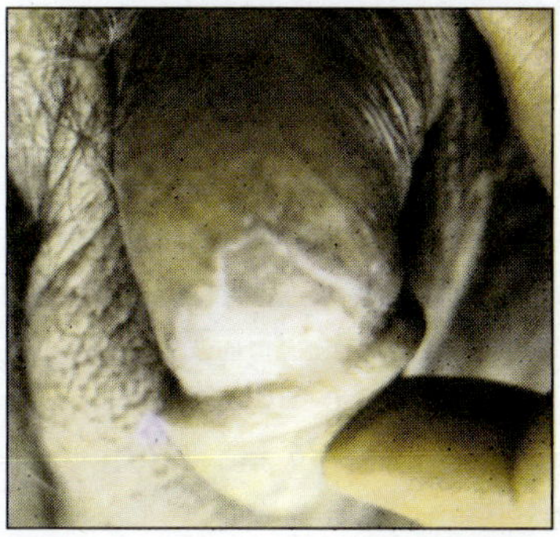

Fig. 25.36 Lichen planus glans: circinate lesion

- Lesions may be situated in a linear fashion along the scratch mark, called **Koebner's phenomenon** (Fig. 25.32). They are seen in the active phase of disease.

Size

3–5 mm.

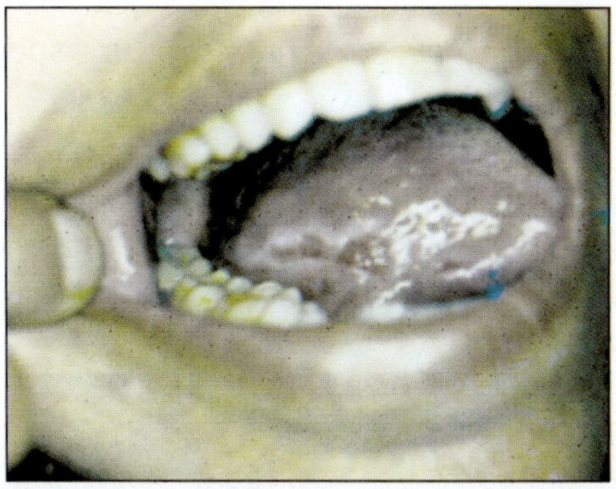

Fig. 25.37 Squamous cell carcinoma on lichen planus ulcer (long standing)

Involvement of Nails

- Slight roughness and thinning of the nail-plate is present.
- Longitudinal ridging is seen.
- Overgrowing of posterior nail-fold on the nail-plate, called **pterygium** (Fig. 25.38).
- Complete disappearance of the nail or/and nail-plate, called **anychia.**

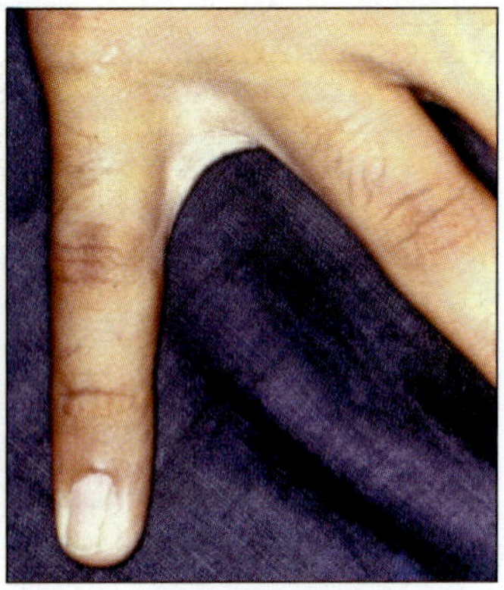

Fig. 25.38 Pterygium unguis: lichen planus

Sites

- Commonly seen in front of the wrists (Figs 25.28–25.31), lumbar region and around the ankles.
- Can occur on any part of the body.
- The face is relatively less involved.
- Mucosal involvement is common and seen as whitish streaks forming lacy pattern or superficial ulcerations.
- Common mucosal sites include lips (Fig. 25.33), tongue (Fig. 25.34), buccal and gingival mucosae (Fig. 25.35) and glan penis (Fig. 25.36).
- Vagina and rectum (occasionally) are involved.
- Mucosal lesions may or may not be associated with the skin lesions, sometimes only mucous membranes are involved without any skin lesions.

Course

- The disease has a tendency for spontaneous remission within 2–3 years.
- Some cases may persist for many years.
- Chronic variants may undergo malignant transformation (Fig. 25.37).
- Lichen planus presents as different types (Table 25.12).

Types of Lichen Planus

Different types of lichen planus are presented in Table 25.12.

Table 25.12 Types of lichen planus

- Lichen planus hypertrophicus.
- Lichen planus atrophicus.
- Lichen planopilaris.
- Actinic lichen planus.
- Linear lichen planus.
- Bullous lichen planus.
- Lichenoid eruptions.
- Lichen aureus.
- Lichen nitidus.

Lichen Planus Hypertrophicus

- Manifests as large, itchy, violaceous, hyperkeratotic papules (Figs 25.39 and 25.40) and plaques.
- Usually seen on the anterior surface of the legs.

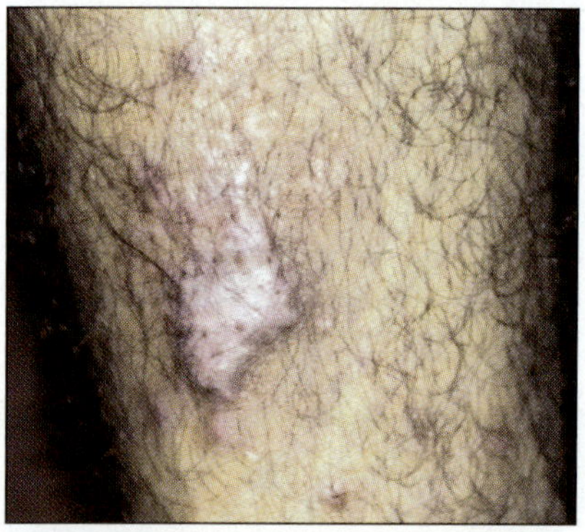

Fig. 25.39 Lichen planus hypertrophicus

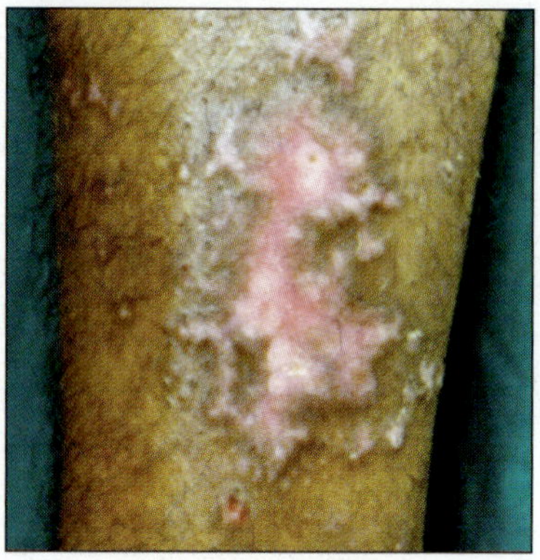

Fig. 25.40 Lichen planus hypertrophicus

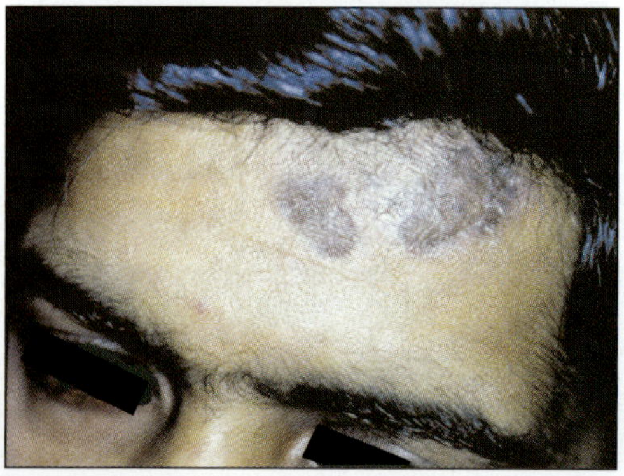

Fig. 25.41 Atrophic lichen planus: forehead

Lichen Planus Atrophicus

- Presents as an annular area having atrophic, hyperpigmented centre and active, erythematous, 1–2 mm thick, raised border (Figs 25.41–25.43).
- Usually seen on the face and dorsum of hands.

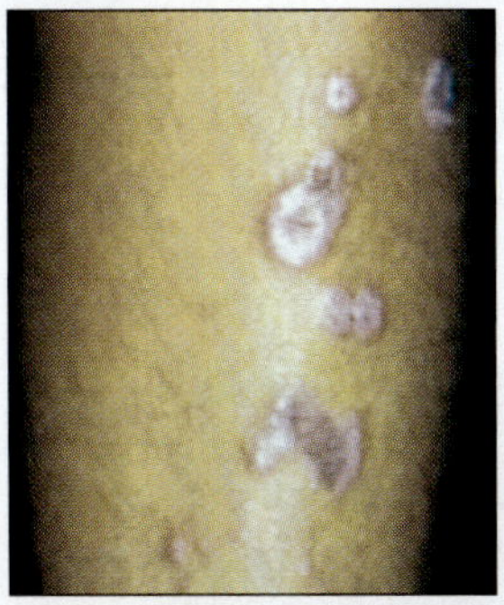

Fig. 25.42 Atrophic lichen planus: leg

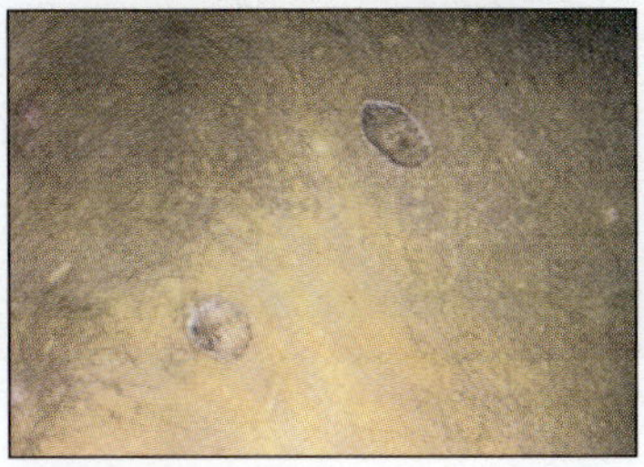

Fig. 25.43 Atrophic lichen planus

Lichen Planopilaris

- Presents as itchy, violaceous papules at the openings of hair follicles (Fig. 25.44).

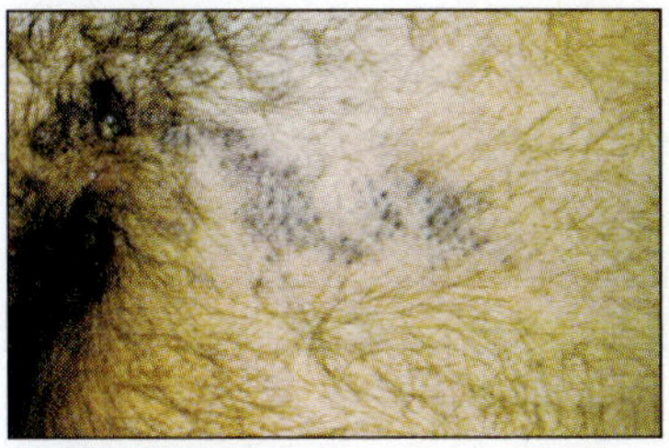

Fig. 25.44 Lichen planopilaris

- It destroys the hair follicle, resulting in the loss of hair.

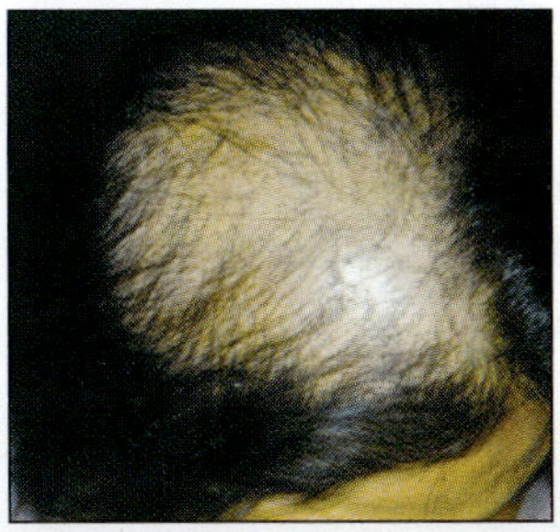

Fig. 25.45 Lichen plano-pilaris: cicatricial alopecia

- On scalp, it causes cicatricial alopecia (Fig. 25.45).
- Presents as an atrophic scar with pigmentation.
- Commonly, seen on the legs and arms.

Actinic Lichen Planus

- Present as annular grouped micropapular lesions.
- Situated on the exposed parts of the body (Fig. 25.46) like extensor surfaces of forearms, hands (Fig. 25.47) and face.
- The lesions get aggravated on exposure to sunlight.

Linear Lichen Planus

The lesions of lichen planus are distributed in a linear fashion.

Bullous Lichen Planus

Bullae are situated on a voilaceous base resembling lichen planus.

Lichenoid Eruptions

Occasionally, certain drugs (Table 25.14) may produce skin lesions resembling lichen planus (Fig. 25.48 and Table 25.15).

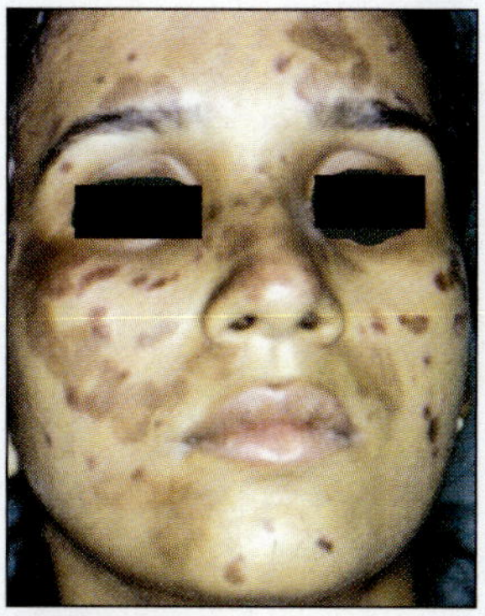

Fig. 25.46 Actinic lichen planus: face

Table 25.13 Management of lichen planus: At a glance

Systemic corticosteroids: • 20 mg prednisolone a day clears the lesions in 6–8 weeks. • Corticosteroids would be tapered-off over the next 3–4 months.
Topical corticosteroids: • For limited lesion.
For residual hyperpigmentation: • Hydroquinone: 2–5% topically.

Table 25.14 Substances causing lichenoid eruptions

Drugs	• Chloroquine. • Gold salts. • Phenothiazines
Contact sensitisers	• Colour photograph developers • Infections • Hepatitis C infection • Graft vs host reaction

Table 25.15 Difference between Lichen planus, Lichenoid eruption and DLE

Lichen planus	Lichenoid eruption	DLE
Violaceous papules.	Lesions are larger and scaly.	Lesions with center scarring, surrounded with erythema.
Scaling minimal or no scaling.	Residual hyperpigmentation is common.	Scaling adherent and prominent.
Wickham's striae present.	Wickhams striae absent.	Follicular plugs present.
Intensely itchy.	Itching present.	Photosensitivity may be present.
Wrists and shins are common sites.	Any part of the body.	Face and ears are common sites.
Mucous membrane frequently Involved.	Mucous membrane involvement is less common.	Mucous membrane is occasionally involved.

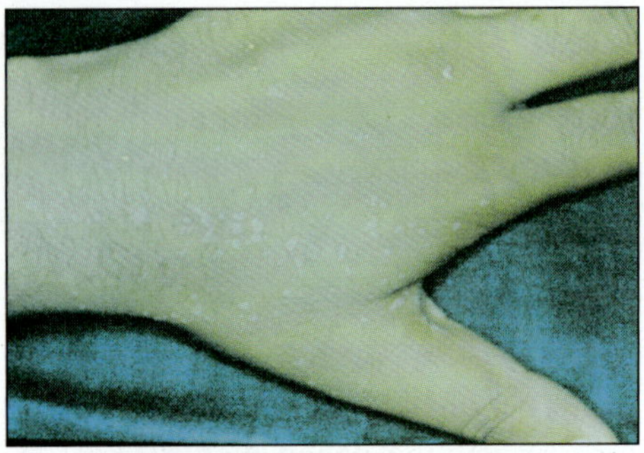

Fig. 25.47 Actinic lichen planus: arm

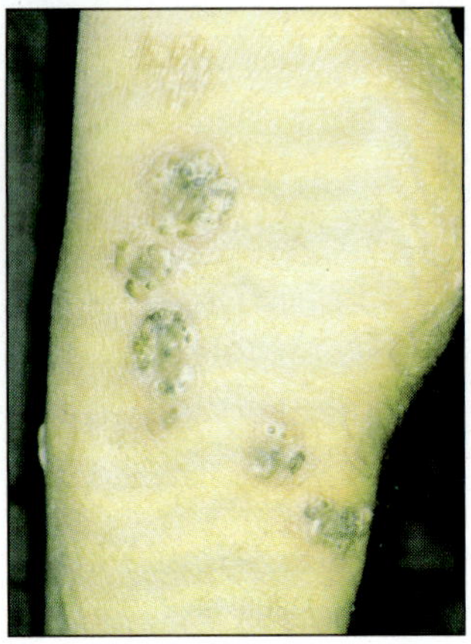

Fig. 25.48 Lichenoid eruption

Lichen Aureus

A variety of pigmented purpuric dermatosis.

Etiology

Remain unknown.

Clinical Feature

- Sudden appearance of one or several golden or red-coloured, closely packed macules or papules.
- Asymptomatic.
- The lesions usually remain unchanged for many years.
- Mostly found on the lower legs.
- The disease in children is more or less self-limiting.

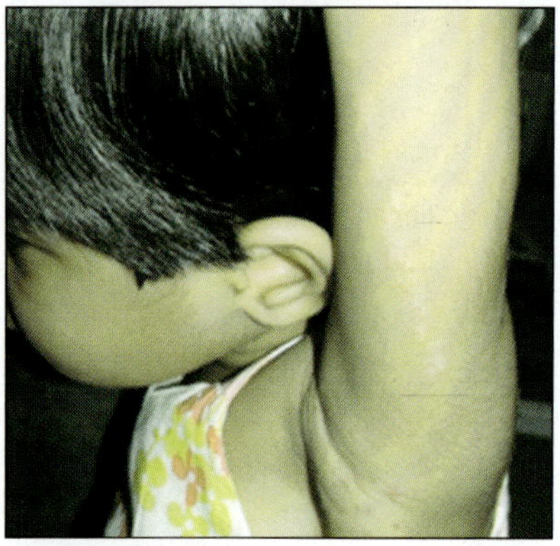

Fig. 25.49 Lichen aureous

Treatment

- Topical corticosteroids.
- Topical pimecrolimus.
- Psorlens-UVA therapy.
- Pentoxifylline + prostacyclin.

Lichen Nitidus

- Asymptomatic, flat-topped, skin-coloured micropapules.
- Occasionally pruritic.
- Mainly affects children and young adults.

Diagnosis

Skin biopsy for histopathological examination.

Treatment

- Topical and systemic corticosteroids.
- Topical tacrolimus.

Prognosis

Spontaneous resolution usually occurs, though it may remain active for several years.

Pompholyx

Etiology

The exact cause is still unknown.

It is believed to be an allergic manifestation to any of the following:

- A septic focus in the body.
- Tinea interdigitale.
- Some food article.
- Some inhalant.
- Some drug.

In several cases, the cause remains untraced.

Clinical Features

Recurrent, extremely itchy vesicles are seen.

Sites

- Both palms (Fig. 25.50) and/or soles (Fig. 25.51).
- Sides of the fingers are frequently involved.
- Occasionally, dorsum of the hands and feet are also involved.

Course

- Lesions heal spontaneously in a few days leaving behind scaling.
- The lesions recur at variable intervals.
- Secondary infection is very frequent.

Treatment

Systemic corticosteroids in a dose of 15–20 mg prednisolone, daily for a few days help to clear the eruptions fast.

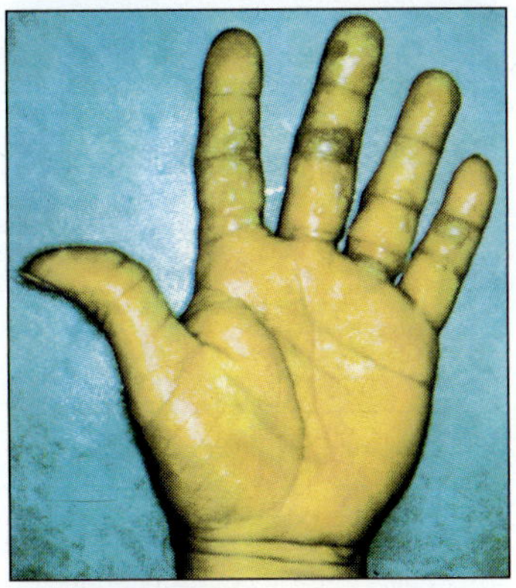

Fig. 25.50 Pompholyx: palm

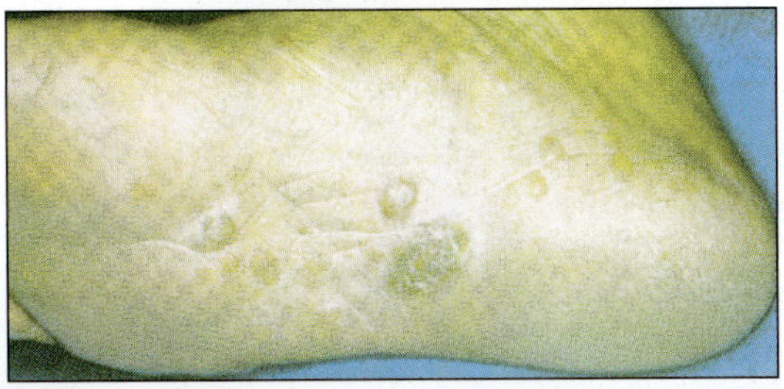

Fig. 25.51 Pompholyx: sole

Table 25.16 Pompholyx: At a glance

Etiology	: Unknown.
Clinical features	: Recurrent severely, itchy vesicles with spontaneous remission.
Sites	: Palms and soles.
Management	: Systemic corticosteroids equivalent to 15–20 mg Prednisolone daily for 4–5 days with or without oral antibiotics Topical steroids and antibiotic ointment

Prevention

For preventing recurrences, the cause should be traced and removed, if possible.

Nummular Eczema

Synonym

Discoid dermatitis.

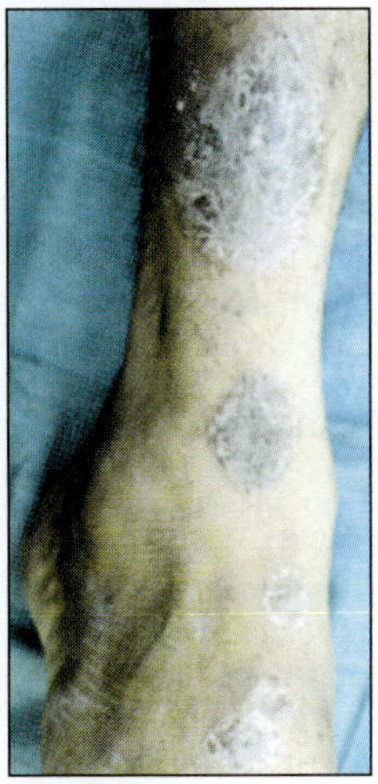

Fig. 25.52 Nummular eczema

Etiology

Unkown.

Age

Common in children and young adults

Clinical Features

- Recurrent, itchy papulovesicles, grouped into **coin-shaped** patches (Fig. 25.52).
- The lesions exude profusely, resulting into heavy crust formation.
- Secondary infections with pyogenic organisms are also common.

Sites

Extensor aspects of the lower and upper extremities.

Course

The disease is punctuated into remissions and relapses.

Treatment

Mild Lesion

Mild lesions may be treated with topical corticosteroids with or without antibiotics.

Severe Lesions

- Systemic corticosteroids must be used to bring fast regression.
- Secondary infections need oral antibiotics.

Lichen Simplex Chronicus

Synonym

Neurodermatitis

Clinical Features

- Severely itchy, flat papules coalescing to form a single patch with prominent skin markings (Figs 25.53–25.57).
- Usually, the skin is brown in colour.
- Older lesions become more lichenified and hyperpigmented.
- The lesions are well-marginated.

Sites

Usually present on the back of the neck, though it can be seen on any part of the body.

Course

- Repeated scratching may result in secondary infection and inflammation.
- Exudation and scaling do not occur.
- In several cases, the lesions persist for a long period.

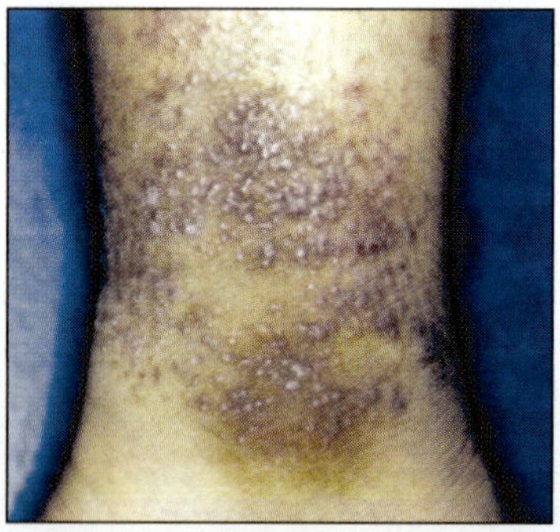

Fig. 25.53 Lichen simplex chronicus: early lesions

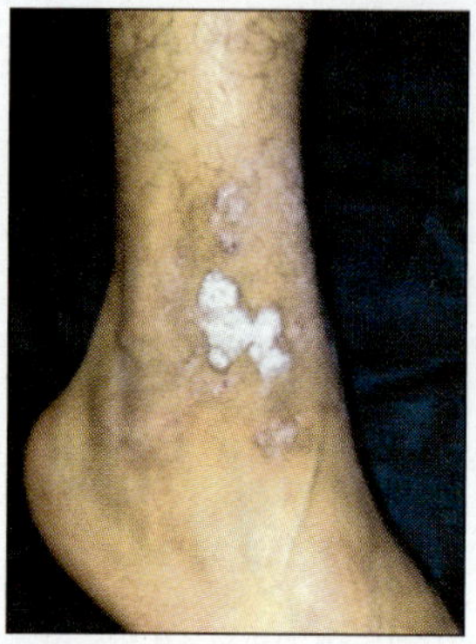

Fig. 25.54 Lichen simplex chronicus: ankle

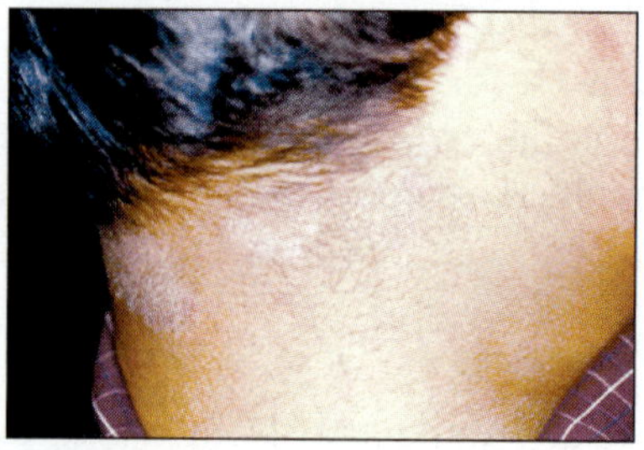

Fig. 25.55 Lichen simplex chronicus: neck

Differential Diagnosis

Secondary lichenification mimicking lichen simplex chronicus occurs in the following conditions:

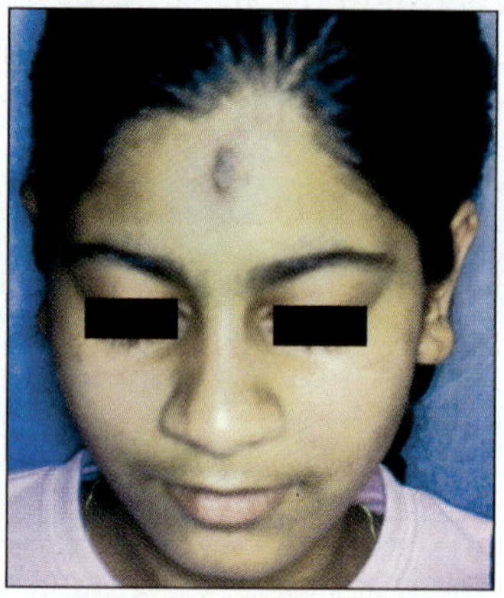

Fig. 25.56 Lichen simplex chronicus: forehead

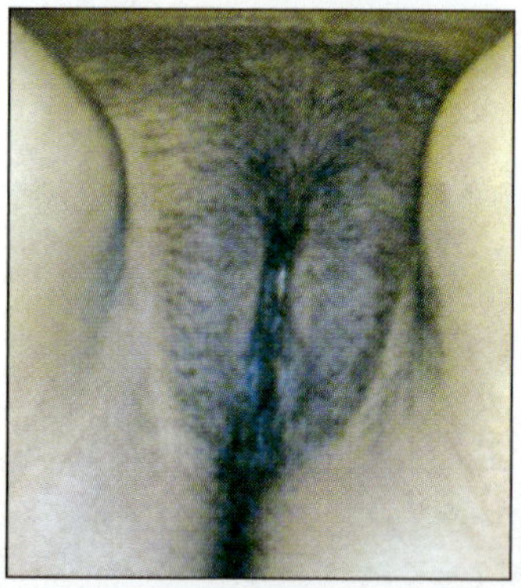

Fig. 25.57 Lichen simplex chronicus: female genital

- Lesions of tinea corporis.
- Insect bites.
- Contact dermatitis.
- Atopic dermatitis.

Here, the lesions will be ill-defined and consist of an area of thickened skin with hyperpigmentation and severe itching.

Scars and Keloids

Pathogenesis

- Scars result when the dermis is damaged. The damaged dermis stimulates proliferation of fibroblasts resulting in the formation of a scar.
- Scar may be depressed or hypertrophic depending upon the degree of fibroblast proliferation in comparison to the amount of the damaged tissue.

Clinical Features

Depressed Scars

Seen in acne, smallpox and chicken pox.

Hypertrophic Scars

Occur from traumatic injuries, infections and surgical procedures (Fig. 25.68).

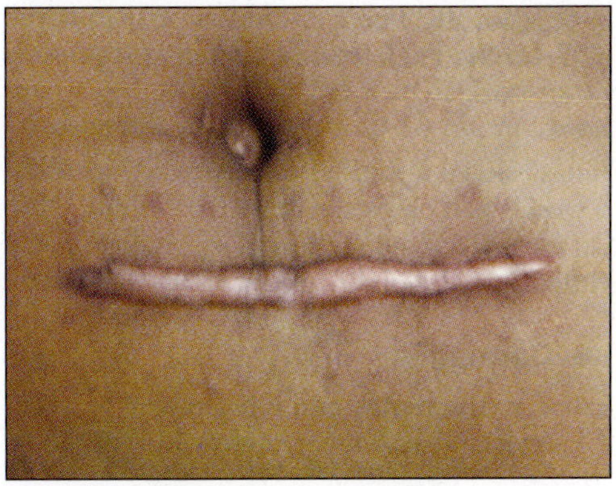

Fig. 25.58 Hypertrophic scar

Keloid

- When fibroblast proliferation continues even after the complete healing of wound, the resulting scar grows beyond the original limit of the lesion and forms a keloid.
- Keloid consists of a firm irregular-shaped mass.
- Keloids of recent origin, or those still growing, are pinkish in appearance, while the older ones look brownish or skin-coloured,
- Severe itching and even pain is frequently felt in active keloids,
- The tendency to develop keloids varies in different individuals in different regions of the body.
- Occasionally, ulceration can occur.

Sites

Located on the front of the chest.

Can occur on any site of the body (Fig. 25.59–25.61).

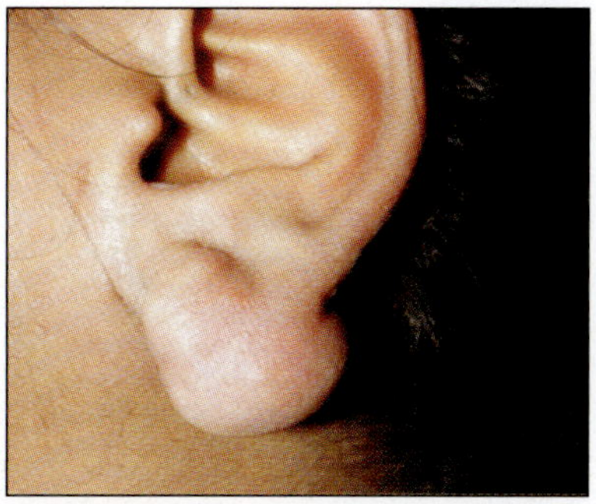

Fig. 25.59 Keloid: earlobe

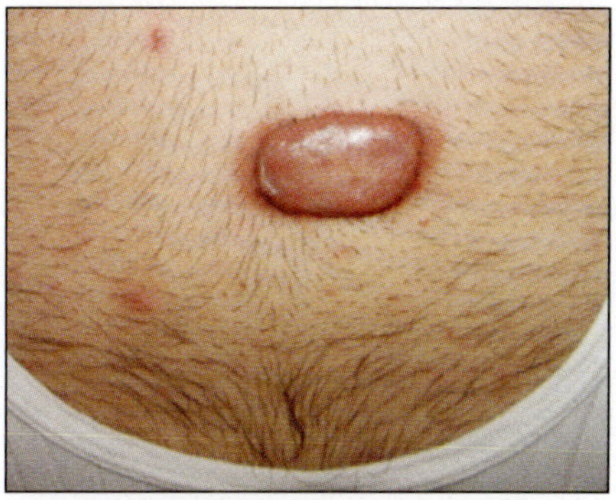

Fig. 25.60 Keloid abdomen

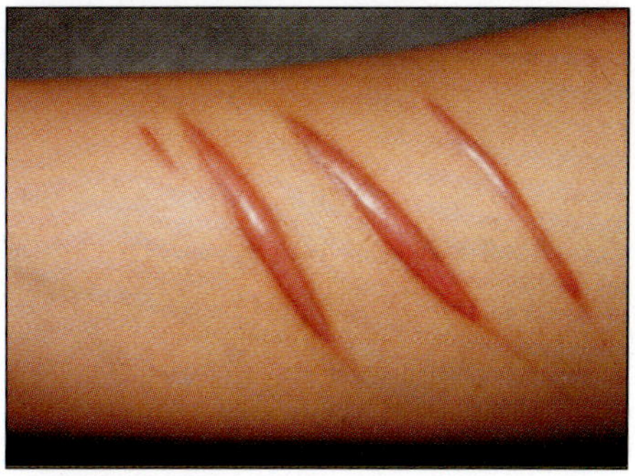

Fig. 25.61 Keloid: arm

Treatment

- Repeated intralesional injections of corticosteroids (triamcinolone: 40 mg/ml) weekly.
- Excision followed by irradiation.
- Cryotherapy with or without intralesional corticosteroids.
- Lasers.

Exfoliative Dermatitis

It is a special type of reaction to a variety of known and unknown causes wherein the skin of whole body becomes erythematous and scaly (Fig. 25.23).

Synonym

Erythroderma.

Etiology

The causes of this disorder are presented in Tables 25.17 and 25.18.

Table 25.17 Causes of exfoliative dermatitis

- Psoriasis
- Lichen planus
- Pityriasis rubra pilaris
- Generalised contact dermatitisSpecially air-borne contact dermatitis
- Atopic dermatitis
- Cutaneous manifestation of internal malignancy, especially lymphomas like Hodgkin's disease
- Injudicious use of local applications
- Drugs (Table 25.20)

Tabel 25.18 Drugs causing erythroderma or exfoliative dermatitis

- Isonicotinic acid hydrazide.
- Para-aminosalicylic acid.
- Thiacetazone.
- Arsenic.
- Gold.
- Mercury.
- Chloroquine.
- Sulphonamides.

Clinical Features

- Exfoliative dermatitis/erythroderma due to drugs or application of topical irritants is usually acute and may be fatal, if not treated quickly.
- Psoriasis generally shows intense erythema as compared to the erythroderma of other origins.
- Intensity of itching is variable in different individuals.
- Lymph nodes may also get enlarged in long-standing diseases, but remain discrete and non-tender.
- Individuals develop hypoproteinaemia due to excessive loss of proteins through the scales.
- May develop chills and rigor due to inability to control temperature secondary to the generalised erythema.
- Prone to develop superadded infections in the form of infection of lungs, indurated nodules of the skin and of other systems.
- Severe cases may develop the loss of hair which is usually temporary.

Treatment

- The patient should be kept in a room with controlled temperature.
- The patient should be given a high-protein diet to compensate for the loss of proteins through the scales.
- Corticosteroids, as 40–60 mg prednisolone, daily.
- Dose may be adjusted according to the clinical response.
- An attempt should be made to find out the cause of the disease to prevent the recurrence.

Pigmented Purpuric Dermatoses (PPD)

Etiology

Not known.

Clinical features

- Irregular, small, brown macules (Fig. 25.62a–25.62b) are seen.
- Occasionally purpuric lesions are present.
- Mostly seen on the lower parts of legs, occasionally on proximal parts of lower-legs.

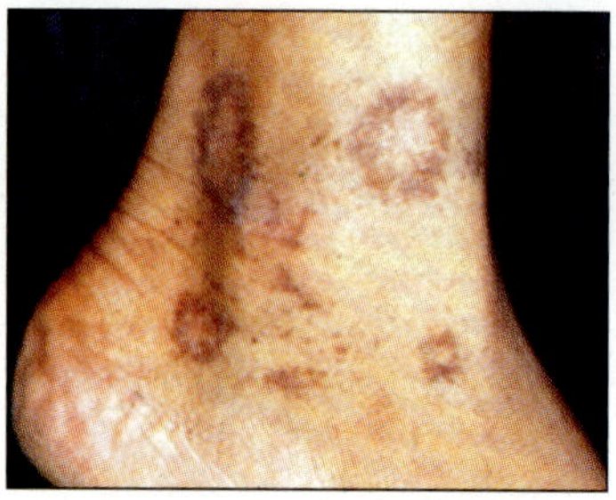

Fig. 25.62 (a) Pigmented purpuric dermatoses

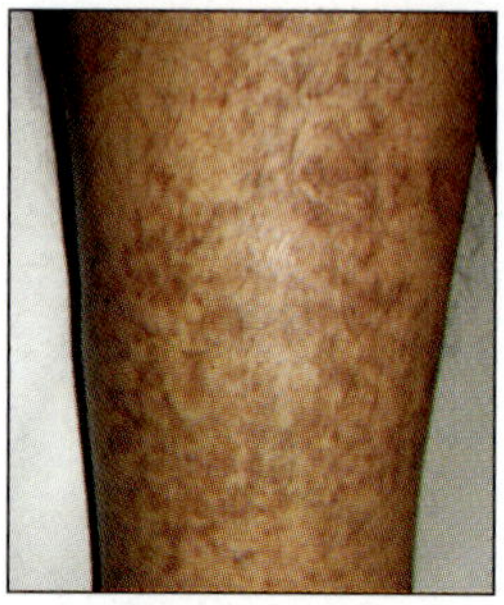

Fig. 25.62 (b) Pigmented purpuric dermatosis: leg

Course

Chronic, relapse is also frequent, lesions appear in crops and persist.

Treatment

- Hydroquinone: 2–5% lotion clears the lesions faster.
- Pentoxifylline (a xanthine derivative): 400 mg, 2–3 times daily, may be helpful.

Lichen Sclerosus Et Atrophicus

Etiology

Unknown.

Sex

More commonly in women.

Clinical Features

Non-Genital Lesions

- The lesions are asymptomatic.
- Trunk (especially around the umbilicus), neck, axillae and flexure surface of the wrists are the commonly affected sites.
- The lesions are small, ivory or porcelain-white in colour, shiny, round macules with yellow or brown follicular hyperkeratosis (Figs 25.63 and 25.64).
- Lesions at later stages aggregate into plaques.

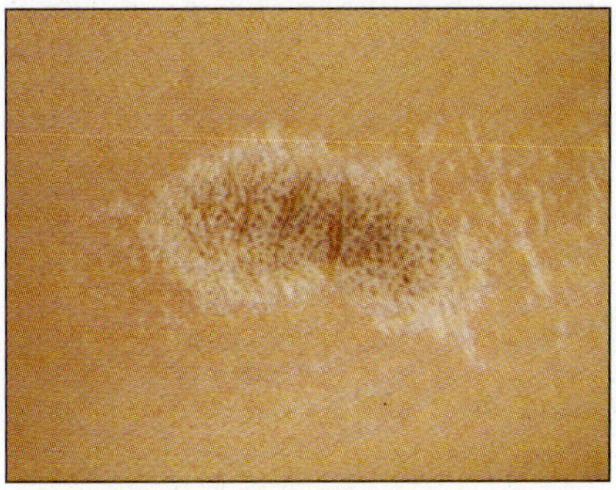

Fig. 25.63 Lichen sclerosus et atrophicus

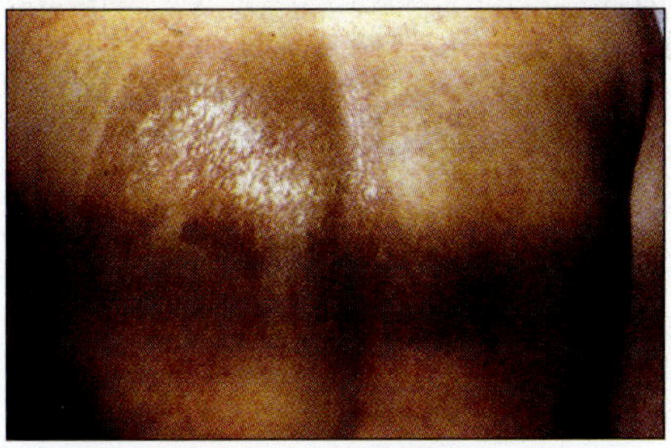

Fig. 25.64 Lichen sclerosus et atrophicus

Genital Lesions: Female

- Lesions occur on vulva and around the anus in females (figure-of-8 appearance).
- Ivory-coloured atrophic plaque with follicular hyperkeratosis and plugging is seen on the vulva.
- The patient may complain of soreness, itching and dyspareunia.
- Atrophy with shrinkage of vulva, especially clitoris and labia minora, with shortening of vaginal introitus may be present.

Genital lesions: Male (Balanitis xerotica obliterans)

- Recurrent balanitis and acquired phimosis are present.
- Prepuce becomes sclerotic and difficult to retract.
- The glans and prepuce become shining and bluish white.

Prognosis

Long-standing, untreated cases may develop leukoplakia and squamous cell carcinoma

Treatment

- Massage with topical corticosteroids, 2–3 times daily.
- Intralesional triamcinolone for sclerotic lesions of balanitis xerotica obliterans.
- Circumcision can be attempted.

Behcet Syndrome

It is a chronic, progressive disease, manifested as recurrent ulcers of the mouth and genitalia associated with iritis.

Etiology

The exact cause is not known. However, it may be caused by virus, may be associated with HLA-B-51.

Sex and Age

More in males between 20–30 years.

Clinical Features

- Recurrent oral and genital ulcers are seen.
- Painful and tender ulcers which are round or oval, sharply demarcated with yellowish floor and bright red areola, are present on the labial mucosa and mouth.
- Genital ulcers are smaller, mainly seen on the scrotum (Fig. 25.65), roof of penis or labia majora.
- Follicular and non-follicular pustules are seen on the trunk and genitocrural flexures.

- Acneform pustules or papules may be formed.
- Sterile pustules are seen at the site of skin-puncture.
- Erythema nodosum like nodules may be present mainly on the legs.
- Recurrent cellulitis may occur.
- Thrombophlebitis can be present in about 20% of cases.

Ocular Manifestations

- Photophobia, irritation and conjunctivitis.
- Uveitis, loss of vision, vitreous opacity.
- Hypopyon.
- Posterior uveitis and optic neuritis.

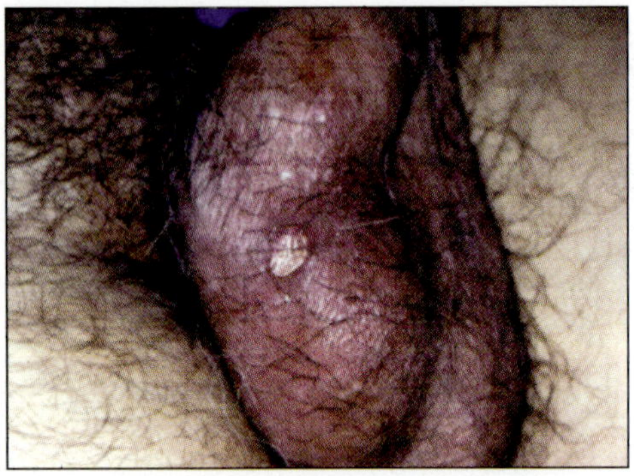

Fig. 25.65 Behcet syndrome: small ulcer on scrotum

Arthritis

Meningoencephalitis

Disseminated sclerosis or a state of organic confusion may be associated with this disease.

Course

- Always a potentially dangerous disease.
- Occurrence of orogenital or ocular lesions ceases after 5–10 years.

Treatment

- No specific treatment.
- Oral colchicine 0.6 mg daily in divided doses.
- Thalidomide: 100 mg, thrice daily.
- Systemic corticosteroids.

Granuloma Pyogenicum

It is a benign, acquired haemangioma.

Clinical features

- It presents as a bright or deep-red, pedunculated (Figs 25.56 and 25.67) or sesile lesion.
- The lesion bleeds easily even on minor trauma.
- A clear cut collar is usually seen at base of the lesion.
- It can be present anywhere on the body, especially at the site of a trauma.

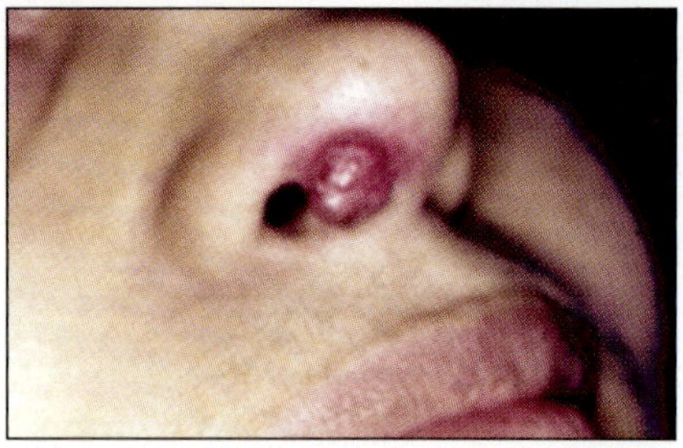

Fig. 25.66 Granuloma pyogenicum

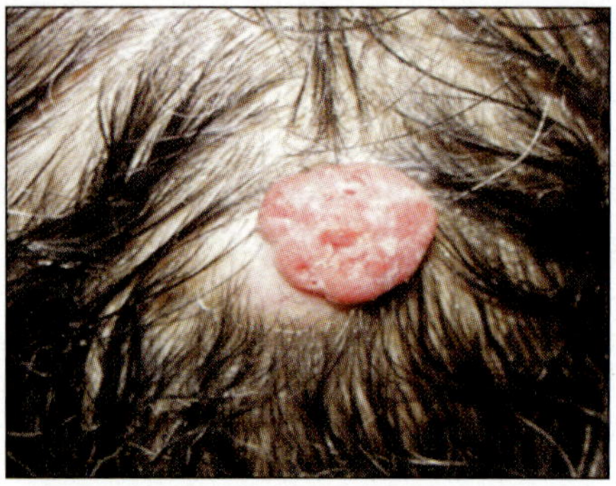

Fig. 25.67 Granuloma pyogenicum: scalp

Treatment

- Curette and cauterisation of the base of the lesion.
- Cryotherapy shows good results.

Prurigo Nodularis

Not a very common disease.

Clinical Features

- Scratching is the main feature, it is paroxysmal and intense.
- Intensely itchy, firm, pigmented, keratotic papules and nodules (Figs 25.68–25.70).
- Lesions are chronic and persistent.

Sites

- Extensors of the arms or legs.
- Usually bilaterally symmetrical.

Treatment

- Avoid scratching.
- Topical corticosteroids with occlusion.
- Recently, modified DCP has been used to cure it.

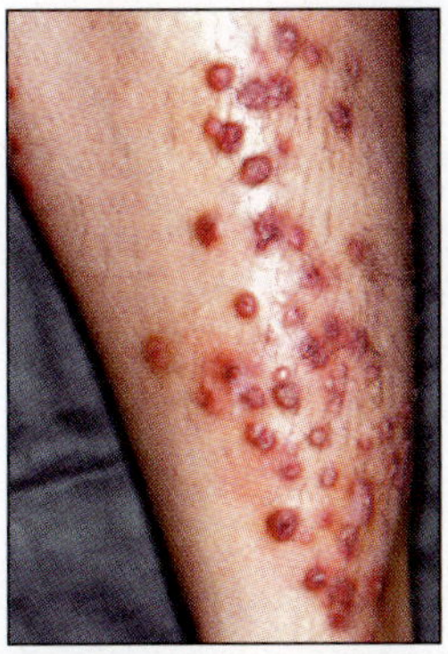

Fig. 25.68 Prurigo nodularis: early lesions

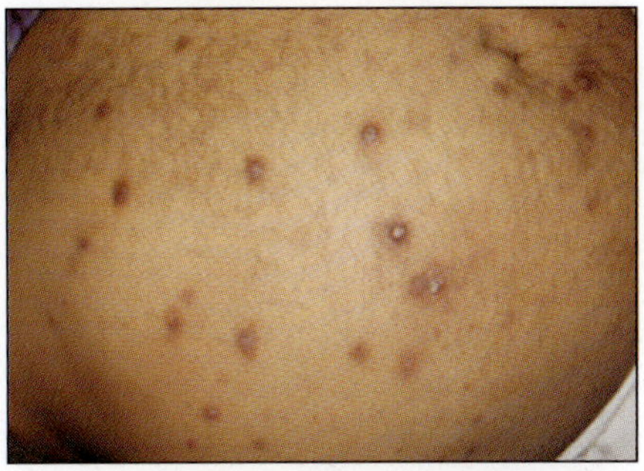

Fig. 25.69 Prurigo nodularis: classical lesions

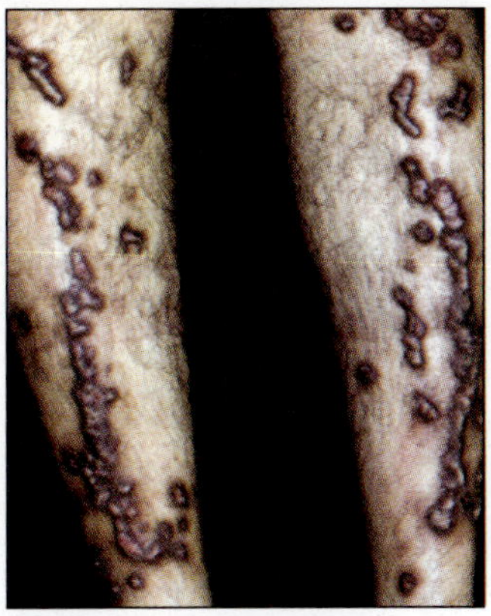

Fig. 25.70 Prurigo nodularis: late lesions

Dermatitis Artefacta

- Occurs in severely emotionally disturbed, often hysterical women.
- Self-inflicted injuries by physical, mechanical or chemical agents.

Clinical Features

- Lesions are uncharacteristic and bizarre in shape and size (Fig. 25.71).
- Appear abruptly and repeatedly with varying periods of remission.
- Not conforming to any disease pattern.
- Inaccessible areas of the body are spared.

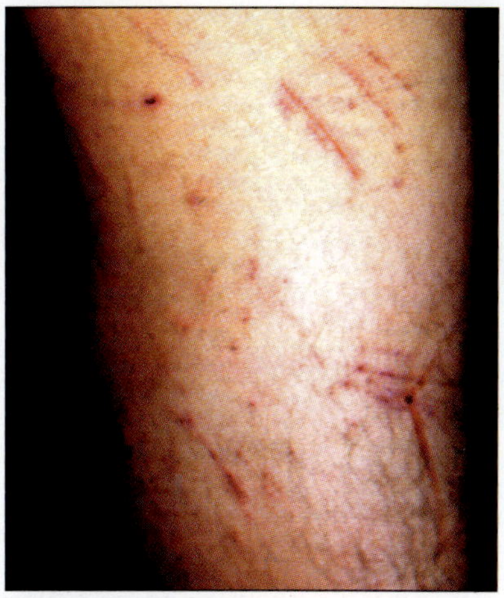

Fig. 25.71 Dermatitis artefacta

Treatment

- Antibiotic—topical and systemic—for the prevention of infections.
- Psychiatric assessment.

Aphthous Ulcer

Commonly presents as recurrent ulceration of oral mucosa (Figs 25.72 and 25.73).

Etiology

Unknown.

Clinical Features

- Present as small, red macules of 1–10 mm diameter.
- Within a few hours, the surface whitens and breaks down to form a shallow, yellow ulcer surrounded by erythematous halo; ulcer is usually painful.
- Heals usually in 7–10 days, without any scar.

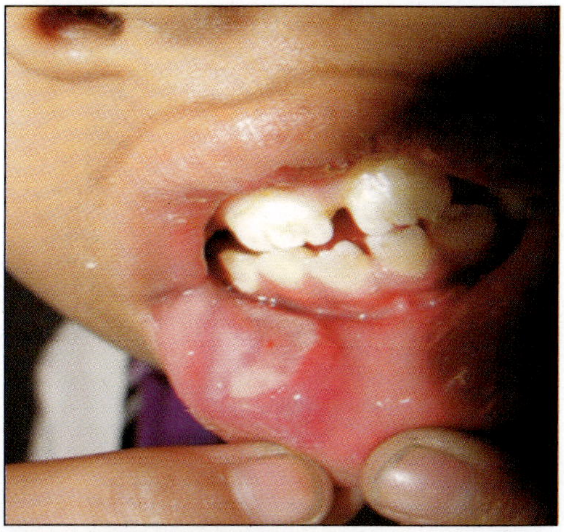

Fig. 25.72 Aphthous ulcer: lips

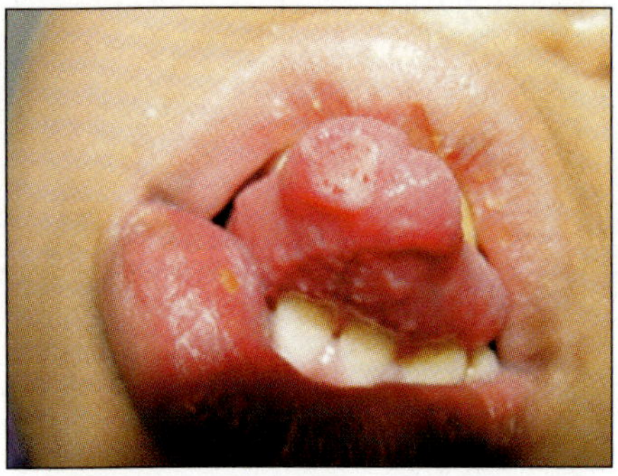

Fig. 25.73 Aphthous ulcer: tongue

Sites

Most commonly affects the lips, buccal mucosa, tongue and the mucobuccal fold.

Differential Diagnosis

Recurrent Herpes Simplex

Clusters of small, superficial ulcers, confirmed by the isolation of virus

Bullous Eruption

Often present as ragged erosion.

Traumatic Ulcer

Usually irregular and related to local dental trauma.

Treatment

- No specific treatment.
- Topical steroid in orabase, 2–3 hourly.
- Painful and large ulcers can be treated with oral corticosteroids. Prednisolone 20 mg, daily for 5–7 days, clears the lesions completely.

Varicose Vein

- Occurs in the long veins of legs (Fig. 25.74).

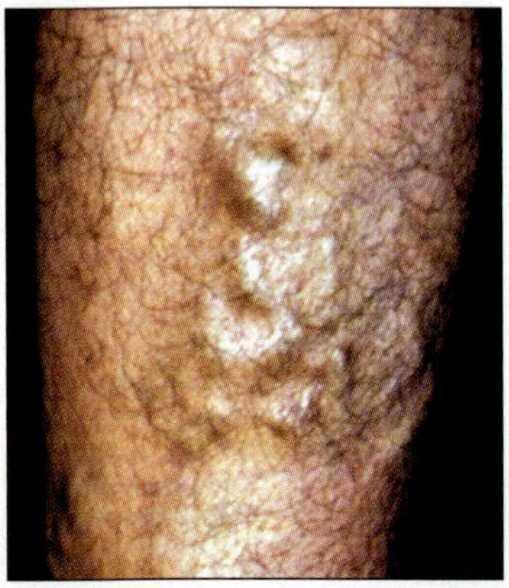

Fig. 25.74 Varicose vein: leg

- Venous valves are faulty and blood leaks back through these faulty valves.
- Venous pressure caused by back pressure is transmitted back to the superficial veins via perforating vein leading to varicosities and telangiectasia.
- Extravasation of RBCs results into brownish pigmentation of the skin.

Clinical Features

- Pitting edema is seen on the ankles.
- Distended superficial long veins are present in the lower legs.
- Network of smaller veins seen around the medial malleolus and foot.
- Discomfort and heaviness of the lower leg.
- Oedema becomes firm due to fibrosis.

Varicose Ulcer

- After a minor injury of the ankle, an ulcer may develop which usually does not heal (Fig. 25.75).
- Ulcers are usually single and seen around the medial malleolus.
- Base is lined with yellowish-grey slough.
- Edges are usually flush with skin surface and are irregular in outline.
- Large ulcers may encircle the leg.

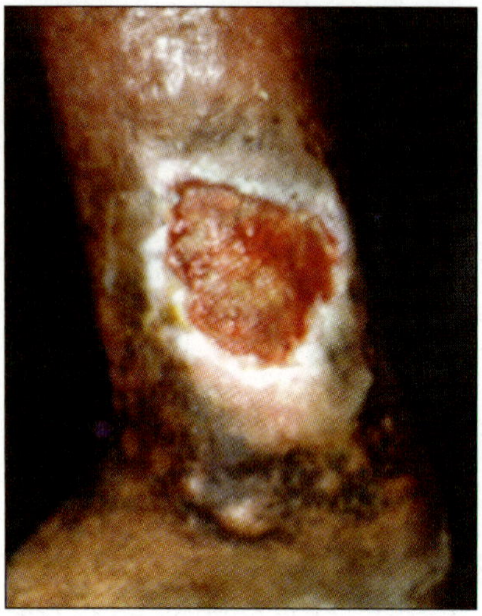

Fig. 25.75 Vericose ulcer: leg

Treatment

- Elevation of leg.
- Compression bandage.
- Gentle regular exercise.
- Weight reduction.
- Systemic antibiotics in full doses.
- Surgical management of the varicose vein.

Pearly Penile Papules

Often assumed to be sexually-transmitted.

Site

Found around the head of penis (Fig. 25.76).

Clinical Features

- Small dome-shaped to filliform, skin-coloured papules are present.
- Located typically on the sulcus or corona of the glans.
- Arranged circumferentially in one or several rows.
- Considered a normal variant.
- Observed more frequently in uncircumcised males.

Treatment

- Regression of papules occurs often after circumcision.
- It is typically asymptomatic and requires no treatment.
- For those who insist on treatment, ablative therapies like surgical excision or carbon dioxide laser resurfacing can be done.

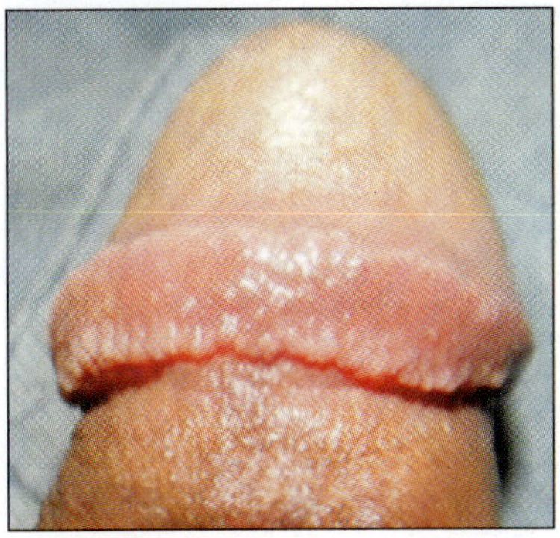

Fig. 25.76 Pearly penile papules

Keratolysis Exfoliativa

Synonym

Lamellar dyshidrosis or recurrent focal palmar peeling.

Etiology

It normally appears during the warm weather. Due to excessive sweating and friction, the skin starts exfoliating.

Clinical Features

It is a harmless, though sometimes painful skin condition that has the following characteristics:

- Focal peeling of palms (Fig. 25.77) and, less often, soles.
- Characterised by dry skin with superficial air-filled blisters which can be peeled-off very easily, leaving behind reddish, tender areas.
- Loss of the horny layer of skin on palms, leaving the skin drier and cracking.
- Often misdiagnosed as contact dermatitis or psoriasis.

Course

- In most cases, the exfoliation resolves spontaneously and no lasting damage is seen.
- Some patients experience cracking and even bleeding in extreme cases.

Treatment

- Usually no treatment is required.
- Creams, especially with urea, silicon and lactic acid are helpful.

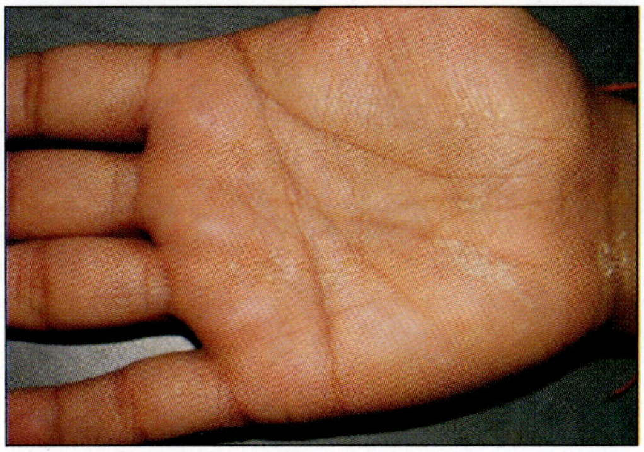

Fig. 25.77 Keratolysis exfoliativa

Appendix

TREATMENT MODALITIES IN DERMATOLOGY

The main components of treatment modalities in dermatology are as follows:

- Counselling.
- Medical options.
- Physical modalities.

Counselling

Counselling of the patient and his/her partner(s) and family is crucial in infectious diseases and STD. Counselling includes explaining the disease and discussing various treatment options. It also includes discussing and explaining the importance of general cleanliness, education about sexual abstinence and use of barrier methods to prevent the transmission of STDs.

Medical Options

Table: Drugs used in dermatology

Emollients like petroleum jelly, liquid paraffin, etc.
Keratolytics like urea, salicylic acid, etc.
Shampoos.
Depigmenting agents like hydroquinone, retinoic acid, tranexamic acid and glutathione.
Sunscreens like zinc oxide, etc.
Steroids.
Various antibacterial, antifungal, antiviral, antiparasitic, antiacne and anti-psoriatic agents.
Miscellaneous drugs like minoxidil, immunomodulators, antiandrogens, biologics and dapsone.

Corticosteroids

The corticosteroids are classified into glucocorticoids, mineralocorticoids and adrenocorticoids. Common corticosteroids used are cortisones which get converted into hydrocortisone in the liver. Equivalent doses of different corticosteroids are:

- Cortisone: 25 mg.
- Hydrocortisone: 20 mg.
- Prednisolone: 5 mg.
- Triamcinolone: 4 mg.
- Betamethasone/dexamethasone: 0.5 mg.

All of these are very potent corticosteroids.

Betamethasone/dexamethasone 0.5 mg are anti-inflammatory, anti-allergic and immunosuppressive agents. Thus, they can be used for allergic and autoimmune disorders. They have to be used in adequate doses. When the disease becomes quiescent, the corticosteroids can be withdrawn. But this should never be done abruptly. All corticosteroids have similar properties and they should be given in equivalent doses. They are equally effective.

Cortisone and hydrocortisone are short-acting, prednisolone and triamcinolone are intermediate-acting, while dexamethasone and betamethasone are long-acting.

A single dose after meals in the morning causes lesser adrenal suppression. Dexamethasone or betamethasone are the longer acting corticosteroids. They commonly cause lesser adrenal suppression if used for a prolonged period. Triamcinolone can cause muscle-wasting. It is soluble in water and fat. It is converted into a water-soluble metabolite after conjugation with glucuronic acid and is excreted in the urine.

Dosage Schedules

Short-Term, High-Dosage Schedule

Diseases like toxic epidermal necrolysis, Stevens–Johnson syndrome, severe forms of erythema multiforme and acute generalised contact dermatitis require a short-term, high-dosage schedule. Once the disease has been controlled, reduction is done gradually.

Long-Term, High-Dosage Schedule

Diseases like pemphigus, pemphigoid exfoliative dermatitis and systemic lupus erythematosus also require higher dosages. But usually these have to be used for relatively much longer periods.

Long-Term, Low-Dosage Schedule

Diseases, like alopecia areata, scleroderma and discoid lupus erythematosus are best treated by giving 10 to 20 mg of prednisolone a day. Continue this treatment for as long as necessary.

Side Effects of Corticosteroid Therapy

When used for prolonged periods or in high dosages, corticosteroids can produce a variety of side effects.

However, all the side effects are not produced in all the patients. There are individual variations in the side effects. Following are the major side effects seen during corticosteroid therapy:

- Electrolyte imbalance.
- Increased susceptibility to infections.
- Increase in body-weight.
- Pitting oedema.
- Peptic ulceration.
- Increased tendency for diabetes mellitus.
- Hypertension.
- Osteoporosis.
- Psychosis.
- Steroid acne.
- Striae atrophicans.
- Increased tendency for bleeding.
- Myopathy.
- Cataract.
- Hypertrichosis.

Antibiotics

Various antibiotics are used for the treatment of infections with pyogenic bacteria. Some act by killing the bacteria and are called **bactericidal drugs** while others only inhibit their proliferation and are called **bacteriostatic drugs**. While most of them have a **broad-spectrum** of activity, a few have a limited range of activity. Some bacteria are originally susceptible to the drug but later on develop resistance to it, more so, if the patient is given sub-therapeutic doses.

Commonly Used Antibiotics

Sulphonamide

These are active against common pyogenic organisms such as *staphylococci* and *E.coli*. The commonly used sulphonamides include sulphadiazine, sulphadimidine, sulphathiazole and sulphamerazine. Long-acting sulphonamides are sulphaphenazole, suphadimethoxone and sulfamethoxazole-trimethoprim.

Side Effects

- Crystalluria.
- Fixed drug eruption.
- Photosensitivity.
- Leucopenia.
- Generalised skin rashes.

Penicillin

This is a bactericidal drug. The drug is effective against gram positive and gram negative cocci and some gram positive bacilli. Penicillins are usually administered by intramuscular route using one of the following options:

- Crystalline penicillin: 500,000 units twice a day.
- Procaine penicillin: 400,000 units once a day.
- Benzathine penicillin: 1.2 to 2.4 mega units once a week or once a fortnight.

Penicillin is also available in the form of tablets for oral use.

Side Effects

- Hypersensitivity reaction.
- Papulovesicular reaction.

As a routine, it is advised to test the patient for hypersensitivity.

Streptomycin

This is a bacteriostatic drug effective against *streptococci, E.coli, Proteus sp., Pseudomonas aeruginosa* and *staphylococci* that are resistant to penicillin. Its main therapeutic value lies in the treatment of tuberculosis and donovanosis.

Side Effects

- Vertigo.
- Dizziness due to the involvement of the eighth cranial nerve.
- Hypersensitivity reaction.

Tetracycline

These contain three closely related compounds, viz., chlorotetracycline, oxytetracycline and tetracycline. These act as bacteriostatic agents towards gram positive and gram negative bacteria. Hence, they are called broad-spectrum antibiotics.

Side Effects

- Development of vitamin B-complex deficiency.
- Candidiasis of the gastrointestinal tract.

Chloramphenicol

It is a broad-spectrum antibiotic that acts as a bacteriostatic agent and is given as 500 mg tablets, twice daily. It is given for those bacterial infections which are resistant to other antibiotics.

Side Effects:

- Aplastic anemia.
- Agranulocytosis.
- Thrombocytopenia.

Erythromycin

This is a bactericidal drug which acts by interfering with the protein synthesis by bacterial ribosomes. Organisms can easily develop resistance to this drug.

Side Effects

- Giddiness.
- Nephrotoxicity.

Ampicillin

It is a modified form of penicillin. It is effective against gram positive and gram negative bacteria. It acts by inhibiting the formation of bacterial cell wall. It can be inactivated by penicillinase.

Cloxacillin

This is a modified penicillin and is useful against penicillin-resistant *staphylococci*.

Amoxicillin

This is another modified penicillin with a broad-spectrum anti-bacterial activity.

Doxycycline

This is a modified tetracycline. High levels in blood are maintained for prolonged periods. It has a wide range of anti-bacterial activity. Doxycycline does not damage the kidneys.

Gentamicin

It is effective against *Pseudomonas aeruginosa*, resistant strains of *staphylococci* and other organisms

Side Effects

- Dizziness.
- Nephrotoxicity.

Cephalosporin

These are a group of antibiotics derived from *Cephalosporium acrimonious*. They have a wide range of antibacterial activity against gram positive and gram negative organisms but have no action on *Pseudomonas aeruginosa*. They can be given intramuscularly or intravenously in an equivalent dose.

Side Effects

- Diarrhoea.
- Candidiasis.
- Nephrotoxicity.

Different Types of Drug Delivery Systems

- Lotions.
- Creams.
- Ointments.
- Pastes.
- Microspheres.

These formulations are used, based on the morphology of the lesions and the site affected:

- Lotions are helpful in inflamed, exudative lesions that are present in the scalp.
- Creams are effective in both, dry and exudative lesions.
- Ointments are used more commonly for dry and lichenified lesions.

Physical Modalities

Different physical modalities used in dermatology are as follows:

- Electrocautery.
- Cryotherapy/cryosurgery.
- Intralesional therapy.
- Phototherapy.
- Chemical peeling.
- Photochemotherapy.
- Surgical excision and incision.
- Fulguration.
- Electrocoagulation.
- Electrodessication.
- Laser therapy.
- Electrolysis.

Chemical peeling and phototherapy have been detailed in the respective chapters.

Electrocautery

The tissue is destroyed by the heat that is generated from conversion of electric current due to the resistance of platinum loops.

Cryotherapy or Cryosurgery

Skin lesions such as warts, molluscum contagiosum, cutaneous tags or seborrhoeic keratosis can be destroyed by freezing. The agents commonly used for this purpose include carbon-dioxide snow (boiling point, –80°C) and liquid nitrogen (boiling point, –180°C). The duration of application varies from 5 to 30 seconds for small lesions and 30 to 90 seconds for deeper lesions. The white zone of freezing should become visible for 1–3 mm beyond the margin of the lesion. This treatment, as a rule, results in a blister within six to eight hours. Later on, this blister dries-up and forms a crust. Complete healing occurs in two to three weeks and generally there is no scarring.

Intralesional Therapy

By an intralesional injection, a drug can be deposited directly at a place where it is required to act. For this, a high concentration of the drug is to be used so that a large dose of the drug can be deposited by injecting in a small volume. Such injection needs to be injected only once a week and can be continued till the desired effect has been achieved. This mode of treatment can be used for a few lesions only. Corticosteroids are the most commonly used drugs for intralesional therapy. They have been used for the treatment of resistant psoriasis, hypertrophic scar, lichen planus, lichen simplex chronicus, alopecia areata and keloid. However, repeated injections of corticosteroids sometimes result in atrophic changes in the skin.

Photo Chemotherapy

This is used in the treatment of psoriasis and dermatitis of nails. If given in large enough doses (20–30 Joules/cm^2), it was found beneficial in psoriasis. Other uses of PUVA therapy are in treating pityriasis rosea and pityriasis lichenoides chronica. The term PUVA (psoralens + ultra violet A = PUVA) is used in the treatment of various types of psoriasis. The psoralens include 8-methoxypsoralen (8-MOP), methoxypsoralen and 4, 5, 8 trimethoxypsoralen (TMP). They inhibit the epidermal DNA synthesis. Sunlight is a potent source of UVA light. Side effects include carcinoma and fibrosarcoma.

Surgical Excision

Small tumors or cysts can be easily taken out by surgical excision. The area of skin bearing the lesion should first be thoroughly cleaned with spirit and then anaesthetised by injecting xylocaine under and around the lesion. Within one to five minutes of the injection, the skin becomes anaesthetised. This can be confirmed by testing with a sterile needle. Once the area is anaesthetised, an elliptical incision should be given around the lesion, the long axis of which should correspond to the imaginary lines of Langer. The margin of wound is appropriated by stitches using silk or cotton, this leads to the stoppage of any further bleeding. In case some oozing persists, a pressure bandage on the wound is usually sufficient. The patient should be instructed to keep the part dry. Generally, there is no need for further dressing.

Surgical Incision of Abscesses

Abscesses due to pyogenic infection or cystic acne need to be incised to drain out the pus, otherwise pus interferes with the healing process. After anesthesia with ethyl chloride, a sterilised nail should be inserted through the surface of the abscess. For cystic acne, one should make a very small incision so that it does not leave a scar. After the pus is drained out, an antiseptic dressing can be applied. Depending upon the etiology, systemic antibacterial agents are given to promote proper healing.

Fulguration

Spark action is used in fulguration. If the tip of the needle is kept slightly away from the lesion, a spark is generated between the needle and the lesion resulting in destruction of the lesion. This procedure is useful when only superficial destruction is required or if the lesions are of the size of a pin-point.

Electrocoagulation

The tissue charring is achieved due to the intense heat produced by a bi-terminal spark gap.

Electrodessication

In electrodessication, a needle is inserted into the lesion and is kept as long as the cell is dried up and shrunken.

Laser

The **laser** (light amplification by stimulated emission of radiation) technology is enormously destructive and penetrative. Commonly used lasers are Nd: YAG laser, **intense pulsed light** (IPL), etc. Various indications include removal of tattoos and small port wine naevi, multiple basal cell carcinomas, small anglosarcoma, melanomas, hirsutism, etc.

Electrolysis

Destruction of tissues utilising electric currents directly causes the liberalisation of electrolytes around the electrodes. It is commonly used to remove hair in hirsutism.

Botox

It is a neurotoxin protein produced by bacterium *Clostridium botulinum*. It is considered safe and effective for the reduction of facial wrinkles, especially on the upper third of the face. Injection of botox into the muscles under facial wrinkles causes relaxation of the muscles resulting in smoothening of the overlying skin. Smoothening of the skin usually appears 3 days after the treatment and is maximally visible for two weeks after the injection. The treated muscles regain their function gradually. They generally return to their normal appearance 3–4 months after the treatment. Muscles can be treated repeatedly to maintain the smoothness of skin.

Side Effects

Unintended paralysis of the facial muscles may occur. Other side effects include partial facial paralysis, muscle weakness and troubled swallowing. Headache, flu-like syndrome and allergic reactions may also occur.

Index